D1709144

Toxicology
of
Pesticides
in
Animals

Editor

T. S. S. Dikshith, Ph.D.
Scientist-in-Charge
Pesticide Toxicology Division
Industrial Toxicology Research Center
Lucknow, India

CRC Press
Boca Raton   Boston   Ann Arbor

Library of Congress Cataloging-in-Publication Data

Toxicology of pesticides in animals/editor, T. S. S. Dikshith.
    p.   cm.
    Includes bibliographical references and index.
    ISBN 0-8493-6907-X
    1. Pesticides—Toxicology. I. Dikshith, T. S. S., 1932-
RA1270.P4T668   1990
615.9′02—dc20   90-40861
                                                                              CIP

Direct all inquiries to CRC Press, Inc., 2000 Corporate Blvd., N.W., Boca Raton, Florida 33431.

© 1991 by CRC Press, Inc.

International Standard Book Number 0-8493-6907-X

Library of Congress Card Number 90-40861
Printed in the United States

To
My Parents
and to
Saroja, Pratibha and Prerana

ACKNOWLEDGMENT

The editor is grateful to the contributors whose valuable expertise and patience made this work possible. Grateful thanks are also due to several publishers who generously permitted copyrighted material to be reproduced.

The editor expresses sincere thanks to all his colleagues because of whose cooperation and meaningful discussions this work could be completed. Sincere appreciation of the editor goes to Mrs. Syamala Das for her technical assistance. Thanks are due to the Editorial Board and Publication Unit of CRC Press for providing an opportunity to complete this work and for all encouragement and patience.

T. S. S. Dikshith

FOREWORD

Pesticides have become an important aspect of modern agriculture and public health management. The potential toxicity of pesticides has acted as a double-edged sword both in saving the millions of people from hunger and disease and also in causing poisoning and death to an equally large number of people around the world. Effective procedures have been introduced in the registration and management of pesticides by different countries. The generation of toxicological data in species of animals has been considered as one of the most important requirements in the correct understanding of potential toxicity and health effects of pesticides in animals and humans. The comprehensive coverage by Dr. Dikshith on various aspects of pesticides has added valuable information to our present knowledge in this area. I am glad that he has succeeded in adding a number of useful contributions from his own laboratory and also from outstanding scientists from Bulgaria, France, and The Netherlands.

Besides being an active worker in the area of pesticide toxicology over the years, Dr. T. S. S. Dikshith has also presented on different occasions articulated overviews on many aspects of pesticide research. He also has served on the committees and expert panels concerned with the regulation of pesticides in India, under the Insecticide Act of India on behalf of the Central Insecticide Board, Government of India. Presently, he is a member of the Apex Expert Committee on the Toxicology of Pesticides, Government of India and also a member of the Scientific Advisory Committee of a pesticide manufacturing company in India. He has also been exposed to the international trends of research in the toxicity of pesticides by participating in the bilateral scientific programs of WHO, CNRS, and INSERM, France. It is therefore only fitting that Dr. Dikshith was asked to be the Editor of *Toxicology of Pesticides in Animals* for CRC Press. I do hope that the volumes will be welcomed by research workers and concerned scientists as a timely reference tome on several important aspects of pesticide toxicology in animals.

C. R. Krishna Murti
Chairman
Scientific Commission for Continuing
Studies on Effects of Bhopal Gas Leaking on
Life Systems, Government of India

THE EDITOR

Dr. Turuvekere Subrahmanya Shanmukha Dikshith had his early education at Central College, Bangalore, India. He received has M.Sc. and Ph.D. degrees in Zoology from the University of Mysore, Mysore. Dr. Dikshith is presently working as a Senior Scientist and Scientist-In-Charge of the Pesiticide Toxicology Laboratory at the Industrial Toxicology Research Centre, Lucknow, one of the laboratories of the Council of Scientific and Industrial Research, India. Dr. Dikshith is also the leader of the Pesticide Toxicology Group of the research centre.

In 1968, Dr. Dikshith was called upon to start the first Pesticide Toxicology Laboratory at the Industrial Toxicology Research Centre, Lucknow. He organized the laboratory and initiated studies to unravel the effects of pesticides in animals. Dr. Dikshith was also responsible for the organization, development of capabilities, and creation of facilities at Gheru, an extension centre of the Industrial Toxicology Research Centre in 1978. The focus of this centre is to conduct studies on the safety evaluation of pesticides and other chemicals. Dr. Dikshith has been actively engaged over the last two decades in programs and management of pesticide toxicology.

Dr. Dikshith is an awardee of a World Health Organization fellowship. He worked at the Centre for Comparative Pathology and Toxicology, Albany Medical College, Albany, New York and at the International Centre of Environmental Safety, Holloman, New Mexico. He has visited laboratories in France, West Germany, and Canada. He has also worked as a visiting scientist and was awarded an INSERM fellowship by the government of France.

Dr. Dikshith has published over 70 original research papers, review articles, and book chapters. He has to his credit several project reports on the toxicology of pesticides, synthesized and formulated in the country. These have supported the research and development work of various pesticide manufacturing industries in India, and laboratories of CSIR and other agencies. Dr. Dikshith has worked as a member of several expert committees and panels such as the Sub-Committee on Pesticide Toxicology (Gaitonde Committee); Panel on Toxicology of Antibiotics and Biocides, Ministry of Agriculture, Government of India; Advisory Committee on Pesticide Environmental Pollution; Central Insecticide Board; Committee on Health Effects of Pesticides of the Indian Council of Medical Research; Central Board for Prevention and Control of Water Pollution, Government of India; Research & Development Coordination Committee, Hindustan Insectide Ltd., Government of India; and the Sub-Group on Science, Technology, Environment and Pesticides, Ministry of Chemicals and Fertilizers, Government of India. Presently Dr. Dikshith is a member of the Expert Committee on Identification, Use and Import of Pesticides; Expert Panel on Toxicology Data Requirement on Household Pesticides; and Expert Panel on Toxicology, Registration Committee, Ministry of Agriculture, Government of India. Dr. Dikshith also provided an overview on Approaches to Manpower Development and Training in the Field of Chemical Safety in India to the World Health Organization, Geneva.

Dr. Dikshith has participated in several group discussions at national and international conferences on pesticides. He organized the India-United States Workshop on Biodegradable Pesticides in 1979 at the Industrial Toxicology Research Centre. He was also the General Secretary of the International Conference on Pesticides, Toxicity, Safety and Risk Assessment held at the Industrial Toxicology Research Centre, Lucknow in October 1985. Dr. Dikshith also organized workshops on Development, Toxicity and Safe Use of Pesticides in India during 1989 and 1990.

CONTRIBUTORS

B. J. Blaauboer, Ph.D.
Department of Veterinary Pharmacology,
  Pharmacy and Toxicology
University of Utrecht
Utrecht, The Netherlands

G. Carrera, Ph.D., D.Sc.
Toxicologie des Aliments
Institut de Physiologie
INSERM Unit 87
Toulouse, France

Fina Petrova Kaloyanova-Simeonova
Department of Toxicology
Institute of Hygiene and
  Occupational Health
Sofia, Bulgaria

S. Mitjavila, Ph.D., D.Sc.
Department of Food Toxicology
INSERM Unit 87
Toulouse, France

A. Periquet, Ph.D., D.Sc.
Department of Food Toxicology
INSERM Unit 87
Toulouse, France

T. A. Popov, M.D., Ph.D., D.Sc.
Department of Toxicology
Institute of Hygiene and
  Occupational Health
Sofia, Bulgaria

R. B. Raizada, Ph.D.
Pesticide Toxicology Division
Industrial Toxicology Research Centre
Lucknow, India

TABLE OF CONTENTS

Chapter 1

PESTICIDES

T. S. S. Dikshith

TABLE OF CONTENTS

I. INTRODUCTION

Pesticides are chemicals used for the control of a variety of organisms, for example insects, weeds, fungi, and rodents. In fact, to a large extent these organisms have been identified as man's competitor for food. Before the 1940s, development of pesticides was slow; however, in later years a large number of pesticidal chemicals entered the world market.

The majority of the pesticides used before the 1940s were mostly inorganic compounds and inhibitors of the carbohydrate oxidation. The first synthetic organic pesticides which became public during the 1930s, for example, were the dinitro compounds and thiocyanates. However, the evolution of synthetic pesticides, with three major groups, namely, the organochlorine (OC), organophosphorus (OP), and the carbamate insecticides, essentially began with the introduction of DDT. Interestingly, although DDT was first synthesized by

TABLE 1
Classification of Pesticides on the Basis of Chemical Nature

		Pesticides		
Insecticides	Herbicides	Fungicides	Rodenticides	Fumigants
Organic Compounds		Inorganic compounds		Natural products

Organochlorine		
Aldrin, DDT, HCH	Arsenicals	Rotenoids
Organophosphorus	Mercurials	Pyrethrum
Diazinon, malathion, parathion		Nicotine
Carbamates		
Aldicarb, carbaryl		
Thiocyanate		
Thanite		
Nitrophenols		
Binapacryl		
DNOC		
Pentachlorophenol		

Zeidler as early as 1874, it was not used until its insecticidal properties were discovered by Paul-Muller in 1939. This discovery of DDT and its effectiveness against a variety of insect pests earned a Nobel Prize for Muller in 1948.[1] Several other OCs were synthesized in later years, for example, hexachlorocyclohexane (HCH, BHC) aldrin, dieldrin, endrin, and chlordane.

The other important group of pesticides, namely the OPs, first appeared in 1945. In fact, this was the result of German industry finding modifications of chemical warfare agents useful for insect pest control. The singular contribution of Gerhard Schrader, pioneer in chemistry, helped the use of organophosphorus insecticides such as TEPP, EPN, parathion, malathion etc. for pest control.[2] In contrast, the carbamate group of compounds is relatively of recent origin with the introduction of carbaryl during 1958.

II. CLASSIFICATION AND USES

Invariably the term *pesticide* is equated and considered as a synonym to *insecticide*. It need not be emphasized that while the former is a general term, the latter denotes to a particular group of chemical under pesticides, for instance insecticide, weedicide, acaricide, rodenticide, fungicide etc. The raionale behind the classification of pesticides, however, is in terms of their use, chemical nature, and the mode of action. (Table 1).

The inorganic chemicals dominated the pest management before World War II. For instance, the arsenicals, fluroides, thiocyanates, and salts of copper and sulfur were the major chemicals which helped man to protect his farm produce. After World War II a host of synthetic compounds came into use to control insects, weeds, rodents, ticks, mites, fungi ets. Use of natural products in the management of crop pests is not new. In fact, products of plant origin such as nicotine, pyrethroids, neem, rotenoids, and pine resin have been used during the centuries. Azadirachtin, a product from neem tree (*Azadirachta indica*) is known to possess insect repellent properties.

A. USES

The largest use of pesticides is for agriculture followed by vector control. Millions of hectares of farm and forest land all over the world have been sprayed and dusted with pesticides to contain insect pests and weeds. For instance, about 119 million acres of land in the U.S. were sprayed with herbicides, 97 million acres with insecticides, and 25 million acres with fungicides. In a similar fashion, a major part of fertile land in Asia and Europe is sprayed with pesticides to contain pests of different food crops.

In India, the average consumption of pesticides is more in the agricultural sector (about 63%) than in the nonagricultural sector (37%). In fact, the requirements of pesticides in the country are closely related to the plant protection coverage programs. According to the Ministry of Agriculture, Government of India, the covered area in hectares for plant protection was around 70 million during 1977-1978, 75 million during 1978-1979, and 100 million in 1982-1983.

The total production of pesticides in India during 1985-1986 was about 54,919 tons, of which 30,887 tons (56.2%) were HCH and DDT and 24,032 tons (43.8%) were other pesticides. In India more than half of all pesticide usage in agriculture is on cotton (42%) while the remaining share of pesticides is used for the control of pests on pulses, cereals (24%), fruits and vegetables (18%), oil seeds and pulses (3%), and plantation crops (8%).[3]

The effectiveness of the pesticide in agriculture is very spectacular. In fact, pesticides have become the material of choice for a majority of insect problems and for the elimination of unwanted weeds. In yields of important food crops, for example, wheat and barley in the United Kingdom were recorded to increase twofold between 1950 and 1975. These increases have been due to the use of pesticides along with fertilizers and other agricultural inputs.

The judicious use of pesticides also helped in improving the quality of cereals and seeds, a very important consideration in relation to E.E.C. marketing standards.

The role of pesticides in the protection of human health during the yester years is no less significant. The annual loss of human health due to vector borne diseases, mainly malaria and typhus, is still staggering. For example, malaria itself involved about 300 million cases and 3 million deaths. This was minimized to 120 million cases and 1 million deaths with the use of pesticides for vector control.

DDT showed spectacular successes in the control of malaria in different countries of the world. For example, in Mediterranean countries, India, Sri Lanka, Java and Bali, the Far East, Central and South America, control of malaria was a partial success. So is the case of Africa which is populated by about 400 million people representing about 10% of the world population. In spite of several setbacks more than 825 million people have been freed from the threat of malaria and the role played by DDT is creditable. In fact, as far as malaria, typhus, and other diseases are concerned the benefits gained by using DDT outweigh the detrimental effect to mankind. However, this is not to ignore the adverse effects caused by the misuse of DDT to a variety of organisms and ecosystems.

B. HAZARDS

There is another side to the story of pesticides which is not always rosy. This is particularly so with OCs and other compounds. For example, DDT and HCH persist in the environment and their local applications result in much wider distribution and bioaccumulation. Some of the persistant pesticides move insidiously within the biomass and the physical environs. Because of the lipophilic and adsorptive properties, the pesticides accumulate in the biomass.

Our concern for the environment today is centered mostly around aquatic ecosystems and the effect of pesticides on the nontarget organisms. This has been exemplified in fish kills, and death of predatory birds. In fact, application of fenitrothion in the northwestern Ontario forest produced adverse effects on predators and other organisms.

1. Fish

The application of OCs to control infestation of the Japanese beetle in Milford, Illinois caused extensive mortalities of the fish in the creek running through the area. Involvement of endosulfan in the die-off of 40 million fish in the Rhine River in 1967 near Borin, Germany is still fresh in our memory.[4]

2. Birds

In the case of some birds of prey, evidence is available showing that the amounts of OCs available to individual birds in the field have been enough to cause death and reproductive failure; these declines in bird population and adverse effects on reproduction were closely correlated with the introduction of the pesticides. In fact, after the withdrawal of the pesticides, some of the studies revealed increases in bird population and reproductive success was noticed.

The far ranging consequences of pesticide contamination have been demonstrated by sea birds which feed on ocean fish. For example, Glaucous gulls on Bear Island in Barnets Sea about 250 miles north of Scandanavia, where the surrounding water comes from the western North Atlantic contained on the average 17 ppm of DDE.[6]

3. Marine Animals

The most alarming aspect of pesticide contamination is the identification of OCs, particularly DDT in the large and long livered aquatic mammals. For instance, the blubber of aquatic mammals such as sea link, Horbor porpoise, fur seal, pilot whale, and long snouted Dolphin contained very high concentrations of DDT. In Horbor porpoises sampled from the Northwest Atlantic in 1970 the blubber (lipid extract) contained 29 to 119 ppm DDT, 26 to 122 ppm DDE, and 13 to 48 ppm DDD.[7] The total DDT residues in the blubber of sea lions sampled on the islands of the California coast were beyond 900 ppm with 94% being DDE.[8,9]

4. Ecological Effects

The abuse as well as the massive military employment of herbicides have inflicted ecological effects. For instance, in the second Indo-China war in South Vietnam extensive use of herbicides, 2,4-D and 2,4,5-T destroyed the flora and fauna of coastal mangroves. Military spraying of pesticides thus caused a drastic impact on the semi-aquatic, tropical and estuarial ecosystem leading to long-lasting socioeconomic problems.

5. Residues in Water Bodies

Residues of OCs are detected in most rivers, lakes, estuaries, and other water bodies. For example, Weaver et al.[10] showed that water samples from 56 rivers in the U.S. during 1964 had residues of DDT, dieldrin, and endrin. In 1966 to 1968 rivers in the Western half of the U.S. showed 72 samples positive for DDT, as compared to 16 for dieldrin, 10 for lindane, and 3 for endrin. A further survey of 118 American rivers in 1968 indicated 63 as positive for OCs. In fact, the maximum levels found were 316 ppm for DDT (Beaulieu River, Florida) 840 ppt (DDD (Kansas River, Kansas) and 407 PPT for dieldrin (Tombigbee River, Mississippi).

Monitoring studies have shown high levels of OCs in the surface waters and ground waters and sediments particularly from the coasts of Bay of Bengal in India. For instance, analysis of water samples from lakes, ponds, wells, and rivers in some parts of India showed residues of DDT and HCH.[11] The coastal sediments show the presence of ·DDT and its metabolites.[12]

6. Pesticide Poisoning in Humans

Pesticides cause acute and chronic poisoning in animals and humans. Exposure to single or repeated doses of OCs has caused acute poisoning. In a majority of cases the exposure was massive, accidental, or suicidal (Table 2). In fact, such poisonings have occurred in

TABLE 2

Symptoms of Pesticide Poisoning In Man

Pesticides	Nature of poisoning	Symptoms	No.of cases
Aldrin	Accidental	Vomiting, convulsion, death (see dieldrin and endrin)	Several
Carbofenthion	Accidental	Nausea, vomiting, coma	
Chlordane	Accidental	Vomiting	
	Suicidal	Gastrointestinal disorders	Several
		Bronchopneumonia, damage of the renal tubules	
		Tremors, neurological disturbances, convulsion, death	
Chlorfenvinphos	Accidental	Nausea, headache, salivation and vomiting, muscular weakness, convulsion	
2,4-D	Accidental	Headache, nausea, vomiting, muscular weakness	
	Suicidal	Fatigue, vertigo, cardiovascular and hepatic complaints, peripheral neuropathy, degeneration of all ganglionic cells of CNS, acute congestion of all vital organs	Several
DDT	Accidental	Muscular weakness, joint pain	
	Suicidal	Anxiety, nervousness, confusion, death	Several
Demeton	Accidental	Nausea, vomiting, headache, salivation, muscular weakness	Several
Diazinon	Accidental	Dizziness, diarrhea, paralysis	Several
Dieldrin	Accidental	Violent headache, vomiting, muscular pain	Several
	Suicidal	Twitching, vertigo, drowsiness, hyperexcitability tachycardia, convulsions, weight loss, death	
Ediphenphos	Accidental	Vomiting, nausea, dizziness	Several
Endosulfan	Suicidal	Agitation, vomiting, diarrhea, foaming, dyspnea, apnea, cyanosis, coma	Two

Compound	Type	Symptoms	Number of cases
Endrin	Accidental	Nausea, hyperthermia, abdominal discomfort	
	Suicidal	Rolling of eyeballs, dizziness, violent epileptiform convulsions, coma, death	More than 100 cases
	Homicidal		About 70 deaths
EPN	Accidental	Blurred vision, nausea, tremor, dizziness tremors, paralysis	Several
Fensulfothion	Accidental	Vomiting, diarrhea, muscular twitching, pulmonary edema, coma, death	Several
Hexachlorobenzene	Accidental	Pigmentation of the skin, diarrhea, fever, appearance of pink skin-colored papules, liver damage	About 3000
Hexachlorocyclohexane and its gamma isomer (Lindane)	Suicidal		Death of large number of infants
	Accidental	Hyperexcitability, visual and auditory aurea, neurological disorders, myoclonic jerks, cerebral seizures, toxic encephalopathy, aplastic anemia, fatty liver changes, degeneration of cardiac muscles, necrosis of the vessels of the lung, kidney, brain, and death	Several
Leptophos	Accidental	Nausea, headache, weakness, confusion, muscular incoordination, death	Several
Malathion	Accidental	Vomiting, headache, skin irritation, gastrointestinal irritation, cough, chest pain, renal damage, respiratory failure, death	
	Suicidal		
Paraquat	Accidental	Headache, giddiness, miosis, nervousness, diarrhea, salivation, respiratory distress, convulsions, coma, death	Several
Parathion	Suicidal		
	Homicidal		
Parathion methyl	Accidental	Sweating, hyperthermia, rapid pulse, dyspnea, coma, death	Several
Pentachlorophenol	Accidental		Several

TABLE 2 (continued)
Symptoms of Pesticide Poisoning In Man

Pesticides	Nature of poisoning	Symptoms	No.of cases
2,4,5-T	Accidental	Profuse sweating, neurological changes, liver disorders, chloracne, porphyrea cutacarea, pulmonary edema, coma, death	Several
TCDD	Suicidal Accidental	Anorexia, conjunctivitis, nausea, fatigue, diarrhea, dizziness, bronchitis, liver disorders, muscular weakness, loss of memory, psychological disturbances, porphyrea cutanea tarda, mild to severe chloracne, death, stillbirths, infant mortality	Several
TEPP	Accidental spillage	Headache, giddiness, weakness, blurred vision, miosis, tearing, salivation, abdominal cramps, pinpoint pupil, rhinitis, cyanosis, convulsion, coma, death	
Toxaphene	Accidental	Nausea, confusion, jerky movement of limbs, cyanosis, respiratory failure, frequent and violent convulsion, death	About 15 cases

TABLE 3
Involvement of Pesticides In Human Poisoning

Nature of Accident	Pesticides	Medium contamination	Affected	Dead	Country
Spillage during transport or storage	Endrin	Flour	159	0	Wales
	Endrin	Flour	691	24	Qutar
	Endrin	Flour	183	2	S.Arabia
	Dieldrin	Food	202	0	Shipboard
	Diazinon	Doughnut mix	20	0	U.S.
	Parathion	Wheat	360	102	India
	Parathion	Barley	38	9	Malaysia
	Parathion	Flour	200	8	Egypt
	Parathion	Flour	600	88	Columbia
	Parathion	Sugar	300	17	Mexico
	Parathion	Sheets	3	0	Canada
	Mevinphos	Plants	6	0	U.S.
Consumption of contaminated food	Hexachlorobenzene	Seed grain	>73,000	3—11%	Turkey
	Organic mercury	Seed grain	34	4	West Pakistan
	Organic mercury	Seed grain	6,000	450	Iraq(1972)
	Organic mercury	Seed grain	45	20	Guatemala
Contaminated clothing	Phosdrin	Contaminated dress material	—	—	U.S.
Improper use/application	Toxaphene	Collay and orchard	7	0	U.S.
	Nicotine	Mustard	11	0	U.S.
	Parathion	Skin contact	70	11	U.S.
	Parathion	For treatment of body lice	17	15	Iran
	Malathion	Sprayed for controlling mosquitoes	2800	4	Pakistan
Explosion	Pentachlorophenol	Nursery linens	20	2	U.S.
	Dioxin	Environment	Mass		Italy
Leakage	Methyl isocyanate (used for the manufacture of carbaryl and aldicarb)	Air & environment	20,000	2000	Bhopal, India

several countries of the world (Table 3). For example, a large population of Corpus Cristi, Texas was exposed to aerial spraying of malathion during the encephalitis epidemic of 1966. Exposed people showed symptoms of nausea, headache, weakness, and allergic reaction, and contact dermatitis due to malathion.[13,14] In Pakistan several fatalities and a large number of poisoning cases occurred due to malathion among occupational and malaria control workers.[15] Diazinon caused poisoning and as many as 34 cases have been reported in 2 years from Ruby Hospital, Pune, India.[16]

Exposure and contact to pesticides by man are different, particularly in different phases of pesticide development and use (Table 4). In fact, about 90% of the poisonings from pesticides amoung occupational workers have involved OPs.

Data on pesticide poisoning among humans are very scanty. In India, pesticide poisoning has been reported from different states. Some of the pesticides involved are parathion, malathion, sumithion, propoxur, carbaryl, endrin, chlordane etc. Interestingly more than 90

TABLE 4
Phases of Pesticide Exposure in Man

Stage	Potential exposure to pesticides
Research	Laboratory and field test personnel
Development	Research, development, pilot plant, semiscale production personnel.
Production	Production and formulation plant, packaging plant, and engineering maintenance personnel. Community aspects of local waste disposal effluents, plant emergencies, transportation in bulk. Package by road, rail, sea or air.
Distribution	Local formulation plant operators, repackaging personnel, and sales personnel.
User	Professional, large-scale contract users by ground or air, private users in agriculture and horticulture, large scale users, e.g., government insect control campaigns.
	Small scale private users, e.g., homes, gardens, institutions, shops, stores, industrial users, e.g., for preservation of materials, transport and communications systems.
Exposure of public during use or as food consumers	Accidental exposures, e.g., during transportation or while in use, accessibility to children; disposal of wastes and used containers, consumption of contaminated fruits, vegetables, and food products etc.

cases of pesticide poisonings have been recorded in the Mississippi delta area in the U.S. as early as 1977. Reich et al.[17] also reported 129 well-documented cases of poisoning from south Texas. He observed that teenage boys had occupational exposure through skin absorption to parathion and methylparathion.

While some of the human poisonings from pesticides are direct as during manufacture, formulation, and spraying etc., others are indirect for instance, by eating contaminated flour and through drinking water etc. In fact, poisoning cases reported from India, Colombia, Mexico, and other countries have amply demonstrated the involvement of food contamination.

Gross negligence in industrial hygiene resulted in poisoning of workers engaged in the manufacture of chlordecone and leptophos. The recent human tragedy in Bhopal, India is yet another example of negligence and industrial accident. It has opened new dimensions in the management of toxic chemicals and particularly in the manufacture of pesticides.

III. TOXICITY

Pesticides are toxic chemicals and cause injury to animals and humans. Interaction of pesticides and its manifestation in a given biological system is dose dependent. In fact, the toxicity of a given pesticide after a single dose to a particular species of animal is normally expressed in terms of the LD_{50} value. This is a statistical estimate of the dosage necessary to kill 50% of a very large population of the test species under standard conditions. While this value gives little or no information on the possible cumulative effects of the pesticide, it is useful in making an objective comparison of the inherent toxicity of different pesticides to species of animals.

However, several complex reactions occur in the test animal from the time of dosing till the appearance of toxic manifestations. This will involve, for instance, the interaction of the pesticide with a molecular or receptor site to produce the response and secondly, the production of a response and the degree of response in relation to the concentration of the chemical at the reactive site. One of the important steps in the evaluation of pesticide toxicity is to observe the physical and behavioral responses of the test animal which form the basis for an important pharmacological classification of pesticides.

In the following pages only selected examples of different categories of pesticides will be discussed.

A. ORGANOCHLORINE INSECTICIDES

The mode of action of OCs in animals is not clearly known. From the toxicity point of view the OCs are mainly the poisons of the central nervous system eliciting CNS-related neuromuscular and behavioral symptoms.

1. DDT

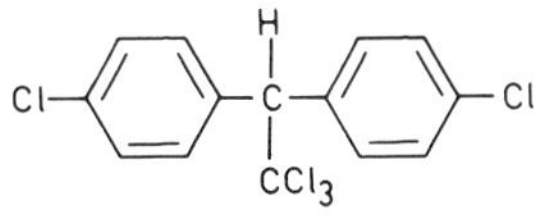

DDT (mixed isomers)

FIGURE 1.

One of the most important insecticides ever to challenge mankind is DDT. No other insecticide has received so much praise or severe condemnation as DDT. Sir Winston Churchill hailed it as a *miraculous DDT powder* when it saved the lives of millions of people affected by the outbreak of louse borne typhus in Italy in 1943. However, DDT was termed *elixir of death* by Rachel Carson[10] 2 decades later, because DDT persisted in the environment and caused damage to the environment and nontarget organisms.

Technical DDT is a white or cream colored powder. DDT is insoluble in water (less than 1 ppm) but soluble in most apolar solvents and petroleum oils. DDT is stable and does not decompose by UV or sunlight.

Variations are observed in the acute oral toxicity of DDT in species of animals. For example, mouse, rat, and cat showed different LD_{50} values. In fact, rats are more susceptible to DDT than other species of mammals.

There is no evidence to demonstrate that DDT is more toxic to young animals than adults. For instance, reports of Henderson and Woolley[19] and also of Harrison[20] show that a 2-month-old rat and adult rat have similar oral LD_{50} values (250 and 225 mg/kg respectively). Also the p,p'-DDT seems to be more toxic than the o,p'-DDT. For instance, an oral dose of 150 mg/kg p,p'-DDT produces severe illness and death in rats but o,p'-DDT at the same dose produces no illlness.

2. TDE (DDD)

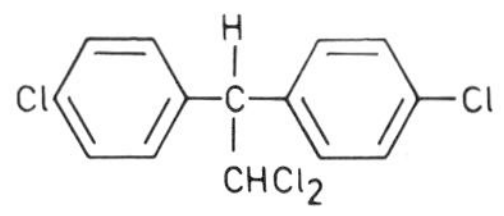

TDE (mixed isomer)

FIGURE 2.

TDE is an important analog of DDT. Pure TDE is a white crystalline solid and has a sweet odor. The oral LD_{50} value for rabbit is 3400 mg/kg and the dermal LD_{50} value for rabbits is 1200 mg/kg.

3. Dicofol

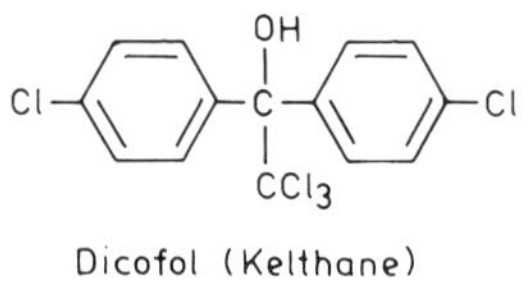

Dicofol (Kelthane)

FIGURE 3.

Dicofol is a brown, viscous oil and is soluble in organic solvents. The oral LD_{50} value for rat is 640 to 842 mg/kg and the dermal LD_{50} value for rabbit is 1870 mg/kg. Dicofol is persistent and is not affected by light or moisture. As an acaricide it is widely used for mite control on a variety of agricultural and ornamental crops.

4. Methoxychlor

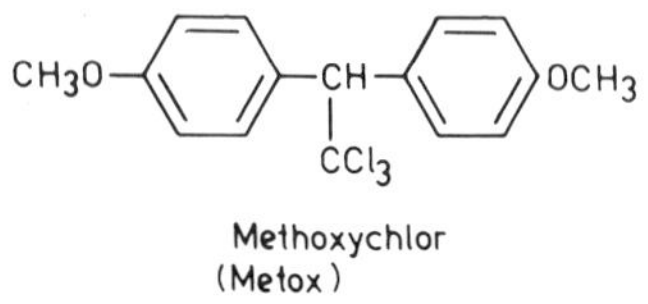

Methoxychlor
(Metox)

FIGURE 4.

Methoxychlor is another important analogue of DDT. It is a white crystalline solid. Methoxychlor is relatively less toxic to animals, the oral LD_{50} value for rat is about 6000 mg/kg. Methoxychlor is relatively less persistent, and does not accumulate in fatty tissue. Because of this property, methoxychlor is used preferentially on products near harvest, in animal feed, and in the dairy barn.

5. Hexachlorocyclohexane (HCH, BHC)

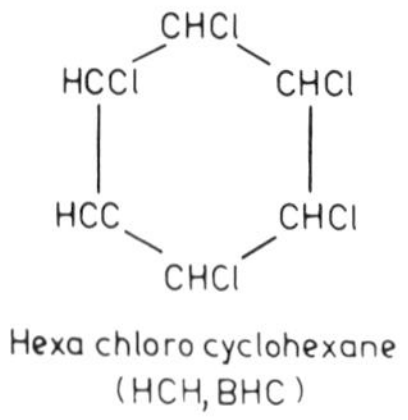

Hexa chloro cyclohexane
(HCH, BHC)

FIGURE 5.

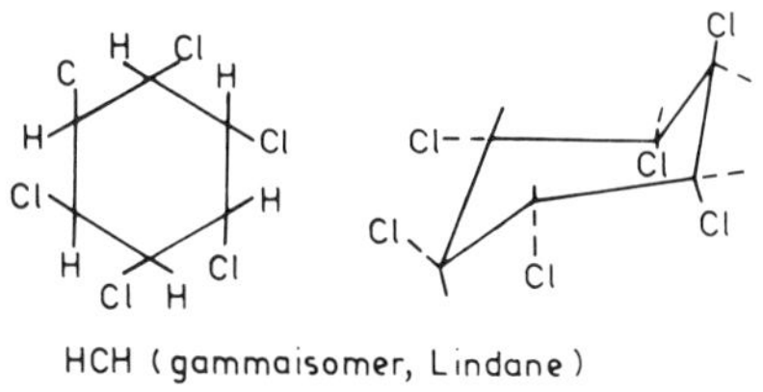

HCH (gammaisomer, Lindane)

FIGURE 5A.

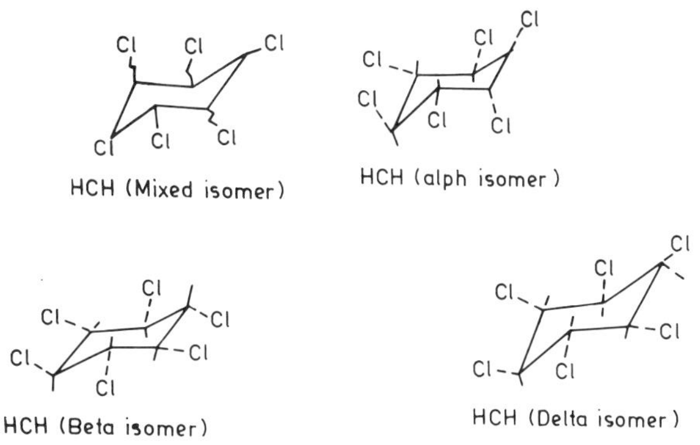

HCH (Mixed isomer)   HCH (alph isomer)

HCH (Beta isomer)   HCH (Delta isomer)

FIGURE 5B.

Technical HCH is a mixture of five chemically distinct isomers with the following composition; alpha, 65 to 70%, beta 6 to 8%, gamma 12 to 15%, delta 2 to 5%, epsilon 3 to 7%, and others 2 to 3%. It is a grayish brown colored amorphous solid. HCH is soluble in most aromatic hydrocarbons, but sparingly in water (10 to 32 ppm).

Technical HCH is toxic to animals and the toxicity is proportional to the percent content of the gamma isomer. Pure gamma isomer (99%) is called *lindane*. The acute oral and dermal LD_{50} value for rat is 1752.8 mg/kg and more than 8000 mg/kg respectively. Rabbit is more sensitive than rat to technical HCH. The acute oral and dermal LD_{50} value for rabbit is 1362.5 mg/kg and 1786.3 mg/kg respectively.[24a]

6. The Cyclodienes

The cyclodienes are an important group of chlorinated cyclic hydrocarbons containing an endomethylene bridge. The group is exemplified by such important insecticides as chlordane, heptachlor, aldrin, dieldrin, endrin, and endosulfan. There are two pairs of stereoisomers namely aldrin and isodrin, dieldrin and endrin. In fact, aldrin is rapidly metabolized to its isomer, dieldrin and hence the toxicity of aldrin is essentially that of dieldrin, likewise isodrin is metabolized to endrin.

a. Chlordane

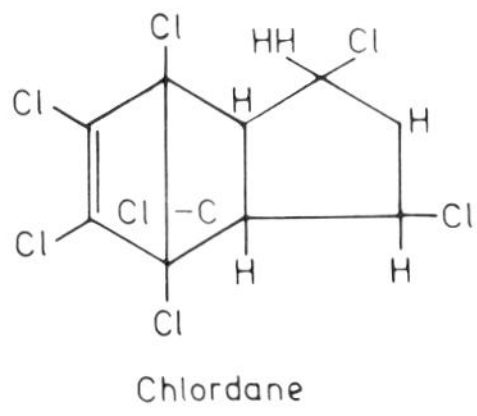

Chlordane

Chlordane (alpha isomer) (cis–chlordane)

Chlordane (gamma isomer) (trans–chlordane)

FIGURE 6. 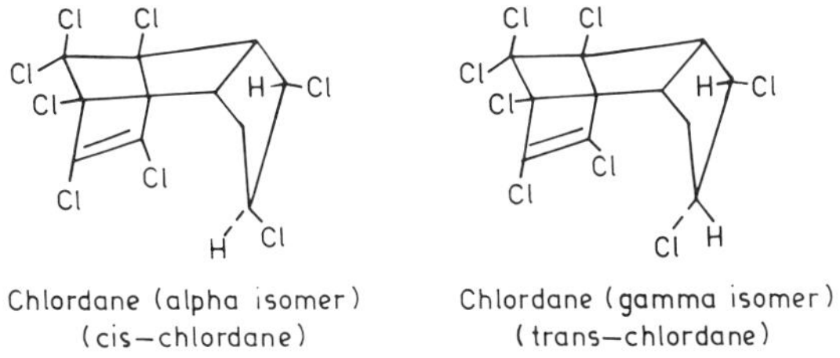   FIGURE 6A.

Technical chlordane is a brownish, viscous liquid. It is insoluble in water but soluble in most organic solvents and petroleum oils. Chlordane is stable in normal temperatures but undergoes degradation when exposed to high temperature and strong light. Chlordane has two isomers, namely cis and trans. The latter is less toxic (about 10 times) than the former. Chlordane is toxic to animals, and is absorbed by the gastrointestinal tract and skin. The oral and dermal LD_{50} values for rat are 336 to 700 mg/kg and 800 mg/kg respectively.

b. Heptachlor

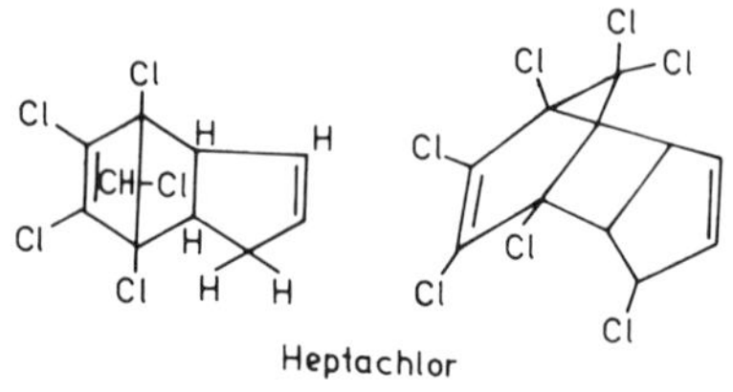

Heptachlor

FIGURE 7.

Heptachlor is a white crystalline solid. It is isolated from technical chlordane. However, heptachlor is 4 to 5 times more toxic than chlordane to mammals. It is sparingly soluble in most organic solvents and least soluble in water. The acute oral and dermal LD_{50} value of heptachlor for rat is 100 to 163 mg/kg and 195 to 250 mg/kg respectively.

c. Aldrin

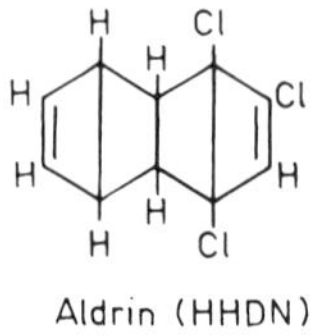

Aldrin (HHDN)

FIGURE 8.

Technical aldrin is a tan brown solid and insoluble in water (0.2 ppm) however, it is soluble in most organic solvents. Aldrin is quickly metabolized into its epoxide form, dieldrin, by a wide range of organisms.

The oral and dermal LD_{50} values in aldrin to rats are 39 to 60 mg/kg and 98 mg/kg respectively. The epoxidation of aldrin into dieldrin is more rapid in the male rat than in the female.

d. Dieldrin

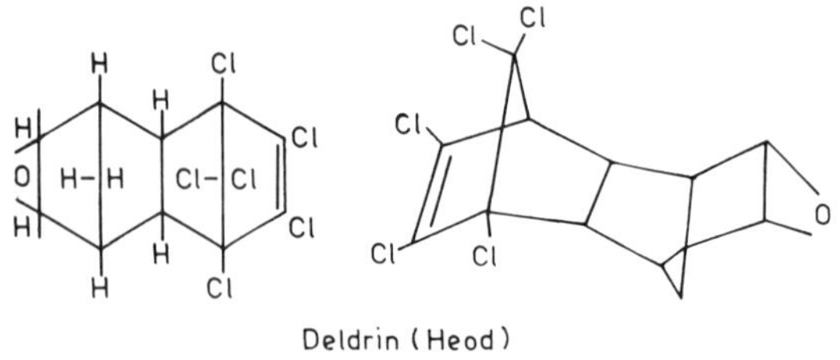

Deldrin (Heod)

FIGURE 9.

Dieldrin is the epoxy form of aldrin. Technical dieldrin is a tan-colored solid. Like aldrin it is insoluble in water but less soluble in organic solvents.

The oral and dermal LD_{50} value for rat is 46 mg/kg and 60 to 90 mg/kg respectively. Dieldrin is rapidly absorbed through the skin. The photo conversion isomer of dieldrin is much more toxic than the parent compound to experimental animals. Toxicity of dieldrin to animals is comparable with that of aldrin.

15

e. Endrin

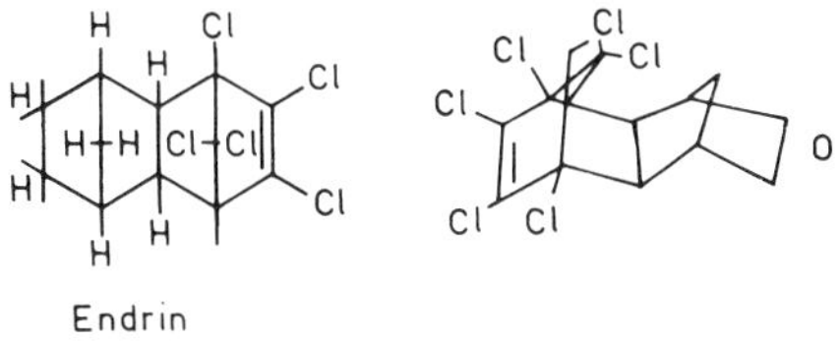

Endrin

FIGURE 10.

Endrin is the end-endo isomer of dieldrin and differs only in the spatial arrangement of the two rings. Among the cyclodienes endrin ranks as the most toxic compound.

Technical endrin is a light tan-colored powder. Although chemically endrin is very similar to dieldrin, it is degraded by light and heat. Endrin is highly toxic to rats and has oral and dermal LD_{50} value of 7.5 to 17.8 and 15 mg/kg, respectively. Young rats are less susceptible than adults, but females are more vulnerable than males to endrin-induced toxicity. Chronic exposure of animals to endrin has caused severe toxicity.[22]

f. Endosulfan

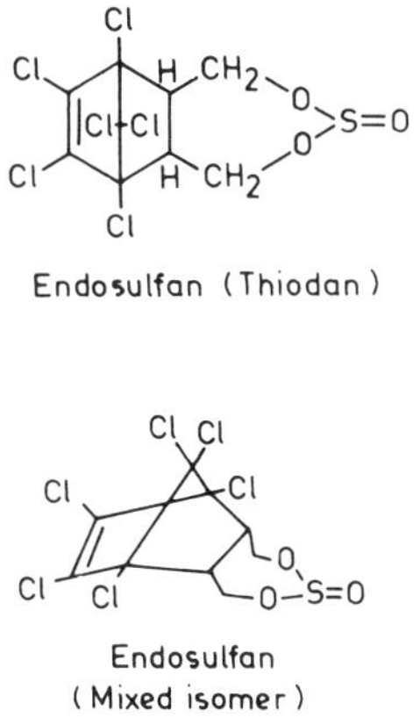

Endosulfan (Thiodan)

Endosulfan
(Mixed isomer)

FIGURE 11.

Technical endosulfan is a brown, crystalline solid and is a mixture of two isomers. It is soluble in organic solvents and highly insoluble in water. Endosulfan is hydrolyzed slowly by water and acids.

The acute oral and dermal LD_{50} value of technical endosulfan for rat is 18 to 43 mg/kg and 78 to 130 mg/kg. Mouse is more susceptible to endosulfan than rat. Experimental studies in rats showed that toxicity of endosulfan doubles with moderate deprivation of protein.[23,24]

7. Mirex and Chlordecone (Kepone)

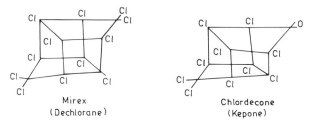

FIGURE 12.   FIGURE 13.

Chlordecone is the product of degradation of mirex. Technical chlordecone is a solid substance of white to tan color. Chlordecone is relatively soluble in water and in most organic solvents.

Mirex is a white crystalline solid. It is virtually insoluble in water but soluble in some organic solvents like benzene and xylene. The oral LD_{30} value of chlordecone for rat is 126 to 132 mg/kg and in rabbits has 410 mg/kg as the dermal LD_{50}. In contrast, mirex has an oral LD_{50} value of 600 mg/kg for rat. Both compounds cause adverse effects to liver of animals. For example, treatment of rats with chlordecone and mirex produces significant liver enlargement, and hepatobiliary disfunction.

8. Toxaphene

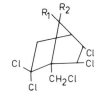

Toxaphene (Camphechlor)

FIGURE 14.

Toxaphene is a product obtained by the chlorination of bicyclic terpenes. Toxaphene is a yellowish wax and is soluble in most organic solvents. It is sparingly soluble in water (3 ppm). The oral and dermal LD_{50} value of toxaphene for rat is 80 to 90 mg/kg and 780 to 1075 mg/kg respectively. As is evident, absorption of toxaphene by the gastrointestinal tract is rapid and hence more toxic by the oral route than through skin absorption. Mouse and dog are more susceptible to taxaphene than rat.

B. ORGANOPHOSPHOROUS INSECTICIDES

The large scale synthesis and development of the phosphoric acid esters are closely associated with their role as insecticides in crop protection, particularly after World War II. Small stocks of two potential war gases *serine* and *tabum* were changed into weapons and this has lead to the identification of the compounds as insecticides, because they were more lethal to insects than to humans.

The number of OPs is very large, but forms a well-recognized class. In fact, the mode of action, chemical structure, and reactivity of the members of this group are well documented. For instance, whether they are true phosphates or other types of OP compounds, these chemicals possess the common characterstic that they are or can become good inhibitors of cholinesterases.

The OPs act on the nervous system by inhibiting acetylcholinesterases (AchE) at the synapse. For the proper function of neurotransmission in animals, there must be proper release of acetylcholine (Ach). When the impulse is passed, AchE acts on the Ach to return to an active ionic state. The manner of action and kinetics of the reactions associated with the OPs are discussed by several workers.[25-28] The following pages will describe some of the important OP compounds.

1. Azinphosmethyl

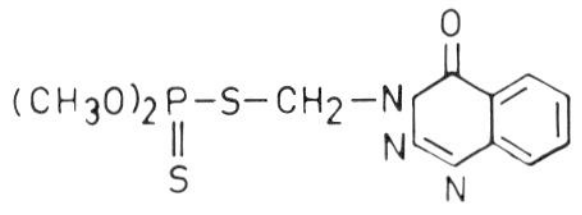

Azinphos methyl (Guthion)

FIGURE 15.

Azinphosmethyl is also known as Guthion. It is a white solid soluble in organic solvents but sparingly soluble in water. Azinposmethyl is highly toxic to animals. It has an oral LD_{50} value of 15 mg/kg for rat and a dermal LD_{50} value of 225 mg/kg.

2. Bromophos

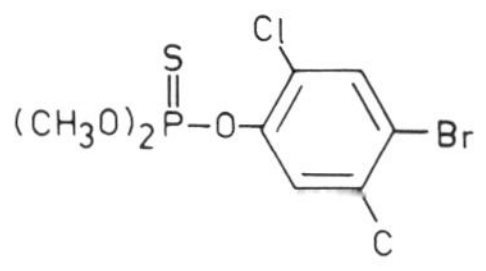

Bromophos (Nexion)

FIGURE 16.

Bromophos is a yellowish crystal. It is appreciably soluble in water (40mg/l) and soluble in most of the organic solvents. The acute oral LD_{50} value for rat is 3750 to 7700 mg/kg, while acute dermal LD_{50} value for rabbit is 2181 mg/kg. Mouse and rabbit are more susceptible than rat. Rats and dogs showed no long term toxicity at doses of 35 mg/kg and 44 mg/kg respectively.

3. Carbophenothion

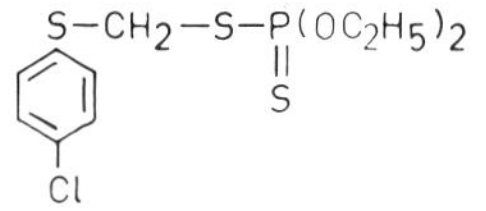

Carbophenothion (Trithion)

FIGURE 17.

Carbophenothion is a colorless to amber colored liquid. It is less soluble in water (40 mg/l of water) and soluble in most organic solvents. The acute oral LD_{50} value for rat is 32.3 mg/kg, while the acute dermal LD_{50} value for rabbit is 1270 mg/kg. In association with malathion carbophenothion causes severe toxicity and the potentiation effect is about threefold.

4. Chlorpyrifos

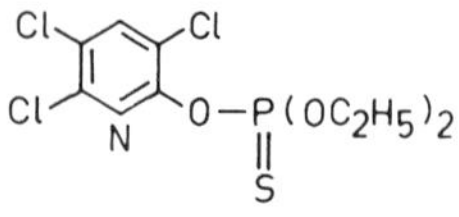

Chlorpyrifos (Dursban)

FIGURE 18.

Chlorpyrifos is a colorless crystal and sparingly soluble in water; however it is readily soluble in several organic solvents. The acute oral LD_{50} value for rat is 135 to 163 mg/kg while the dermal LD_{50} value for rabbit is about 2000 mg/kg. Chlorpyrifos undergoes rapid detoxification in animals.

5. Chlorpyrifos-Methyl

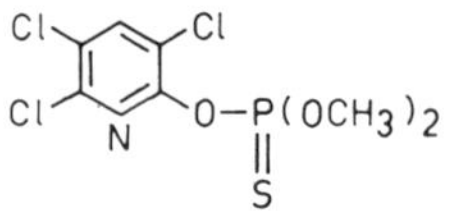

Chlorpyrifos methyl (Reldan)

FIGURE 19.

Chlorpyrifos-methyl is a colorless crystal and soluble in most of the organic solvents. The acute oral LD_{50} for rat is 1630 to 2140 mg/kg while the acute dermal LD_{50} value is more than 2000 mg/kg.

6. Demeton

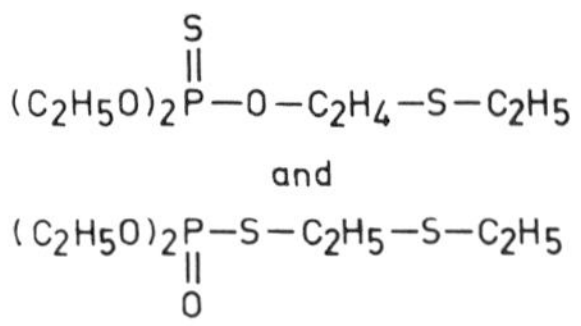

Demeton (mixed isomers) (systox)

FIGURE 20.

Demeton is a mixture and occurs in two forms as Demeton-O and Demeton-S. It is a colorless oil and soluble in most organic solvents and to a less extent in water. Demeton is extremely toxic to animals. The acute oral LD_{50} for rat is 6 to 12 mg/kg. It is more toxic to female rat than to male.

7. Diazinon

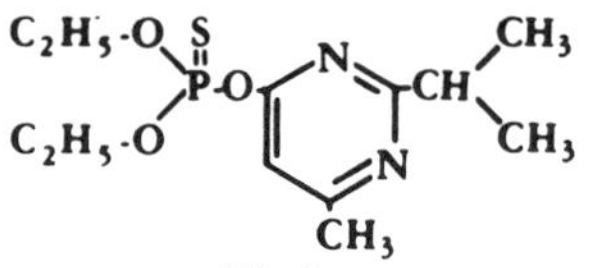

Diazinon

FIGURE 21.

Diazinon is a reddish-brown liquid miscible in several organic solvents, but slightly soluble in water. It decomposes in high temperature. Diazinon has an acute oral LD_{50} value for rats as 600 mg/kg and dermal LD_{50} value as 380 to 200 mg/kg. Diazinon is converted in the animal body to diazoxon, a more potent product.

8. Dichlorvos

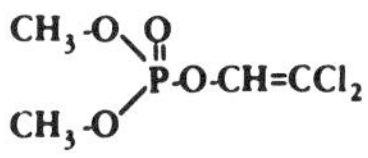

CH$_3$-O O
         ⫽
          P-O-CH=CCl$_2$
CH$_3$-O

Dichlorvos
(DDVP, Vapona)

FIGURE 22.

Dichlorvos is a colorless to amber colored liquid. It is miscible with most organic solvents and to a slight extent with water. Dichlorvos is highly toxic to animals. The acute oral and dermal LD_{50} value for rat is 56 to 108 mg/kg and 75 to 210 mg/kg respectively. It is highly toxic to birds and honey bees.

9. Dimethoate

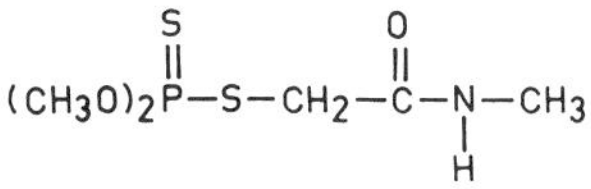

```
        S             O
        ‖             ‖
(CH3O)2P—S—CH2—C—N—CH3
                      |
                      H
```
Dimethoate (Cygon)

FIGURE 23.

Dimethoate is a colorless crystal and soluble in most organic solvents and to a less extent in water. Dimethoate is toxic to animals. The acute oral LD_{50} value for rat is 155 to 500 mg/kg.

10. Disulfoton

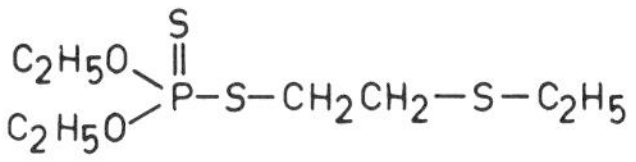

```
          S
          ‖
C2H5O
      P—S—CH2CH2—S—C2H5
C2H5O
```
Disulfoton (Di-Syston)

FIGURE 24.

Disulfoton is a colorless oil with a characterstic odor. It is soluble in most organic solvents and to a less extent in water. Disulfoton is highly toxic to animals. The acute oral and dermal LD_{50} value for rat is 2.6 to 8.6 mg/kg respectively.

11. EPN

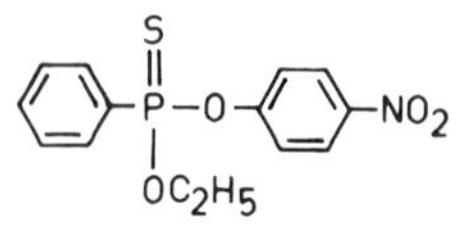

EPN (Santox)

FIGURE 25.

EPN is light yellow colored crystalline powder. It is soluble in most organic solvents but insoluble in water. EPN is highly toxic to animals. The acute oral and dermal LD_{50} value for rat is 14 to 42 mg/kg and 110 to 230 mg/kg respectively. The female rat is more susceptible to EPN than male and the compound is highly toxic to dogs.

12. Ethion

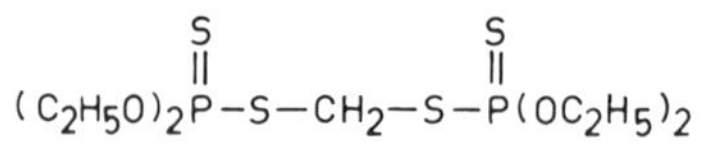

Ethion (Bladan)

FIGURE 26.

Ethion is a colorless to amber colored liquid. It is soluble in most organic solvents including kerosine, but sparingly soluble in water. Ethion is highly toxic to animals. The acute oral LD_{50} value for rat is 24.4 mg/kg and the acute dermal LD_{50} value for rabbit is 915 mg/kg.

13. Fenthion

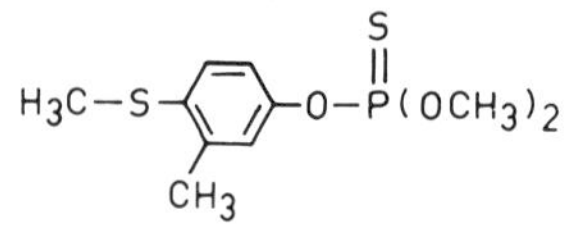

Fenthion (Baytex)

FIGURE 27.

Fenthion is a colorless liquid. The technical product is a brownish oil. It is readily soluble in most organic solvents and less soluble in water. The acute oral and dermal LD_{50} value for rat is 190 to 315 mg/kg and 330 500 mg/kg respectively. The male rat is more susceptible than the female. Fenthion is more toxic to dogs and poultry.

14. Fenitrothion

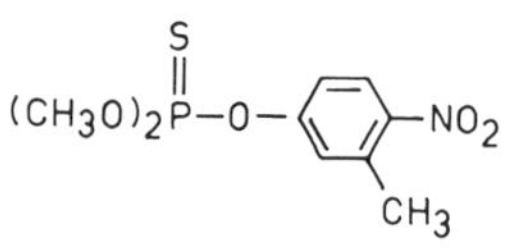

Fenitrothion (Sumithion)

FIGURE 28.

Fenitrothion is a brownish liquid soluble in most organic solvents but sparingly soluble in water. It is moderately toxic to animals with acute oral and dermal LD_{50} values for rats as 250 to 670 mg/kg and 200 to 730 mg/kg respectively. Fenitrothion converts in the body of animals as fenitroxon. The insecticide degrades rapidly into a number of metabolites like p-nitrocresol, demethyl fenitrothion, aminofenitrothion, and dimethyl phosphorothioic acid.

15. Leptophos

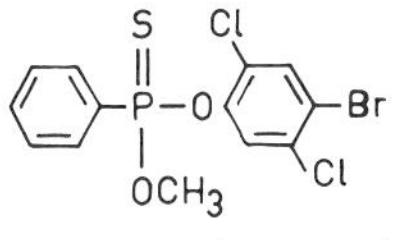

Leptophos (Phosvel)

FIGURE 29.

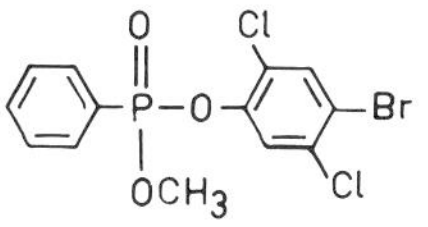

Leptophos oxygen analog (Leptophoxon)

FIGURE 29A.

Leptophos is a colorless, amorphous solid. It is highly soluble in benzene, acetone, cyclohexane and heptane, and sparingly soluble in water. Leptophos is highly toxic to animals. The acute oral LD_{50} for rat is about 50 mg/kg and the acute dermal LD_{50} for rabbit is about 800 mg/kg. Leptophos is known to produce delayed neurotoxicity in animals.

16. Malathion

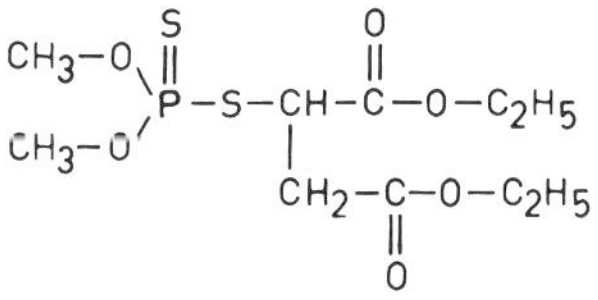

Malathion (Sumitox)

FIGURE 30.

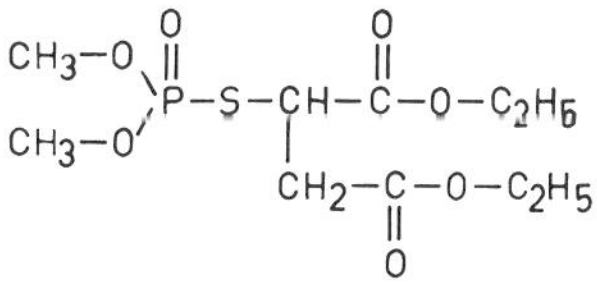

Malathion oxygen analog (Malaoxon)

FIGURE 31.

Malathion is an amber-colored liquid, miscible in organic solvents. It is moderately soluble in petroleum distillates and very slightly soluble in water. Malathion has low toxicity to mammals with oral and dermal LD_{50} values for rat as 1500 mg/kg and 4000 mg/kg respectively. Malathion is converted in the body of animals into malaoxon and degrades rapidly.

17. Methamidophos

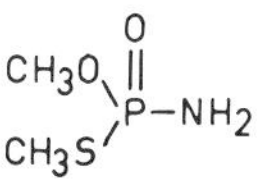

Methamidophos (Monitor)

FIGURE 32.

Methamidophos is a white solid with a pungent odor. It is readily soluble in water and organic solvents. The acute oral and dermal LD_{50} value for rat is 30 mg/kg and 50 to 110 mg/kg respectively.

18. Methylparathion

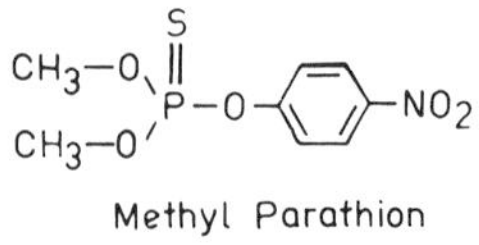

Methyl Parathion

FIGURE 33.

Methylparathion is a white crystalline powder completely soluble in most organic solvents but slightly soluble in petroleum distillates and water. It is highly toxic to animals. The oral and dermal LD_{50} value for rat is 14 to 24 mg/kg and 67 mg/kg respectively. Methyl parathion metabolizes in animal in a manner similar to that of parathion, and forms the highly toxic methyl paraoxon.

19. Oxydemeton-Methyl

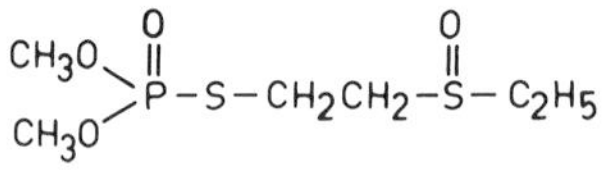

Oxydemeton methyl (Metasystox)

FIGURE 34.

Oxydemeton-methyl is the methyl analogue of the thiol isomer of demeton. It is a clear amber-colored liquid. It is miscible with water and most organic solvents. Oxydemeton-methyl is highly toxic to animals, both as a contact and systemic insecticide. The acute oral and dermal LD_{50} value for rat is 65 to 80 mg/kg and 250 mg/kg respectively.

20. Parathion

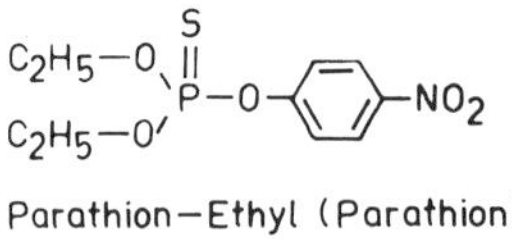

Parathion—Ethyl (Parathion)

FIGURE 35.

Parathion is a dark brown colored liquid miscible in benzene and many other organic solvents. However, pure parathion is a colorless and odorless liquid. It is insoluble in petroleum and mineral oils and partially soluble in water. Parathion is extremely toxic to animals. The oral and dermal LD_{50} value for rat is 3.6 to 15 mg/kg and 6.8 to 21 mg/kg respectively. Parathion converts in the animal body into paraoxon, a powerful anticholinesterase compound. Currently, use of parathion is stopped and less hazardous organophosphorous compounds are advocated. Parathion has a very brief residual life.

21. Phorate

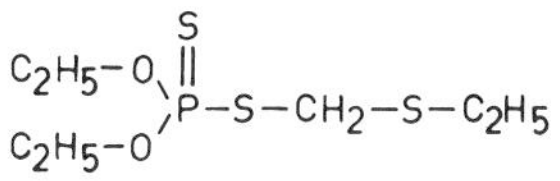

$$C_2H_5-O \quad \overset{S}{\underset{\|}{P}}-S-CH_2-S-C_2H_5$$
$$C_2H_5-O$$

Phorate (Thimet)

FIGURE 36.

Phorate is closely related to demeton. Phorate is a clear liquid. It is miscible with most organic solvents and to a less extent in water. Phorate is extremely toxic to animals. The acute oral and dermal LD_{50} value for rat is 1.6 to 3.7 mg/kg and 2.5 and 6.2 mg/kg respectively. Phorate is a systemic insecticide and miticide.

22. Phosalone

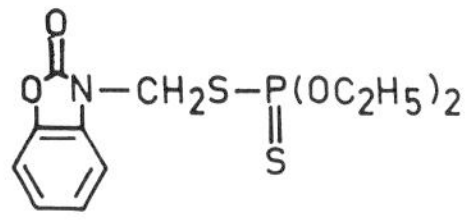

Phosalone (Zolone)

FIGURE 37.

Phosalone is a colorless crystalline powder. It is soluble in acetone and other organic solvents and very sparingly soluble in water. Phosalone is toxic to animals. The acute oral and dermal LD_{50} value for rat is 120 to 170 mg/kg and 1500 mg/kg.

23. Phosphamidon

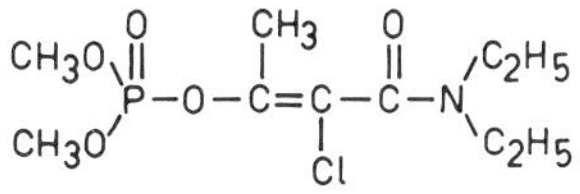

Phosphamidon (Dimecron)

FIGURE 38.

Phosphamidon is a pale yellow liquid. It is soluble in most organic solvents and water. Phosphamidon is highly toxic to animals. The acute oral and dermal LD_{50} values for rat is 17 to 30 mg/kg and 374 to 530 mg/kg respectively.

24. Pirimiphos-Methyl

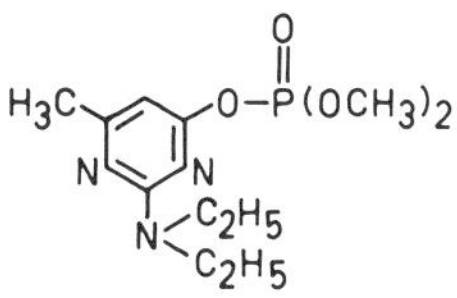

Pirimiphos-methyl (Actellic)

FIGURE 39.

Pirimiphos-methyl is a straw-colored liquid. It is miscible with most organic solvents and less miscible with water. Pirimiphos-methyl is toxic to animals. The acute oral LD_{50}

value for rat is 2050 mg/kg and the acute dermal LD_{50} for rabbit is about 2000 mg/kg. It is more toxic to mouse and dog.

25. Quinalphos

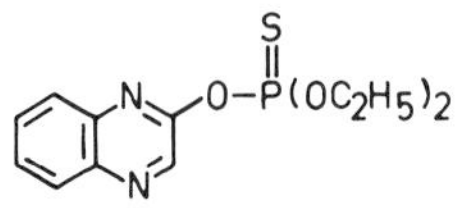

Quinalphos (Bayrusil)

FIGURE 40.

Quinalphos is a colorless crystalline solid. It is soluble in xylene and other organic solvents and slightly soluble in water. The acute oral and dermal LD_{50} value for rat is 62 to 137 mg/kg and 1250 and 1400 mg/kg respectively. It is highly toxic to animals.

26. Schradan

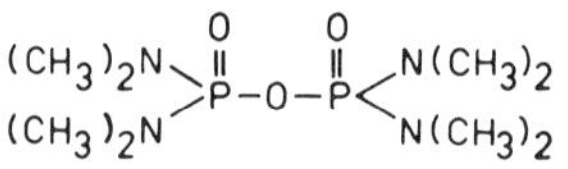

Schradan (OMPA)

FIGURE 41.

Schradan is a colorless viscous liquid. It is miscible with most organic solvents and water. However, it is less soluble in petroleum oils. Schradan is highly toxic to animals. The acute oral and dermal LD_{50} value for rat is 9.1 to 42 mg/kg and 15 to 44 mg/kg respectively. The male rat is more susceptible to Schradan than female rat.

27. TEPP

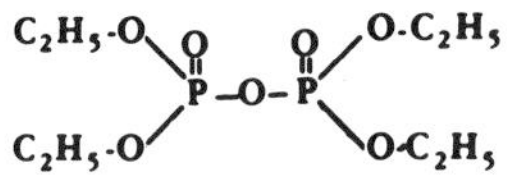

TEPP

FIGURE 42.

TEPP is a colorless, hygroscopic liquid. It is miscible with water and most organic solvents, but sparingly soluble in petroleum oils. TEPP is extremely toxic to animals. The acute oral and dermal LD_{50} value for rat is 1.2 mg/kg and 2.4 mg/kg respectively. TEPP undergoes rapid metabolism in animals.

28. Trichlorfon

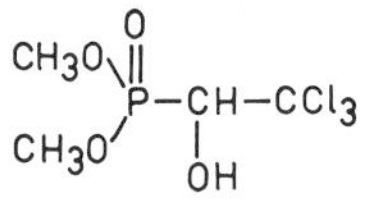

Trichlorfon (Dylox)

FIGURE 43.

Trichlorfon is a colorless crystalline powder. It is soluble in organic solvents and in water. It is insoluble in petroleum oils. The acute oral and dermal LD_{50} value for rat is 560 to 630 mg/kg and more than 2000 mg/kg respectively. Trichlorfon undergoes metabolic conversion to dichlorvos.

C. CARBAMATES

Carbamate compounds as pesticides are of relatively recent origin. They have been used for plant protection purposes since 1958 and onwards. The biological activity of carbamates has a closer relationship with that of OPs. This has been ascribed to the structural similarity with Ach and the attraction of the C=O group to the OH site of the enzyme AchE.

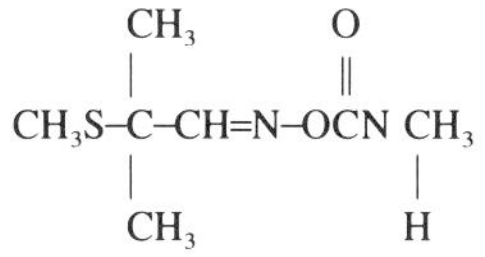

FIGURE 44.   FIGURE 44A.

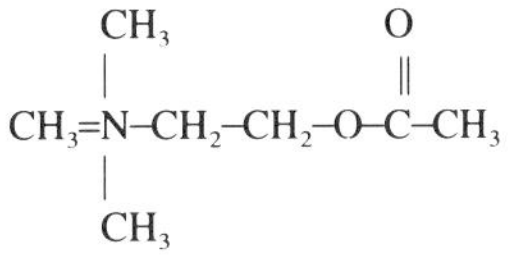

Carbamates have a large range of toxicity to animals and have broad spectrum effects. There are three major classes of carbamates: (a) N-methyl carbamates of phenol and carbaryl are members of this class; (b) N-methyl carbamates of oximes as examplified by aldicarb and methomyl, and (c) N-methyl carbamates and N,N-dimethyl carbamates of hydro heterocyclic compounds such as carbofuran, bendiocarb, and pirimicarb.

1. Aldicarb

Technically pure aldicarb is a white crystal, and sparingly miscible in water and most organic solvents. For instance, the solubility of aldicarb in acetone is 34%, in ethanol 25%, and in toluene 10%. Aldicarb is extremely toxic to animals. The acute oral and dermal LD_{50} value for rat is 0.6 to 0.8 mg/kg and 2.5 to 3.0 mg/kg respectively. The female rat is more sensitive than the male rat.

2. Carbaryl

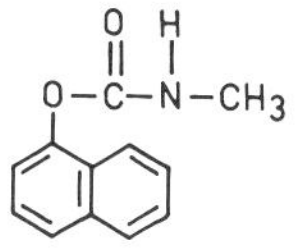

Carbaryl (Sevin)

FIGURE 45.

Pure carbaryl is a white crystalline solid, moderately soluble in most organic solvents and very sparingly soluble in water. Carbaryl is relatively less toxic to animals. The acute oral and dermal LD_{50} value for rat is 500 to 850 mg/kg and more than 4000 mg/kg respectively. Mouse and dog are more susceptible to carbaryl.

3. Carbofuran

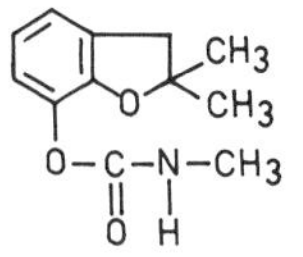

Carbofuran (Furadan)

FIGURE 46.

The pure carbofuran is a white crystalline solid and moderately soluble in most organic solvents and not very soluble in water (700 ppm). Carbofuran is highly toxic to animals. The oral and dermal LD_{50} value for rat is 8.0 to 8.7 mg/kg and more than 1000 mg/kg respectively.

4. Methomyl

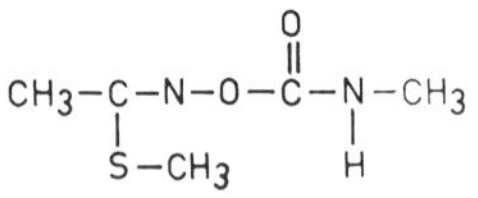

Methomyl (Lannate)

FIGURE 47.

The pure methomyl is a white crystalline solid. It is relatively more soluble in several organic solvents and in water. Methomyl is toxic to animals. The acute oral LD_{50} value for rat is 17 to 23.5 mg/kg. The acute dermal LD_{50} for rabbit is more than 5000 mg/kg.

5. Propoxur

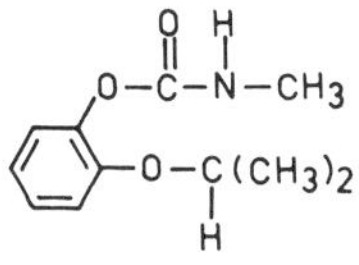

Propoxur (Baygon)

FIGURE 48.

The pure propoxur is a white crystalline powder and soluble in most organic solvents. Its solubility in water is 2 g/l. Propoxur is toxic to animals. The acute oral LD_{50} value for rat is 90 to 128 mg/kg while the acute dermal LD_{50} is more than 2 g/kg. It has a rapid knockdown effect and long residual life. It is used extensively for the control of household pests. More information on the toxicity of several carbmate compounds may be found in other reviews.[28a]

D. OTHER COMPOUNDS
1. Herbicides

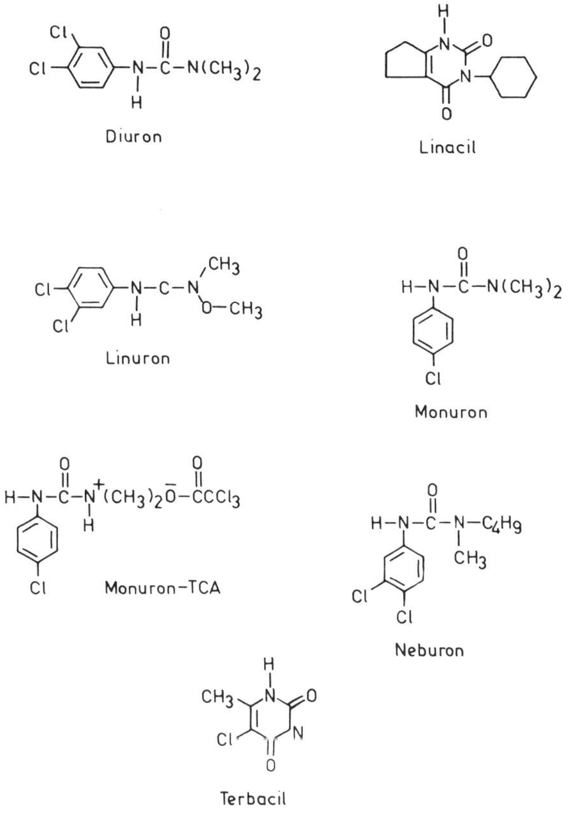

FIGURE 49.

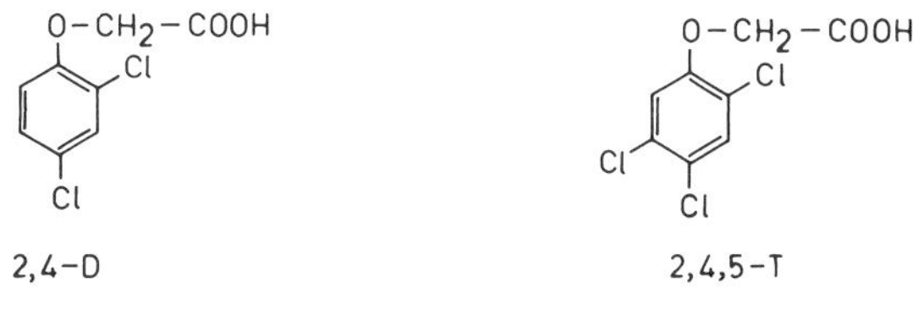

FIGURE 49A.

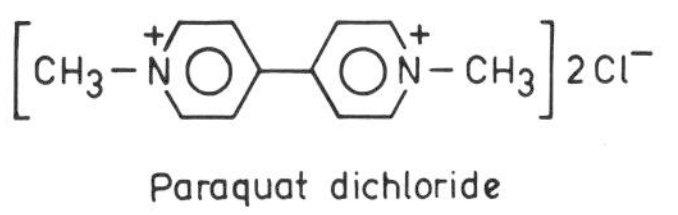

FIGURE 49B.

Herbicides comprise several categories of chemicals, for example, substituted ureas, phenoxy acids, bipyridyliums, triazines, dinitrophenols etc. (Table 5). Herbicides generally have low solubility and high LD_{50} values for animals. For instance, the oral LD_{50} value of monourm and diuron for rat is over 3 g/kg. However, certain compounds do produce strong irritation of skin, eyes, and upper respiratory passages. Also the chronic toxicity studies suggest that monouron has carcinogenic effects on animals.[29,30]

TABLE 5
Chemical Classification of Widely Used
Herbicides

Anilides
Alachlor
Carbetamide
Difenamid
Monilide
Napromid
Pentachlor
Propachlor
Propanyl
Benzonitriles
Bromoynil
Chlorthiamid
Dichlorpheil
Ioxynil
Propyzamide
Carbamates
Asulam
Barbane
Chlorbufam
Chlorpropham
Methiocarb
Pebulate
Phenmedipham
Terbutol
Propham
Diazines
Bentazon
Bromacyl
Brompyrazon
Dazomet
Lenacil
Maleic hydrazide
Terbacil
Toluidines
Benfluralin
Buztalin
Dimethachlor
Ethalfluralin
Fluorodifen
Nitralin
Phenoxaline
Trifluralin
Triazines
Ametryne
Atrazne
Cynatrine
Urea compounds
Chloroxuron
Chloetoluron
Cycluron
Diuron
Isonoruron
Isoproturon
Fenuron
Fluometuron

Dipyridyliums
Bipyridyliums
Diquat
Paraquat
Dithiocarbamates
Butylate
Cycloate
Diallate
Metham
Molinate
Nabam
Tri-allate
Sulfallate
Nitro compounds
Dinoseb
Dinoterb
DNOC
Nitrofen
Cynazine
Desmetryne
Dibrompetryn
Metribuzine
Prometon
Propazine
Simasine
Terbutilazine
Terbutiyne
Phenoxy compounds
2,4-D
2,4-DB
Dichlorprop
Fenoprop
MCPA
MCPB
Mecoprop
Urea compounds
Monolinuron
Monuron
Neburon
Noruron
Phenobenzuron
Siduron
Miscellaneous
Aminotriazole
Benazolin
Dalapn
Dicamba
Dimexan
Ethiofumezate
Flurecol
Glyphosate
Hexaflurate
Naphthalam
oils
Petroleum products
Oxadiazon

TABLE 5 (continued)
Chemical Classification of Widely Used
Herbicides

Anilides	Dipyridyliums
Linuron	Picloram
Methazole	Propazon
Metobromuron	Sodium chlorate
Metoxuron	Sodium metaborate
	Sulfuric acid
	2,3,6-TBA

Paraquat is a well known example of the bipyridyl group of herbicides. Paraquat has been associated with a large number of human fatalities. The oral LD_{50} of paraquat for rat is about 125 mg/kg. However, the range for higher animals like cats and cows is 30 to 50 mg/kg.

2. Fungicides

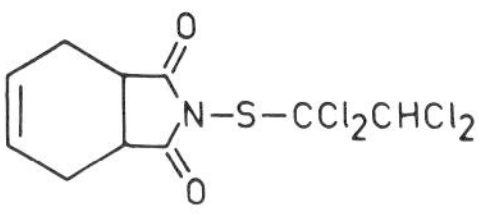

Captafol (Difolatan)

FIGURE 50.

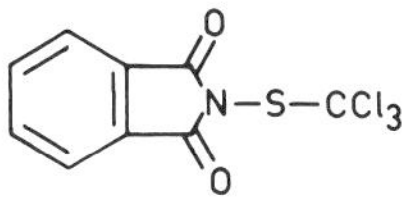

Folpet (Phaltan)

FIGURE 51.

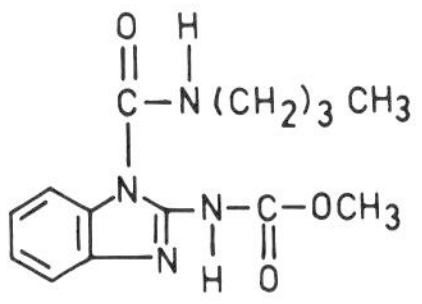

Benomyl (Belnate)

FIGURE 52.

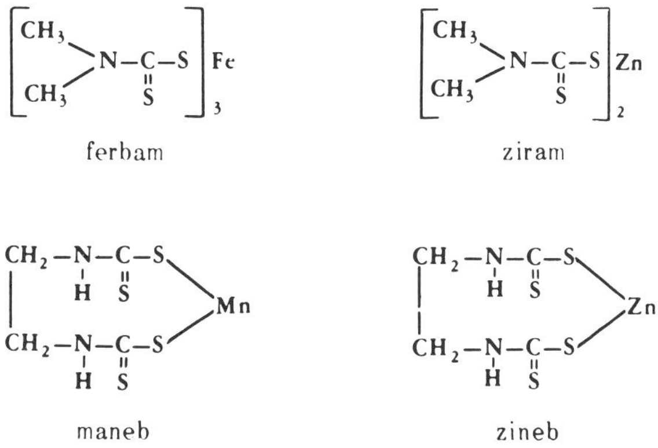

ferbam

ziram

maneb

zineb

FIGURE 53.

Fungicides also encompass a variety of chemical compounds, for example, organomercurial compounds, organotin compounds, phenols, dithiocarbamates, and phthalimides. Barring the organometallic compounds, the acute oral LD_{50} value of several fungicides for rat is very high. For example, compounds like captan, captafol (Figure 50), folpet (Figure 51) and benomyl (Figure 52) have very high LD_{50} values which range between 3,000 mg/kg to 10,000 mg/kg. The dithiocarbamate group of fungicides has been in large use in agriculture (Figure 53). Although the LD_{50} value of several dithiocarbamates like ziram, zineb, maneb, and ferbam range to several grams per kilogram, the compounds convert to more toxic and active products, namely ethylene thiourea (ETU). Some of the dithiocarbamates have been implicated as mutagenic, teratogenic, and carcinogenic agents in laboratory animals.

3. Synthetic pyrethroids

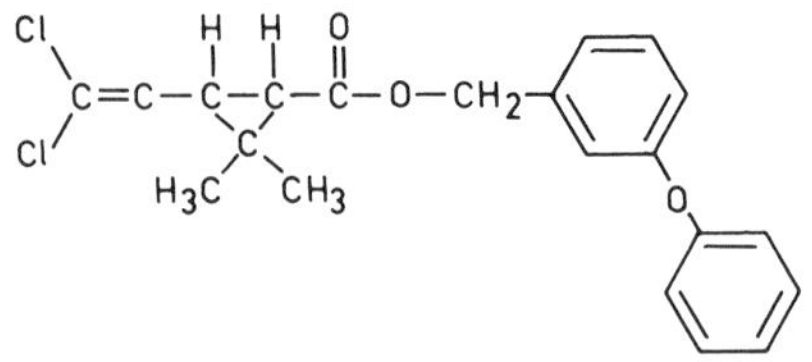

Permethrin (mixed isomers)
(Ambush, pounce)

FIGURE 54.

Research on natural pyrethrins have led to the development of one of the most promising *third generation* pesticides, the synthetic pyrethroids. They are mainly analogues to the most active of the natural pyrethrin I. Allethrin, permethrin, cypermethrin, deltamethrin, resmethrin, and fenvalerate are the few important compounds.

The synthetic pyrethroids have shown remarkable results in the control of pests, and are fast becoming the most potent group of synthetic pesticides ever to enter the pest management program.

4. Rodenticides

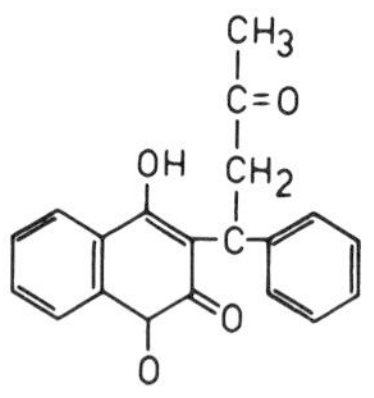

Warfarin

FIGURE 55.

Several chemicals are used in the control of rats and other rodents. For instance, warfarin, sodium fluroacetate, ANTU, and zinc phosphide are a few of the important ones which produce toxicity to rodents as well as to other animals. The rodenticidal selectivity of these compounds is based on the peculiar physiology of rodents.

5. Fumigants

Fumigants are extremely volatile compounds. As such they are used extensively for the control of pests of stored products and food grains. The most important fumigant is phosphine which is released from the aluminum phosphide when it reacts with atmospheric moisture. Phosphine is extremely toxic to animals and humans. The permissible limit of phosphine for man is 0.05 ppm.

Methyl bromide (MB), ethylene dibromide (EDB), and dibromochloropropane (DBCP) are a few more important fumigants used in pest management. These compounds are highly toxic and produce a variety of pathomorphological changes in animals and humans.

In conclusion, it may be stated that pesticides of several kinds are likely to be used on an increasing scale in the years to come. This is required for the control of pests that attack man and his domestic animals, and also for the improvement of crop yields as well as for the preservation of stored food products.

More widespread use of pesticides has resulted in misuse leading to health hazards. The brief outline of each pesticide provides the possible toxicological effects to animals in terms of oral and dermal toxicity and gives a clue to the subsequent chapters, where discussions are in much greater detail.

Pesticides which are in use today cover hundreds of organic molecules. The organo-chlorine compounds are the most persistent ones and are mostly fat soluble, and accumulate in the fat depot and vital tissues of animals and humans. In view of these, they are not metabolized fast enough to facilitate their rapid elimination from the body.

A majority of organophosphorus pesticides are basically of a single chemical nature and are the derivatives of phosphoric acid. These compounds have a uniform mode of action in the inhibition of cholinesterase. The organophosphorus pesticides have the characteristic features of least persistence and rapid biodegradation yet are labeled as highly hazardous compounds. These chemicals present a serious health hazard of acute intoxication.

The carbamates act as inhibitors of cholinesterase in a similar manner as that of the organophosphorus pesticides. Carbamates present a wide diversity with particular reference to mammalian toxicity, while aldicarb is extremely toxic; carbaryl and carbofuran have shown broad spectrum effects to mammals.

A large number of herbicides are used in plant protection. These include amilides, dithiocarbamates, nitrocompounds, triazines, and substituted urea compounds. The toxicity of these chemicals is as diverse as the group itself.

The symptoms of poisoning from pesticides in animals and humans demands greater caution and judicious use. These are economically important compounds required for the benefit of man and for the improvement of quality of life.

APPENDIX A
Pesticides Restricted/Banned from Further Use in Countries

Country	Status	Pesticides
Algeria	Restricted/banned	Heptachlor, Chlordane and dieldrin, Organic mercury (only followed for disinfection of cotton seed)
Argentina	Restricted/banned	Dieldrin, endrin, HCH
Australia	Restricted/banned	HCH and seed dressing mercurials
Austria	Restricted	Hexachlorocyclohexane, lindane, DDT, chlordane, toxaphene, heptachlor, aldrin, dieldrin and endrin
	Banned on vegetable production	Aldrin, dieldrin, endrin, heptachlor
Belgium	Banned/restricted	DDT, chlordane, aldrin, dieldrin, toxaphene, per-thane, methoxychlor, heptachlor, and hexachlorobenzene
Canada	Banned/restricted in registration	DDT, toxaphene, aldrin, dieldrin, endrin, chlordane, heptachlor, 2,4,5-T in some areas
Denmark	Use restricted	Organochlorines
	Banned	Alkyl-mercury
Finland	Banned	DDT, aldrin, dieldrin, chlordane, endosulfan, and Toxaphene (camphechlor)
	Seed dressing	Methyl mercury
France	Banned	Endrin

APPENDIX B
List of Pesticides, Included in the Insecticide Act of 1968 (India)

Pesticides	Chemical name
Aceohate	O,S-Dimethyl-acetyl phosphoramidothioate
Acrolein	2-Propenal or acryladehyde
Acrylonitrile	Propenenitrile

APPENDIX B (continued)
List of Pesticides, Included in the Insecticide Act of 1968 (India)

Pesticides	Chemcial name
Alachlor	Chloro-2',6'diethyl-*N*-(methoxy-methyl) acetanilide
Aldicarb	2-Methyl-2-(methyl thio)propionaldehyde-*O*-(methyl carbamoyl) Oxime
Aldrin	1,2,3,4,10,10-Hexachloro-1,4,4a,5,8,8a-hexahydro-1,4,5,8-dimethanonaphthalene
Allethrin	(Allyl homologue of cinerein I) (±) 3-allyl-2-methyl 4-oxocyclopent-2-enyl (±)-*cis, trans*-Chrysanthemate
Aluminum phosphide	Aluminum phosphide
Amidithion	*S-(N*-2-Methoxyethyl-carbamoyl-methyl)*O,O*-dimethyl Phosphorodithioate
Aminotriazole	3-Amino-1,2,4-triazole
Amiton	*S*-2(Diethylamino)ethyl, *O,O*-diethyl phosphorothioate
ANTU	1 (1 Naphthyl)-2-thiourea
Aramite	2(4-tert-butylphenoxyl)1-methyl ethyl 2 chloroethyl sulfite
Asulam	Methyl [(4-aminophenyl) sulphonyl] carbamate
Atrazine	2-Chloro-4 (ethylamino)-6-(isopropylamino)1,3,5-triazine
Auroefungin	Antibiotic preparation
Azinphos-ethyl	S-(3,4-Dihydro-4-oxobenzo-(*d*)-(1,2,3)-triazin-3-yl methyl) *O,O* Diethyl phosphorodithioate
Bacillus thuringienesis	A microbial pesticide
Barban	4-Chloro-2-butunyl-5 chlorophneyl carbamate
Barium carbonate	Barium carbonate
Barium fluorosilicate	Barium fluorosilicate
Barium polysulfide	Barium polysulfide
Benomyl	Methyl-I (butylamino)-carbonyl [-I H-benzimidazo-2-yl) carbamate
Bensulide	(*O,O*-Di-isopropyl phosphorothiiate) *S*-ester with *N*-(2-mercoptoethyl) benzene sulfonamide
Bentazon	3-Isopropyl-(I H)-2,1,3-benzothiadiazin-4 (3H)-One 2,2-dioxy
Benthiocarb	*S*(4-Chlorobenzyl)-diethylthio carbamate
Binapacryl	2-Sec-buty il-4,6-dinitrophenyl-3-methylcrotonate
Bromacil	5-bromo-6-methyl-3-(1-methylpropyl) 2,4 (IH, 3H)-Pyrimidinedione
Bromophos	*O*-(4-Bromo-2, 5-dichlorophenyl) *O,O*-dimethyl phosphorothioate
Bromophos ethyl	*O*-(4-Bromo-2,5-dichlorophenyl) *O,O*-diethyl phosphorothioate
Bromoxyml	3,5-Dibromo-4-hydroxybenzonitrile
Brompyrazon	5-Amino-4-bromo-2-phenylpyridazion-3 one
Brozone	Methyl bromide + chloropicrin in petroleum solvent
Bufencarb	Mixture of 3-(1-methyl butyl) phenyl methyl carbamate and 3-(1-methyl butyl) phenyl methyl carbamate
Butachlor	N-(Butoxy methyl)2-chloro-2',6' diethyl acetanilide
Buturon	*N*-(4-Chlorophenyl)-*N*-methyl-*N*(1-methyl-2-propynyl) urea
Butylate	*S*-Ethyl-diisobutylthiocarbamate
Calcium arsenate	Calcium arsenate
Calcium cyanide	Calcium cyanide
Campogram M	2,5-Dimethyl-furan 3-carbonic acid anilide and 320 g/kg (Zinc)
Captafol	*N*-(1,1,2,2, Tetrachloro ethane sulfenyl) cyclohex-4-ene-1,2,dicarboximide
Captan	(*N*-Trichlormethane sulfynyl) cyclohex-4-ene 1,2,dicarboximide
Carbaryl	1-Naphtyl-methyl carbamate)
Carbendazim	Methyl-1H-benzimidezol-2-yl carbamate
Carbofuran	2,3-Dihydro,2,2,2-dimethyl-7-benzofuranyl methylcarbamate
Carbon disulfide	Carbon disulfide
Carbonphenothion	*S*(4-Chlorophenylthio)-methyl-*O,O*-diethyl phosphorodithioate
Carbon tetrachloride	Carbon tetrachloride
Carboxin	5,6-dihydro-2-methyl *N*-phenyl-1,4-oxathiin-3-carboxamide
Cartap	1,3-Di-(caramoylthio) 2-dimethylaminopropane

APPENDIX B (continued)
List of Pesticides, Included in the Insecticide Act of 1968 (India)

Pesticides	Chemcial name
Chloramben	3-Amino-2,5-dichlorobenzoic acid
Chloranil	2,3,5,6-Tetrachloro-*p*-benzo quinone
Chlorbenside	(4-Chlorobenzyl-4-chlorophenyl sulfide)
Chlorbufam	1-Methyl-2-propynul-*m*-chlorocarbanilate
Chlordane	1,2,4,5,6,7,8-Octachloro-3a,4,7,7a-tetrahydro-4,7-methanoindane
Chlorfesnon	4-Chlorophenyl-4-chlorobenzene sulfonate
Chlorfenac (Fenac)	2,3,6-Trichloro benzene acetic acid
Chlorfenethol	1,1-Di(4-chlorophenyl)-ethanol
Chlorfenvinphos	2-Chloro-1(2,4-dichlorphenyl)-vinyl diethylphosphate
Chlormequat chloride	(2-Chloroethyl) trimethylammonium chloride
Chlorbenzilate	Ethyl 4,4-dichloro benzilate
Chloroneb	1,4-Dichloro-2,5-dimethoxybenzene
Chlorophacinone	2-(2-4-Chlorophenyl)-2-phenylacetyl-indane-1,3-dione
Chloropicrin	Trichloronitromethane
Chlorothalonil	2,4,5,6-Tetrachloro 1,3-dicyanobenzene
Chlorothion	*O*-(3-Chloro-4-nitrophenyl)*O,O*-dimethyl phosphorothioate
Chloroxuron	*N*-[4(4-Chlorophenoxy) phenyl]-*NN*-dimethylurea
Chlorpropane	Chlorpropane
Chlorpropham	Isopropyl-3-chlorphyenyl carbamate
Chlopyriphos (Dursban)	*O,O*-Diethyl *O*-(3,5,6-trichlore-2-pyridyl) phosphorothioate
Chlorquinox	5,6,7,8-Tetrachloroquinoxaline
Citicide	Chlorinated turpene
Citowett	Alkylarylpolyglycolether
Copper arsenate	Copper arsenate
Copper cyanide	Copper cyanide
Copper hydroxide	Copper hydroxide
Copper naphthanate	Copper naphthanate
Copper oxychloride	Copper oxychloride
Copper sulfate	Copper sulfate
Coumachlor	3-(α-Acetonyl-4-chlorobenzyl)-4-hydroxy coumarin
Coumafuryl	3-[1(2-Furanyl)-3-oxobutyl]-4 hydroxy-2H-I-benzopyran-2-one
Coumaphos	*O*-3-Chloro-4-methyl-coumarin-7 yl-*O,O* diethyl phosphorthicate
Coumatetralyl	4-Hydroxy-3-(1,2,3,4-tetrahydro-I-naphthyl) coumarin
Coyden	3,5-Dichloro-2,6-dimethyl-4-pyridinol
CPAS	4-Chlorophenyl-2,4,5-trichlorophyenyl azosulphide
Cuprous oxide	Cuprous oxide
Cycloate	*S*-Ethyl *N*-ethyl cyclohexane thiocarbamate
Cyclomorph	*N*-Cyclo-dodecyl-*N*-2,6-dimethylurea pholinacetate
Cycluron (OMU)	*N'*pr-Cyclo octyl-*N,N*-dimetylurea
Cypermethrin	Alpha-Cyano-3-phenoxybenzyl-2,2-dimethyl-3-(2,2-dichlorovinyl cyclopropane carboxylate
Dalapon	2,2-Dichloro propionic acid
Daminozide	*N*-Imethylamino succinamic acid
2,4-D	2,4-Dichlorophenoxy acetic acid
2,4-DB	4-(2,4-Dichlorophenoxy) butyric acid
DDD/DDA	2,2-*bis* (*p*-Chloro phenyl) 1,1-dichloroethane
DD Mixture	(Dichloropropane-dichloro propene) mixture
DDT	a mixture of isomer of 1,1,1-trichloro-2,2-bis (*p*-chlorophenyl) ethane
DDVP (Dichlorvos)	2,2-Dichlorovinyl dimethyl phosphate
Decamethrin	(*S*)-Alpha-Cyano-*M*-phenoxybenzyl (IR-3R)-3-(2-2-dibromovinyl 2,2-dimethyl cyclopropane carboxylate
Decarbofuran	2,3-Dihydro-2-methylobenzofuran-7yl-methyl carbamate
Decazolin	1-(alpha, alpha-Dimethyl-beta-acetoxypropionyl)-3-isopropy-2,4-dioxodecahydroquinazoline
DEET	*N,N*-Diethyl-*m*-toluamide
Demeton-*O*	*O,O*-Diethyl-*O*-2-ethylthio-ethylphosphorothioate

APPENDIX B (continued)
List of Pesticides, Included in the Insecticide Act of 1968 (India)

Pesticides	Chemcial name
Demeton-*S*	*O,O*-Diethyl-*S*-2-ethylthio-ethyl phosphorothioate
Demeton-*S*-methyl (Metasystox)	*S*-2-Ethyl thio ethyl *O,O*-dimethyl phosphorothioate
Diazinon	*O,O*-Diethyl-*O*-(2-isopropyl-6 methyl-4-pyrimidinyl) phosphoro-thioate
Dibromochloropropane	1,2-Dibrome-3-chlorophopane
Dicamba	3,6-Dichloro-2-methoxybenzoic acid
Dichlobenil	2,6-Dichlorobenzonitrile
Dichlofenthion	*O*-(2,4-Dichlorphenyl)*O,O*-diethyl phosphorothioate
Dichlone	2,3-Dichloro-1,4-naphthoquinone
Dichlorophen	5,5'-Dichloro-2,2'-dihydroxy phenyl methane
Dicloran	2,6-Dichloro-4-nitroaniline
Dichloropropene	1,3-Dichloro-1-propene
Dicofol	2,2,2-Trichloro-1,1-di-(4-chlorophenyl)
Dicrotophos	Dimethyl phosphate, ester with -3-hydroxy *N,N*-dimethylcrotonamide
Dieldrin	(1,2,3,4,10,10-Hexachloro 7-epoxy-1,4,4a,5,6,7,8,8a-octahydro-1,5,8-dimethanonaphthalene
Dimefox	*bis*-Dimethylamino flurophosphine Oxide
Dimethoate	*O,O*-Dimethyl-*S*-(methylcarbamoyl methyl) phosphorodithioate
Dinobuton	2-Sec-butyl-4,6-dinitrophenyl isopropyl carbonate
Dinoseb	2-Sec-butyl-4,6 butyl dinitrophenol
Dinoseb acetate	2-Sec-4,6-dinitro phenyl acetate
Dioxathion	1,4-dioxan-2,3-diyl *SS*-di-(*O,O*-diethyl phosphorodithioate)
Diphacinone	2-(Diphenylacetyl)-1,3-indanedione
Diphenamid	*NN*-Dimethyl-2,2-diphenylacetamide
Disulfoton	*O,O*-Diethyl-*S*-2-ethylthioethyl phosphorodithioate
Dithianon	2,3-Dicyano-1,4-dithio anthraquinone
Diuron	*N'*-(3,4-Dichlorphyenyl, *N,N*-dimethylurea
DMPA	*O*-(2,4-Dichlorophenyl)*O'*-methyl *N*-isoprophyl-phosphoroamidithi-zate
DNOC	4-6-Dinitro-*O*-cresol
Dodemorph	4-Cyclododecyl-2,6-dimethyl-morpholine
Dodine	Dodecylguanidine monoacetate
DSMA	Disodium methylasonate
EDCT Mixture	Ethylene dichloride carbon 4,3-benzo(*e*)-dioxathiepin-3-oxide
Edifenphos	*O*-Ethyl-*S-S*-diphenyl phosphorodithioate
Endosulfan	6,7,8,9,10-*O*-hexachloro-1,5,5a,6,9,9a-hexahydro-6,9-methano-2,4-3-benzo(*e*)-dioxathiepin-3-oxide
Endothal	7-Oxabicyclo-(2,2,1)-heptane-2,3-dicaboxylic acid
Endrin	1,2,3,4,10,10-Hexachloro-6,7-epoxy-1,4,4a,5,6,7,8,8a-octahydro-exo-1,4-exo-5,8-dimethanonaphthalene
E.P.N.	*O*-Ethyl-*O*-4-nitrophenyl phenyl phosphonothioate
EPTC (Eptam)	*S*-ethyl-diprophylthiocarbamate
Erbon	2-(2,4,5-Trichlorophenoxy)ethyl-2,2-dichloropropionate
Ethepon	(2-Chloroethyl) phosphonic acid
Ethion	*O,O,O',O'*, Tetraethyl *SS'*-methylene-di-(phosphorodithioate)
Ethoprophos	*O*-ethyl *S,S*-dipropyl phosphorodithioate
Ethylene dichloride	Ethylene dichloride
Ethylene dibromide	Ethylene dibromide
Ethyl formate	Ethyl formate
Ethyl mercury chloride	Ethyl mercury chloride
Ethyl mercury phosphate	Ethyl mercury phosphate
Ethyoxy ethylemercury chloride	Ethyoxy ethyl mercury chloride
Fenazaflor	Phenyl 5,6-dichloro-2-(trifluoromethyl) bezimidazon-1-carboxylate
Fenfuram	2-Methyl furan-3-Carboxanilide
Fenitrothion	*O,O*-Dimethyl *O*-(3-methyl-4-nitrophenyl phosphorothioate)
Fenson	4-Chlorophenyl benzene sulfonate

APPENDIX B (continued)
List of Pesticides, Included in the Insecticide Act of 1968 (India)

Pesticides	Chemcial name
Fensulfothion	O,O-Diethyl-4-methyl sulfinyl phenyl phosphorothioate
Fenthion	O,O-Diethyl O-(4-methyl-thio-m-tolylphosphorothioate)
Fentin acetate	Acetyloxy triphenyl stannane
Fentin chlorida	Chloro triphenyl stannance
Fentin-hydroxide	Hydroxy triphenyl stannance
Fenvalerate	Alpha-Cyano-M-phenoxybenzyl-O,O-ixoprophyl-P-chlorophenyl acetate
Ferbam	Ferric dimethyl dithio carbamate
Fluchloralin	N-(2-Chloroethyl)-2,6-dinitro-N-propyl-4-(trifluoromethyl) benzenamine
Fluoturon	1,1-Dimethyl-3-(3-trifluromethylphenyl)-urea
Fonufos	O-Ethyl-S-phenyl ethyl phosphonodithioate
Formothion	S-(N-Formyl-N'-methylcarbamoyl methyl)-O,O-dimethylphosphoroithioate
Fuberidazole	O,O-Dimethyl-S-(methylcarbamoyl methyl) phosphorodithioate
Fujithion	O,O-Dimethyl-S-parachlorophenyl phosphorothioate
Gibberellin	Gibberelic acid
Glyphosate	N-(Phosphonomethyl) glycine
Glyphosine	N,N-bix-(Phosphonomethyl) glycine
Guazatine	1,17-Diguanidino-azahepta decane
Heptachlor	1,4,5,6,7,8,8-Heptachloro-4,7-methano-3a,4,7,7a-tetrahydro-H-indone
Hexachlorobenzene	Hexachlorobenzene
Hexachlorocyclohexane	1,2,3,4,5,6-Hexachlorocyclohexane
Hydrogen cyanide	Hydrogen cyanide
Hydrogen phosphide	Hydrogen phosphide
Indole acetic & butryic acids	Indole acetic acid, indole butyric acid
Ioxynil	3,5-Diodo-4-hydroxy benzonitrile
Isobenzan	1,3,4,5,7,8,8-Octachloro-1,3,3a,4,7,7-a hexahydro-4,7-methanoisobenzofuran
Isobornyl thio cyano acetate	1,7,7-Trimethylbicyclo (2,2,1) hept-2-yl thiocyanato acetate
Isofenphos	1-methyl ethyl 2-[ethoxy (1-methyl ethyl) amino phosphinothioyl oxy] benzoate
Isonoruron	Mixture of 3'-(hexahydro-4,7-methanoidan-1-yl) 1,1-dimethylurea and 3-(hexahydro-4,7-methanoidan-2yl)-1,1-dimethylurea
Isoprocarb (MIPC)	2-Isopropypheyl-N-methyl carbamate
Isoproturon	N,N-dimethyl-N'[4(1-methyl ethyl)-phenyl] urea
Kitazin	O,O-di-Isopropyl-S-benzyl phosphorothioate
Lead arsenate	Diplumbic hydrogen arsenate
Lenacil	3-Cyclohexyl-5-6-trimethyleneuracil
Leptophos	O-(4-Bromo-2,5-dichlorophenyl)-O-methyl phenyl phosphonothieate
Lime sulfur	Calcium polysulfide, water free sulfur, calcium thiosulfate mixture
Lindane	Gamma isomer of hexachloro cyclohexane
Linuron	N-(3,4-Dichlorophenyl) N-methoxy-N-methylurea
Magnesium phosphide	Magnesium phosphide
Malathion	O,O-dimethyl-S-(1,2-carbethoxyethly) phosphorodithioate
Maleic hydrazide	1,2-Dihydropyridazine 3,6-dione
Mancozeb	Complex of zinc and maneb containing 20% manganese and 2,5-zinc
Maneb	Polymeric manganese ethylene bisdithiocarbamate
MCPA	(4-Chloro-2-methyl phenoxy) acetic acid
MCPB	4-(4-Chloro-2-methylphenoxy) butyric acid
Menazon	S-(4,6-Diamino-1,3,5-triazin 2-yl methyl) O,O-dimethylphosphorodithioate
Mephosfolan	2-(Diethoxy phosphinylimino)-4-methyl-1,3-dithiolane
Mercuritrichloride	Mercuric chloride
Merphos	Tributyl phosphoroasothioate

APPENDIX B (continued)
List of Pesticides, Included in the Insecticide Act of 1968 (India)

Pesticides	Chemcial name
Metaldehyde	2,4,6,8-Tetramethyl-1,3,5,7-tetrasoecane
Methabenathiazuron	N-2-Benzothiazoyl-N,N-dimethylurea
Metham sodium	Methyldithiocarbamic acid sodium salt of
Methamidophos	O,S-Dimethyl phosphoroamidothioate
Methomyl	Methyl-N-[methyl amino)-carbonyl)] oxyethanimidothioate
Methoxychlor	1,1,1-Trichloro-2,2-di-4-methoxy-phenylethane
Methoxyethylmercuric chloride	Methoxy ethyl mercury chloride
Methyl bromide	Methyl bromide
Methyl mercuriochloride	Methyl mercuric chloride
Methylmetiram	Ammonium complex with zinc (N,N'-1,2-propylenebis(dithio-carbamate) and N'N-poly-1,-propylene-*bis* (thiocarbamoyl di-sulfide
Methyl parathion	(O,O dimethyl-O-(4-nitrophenyl) phosphorothioate
Metiram	Mixture of (ethylene thiuram disulfide([1,2-ethanedityl *bis*-(carbamedithioate) (2)] zinc
Metobromuron	3-(4-Bromophenyl)-1-methoxy-i-methylurea
Metoxuron	N-(3-Chloro-4-methoxyphenyl)-N,N-dimethyl urea
Metribuzin	4-Amino-6-butyl 4,5 dihydro 3-(methylthio)-1,2,4-triazin-5-one
Mevinphos (Phosdrin)	2-Methoxy carbonyl-1, methylvinyl dimethyl phosphate
Mexacarbate	4-(Dimethylamino)-3,5-dimethyl phenyl methylcarbamate
Molinate	S-Ethyl-hexahydro-1-H-azepine 1-carbothioate
Monocrotophos	3-Dimethoxy phosphinyloxy) N-methyl 1-isocrotonamide
Monolinuron	N-(4-Chlorophenyl) N-methoxy-N-methyl urea
Monuron	3-(4-Chlorophenyl)-1,1-dimethyl urea
MSMA	Monosodium methanearsonate
Nabam	Disodium ethylene-*bis*-dithiocarbamate
Naled	1,2-Dibromo-2,2-dichloroethyl dimethyl phosphate
Naphthylacetic acid	Naphthylacetic acid and its derivatives
Neburon	1-Butyl-3-(3,4-dichlorophenyl)1,1-methyl urea
Nickel chloride	Nickel chloride
Niclosamide	2',5-Dichloro-4, nitro-salicylanilide
Nicotine sulfate	Nicotine sulfate
Nitrofen	2,4-Dichlorophenyl p-nitrophenyl ether
Norvron (Herban)	3-(Hexahydro)-4,7-methanoindan-syl) 1,1-dimethylurea
Omethoate	O,O-Dimethyl-S-(methyl-carbamoylmethyl) phosphorothioate
Osbac (BPMC)	2-Secondary-butylphenylmethylcarbamate
Oxapyrazon	5-Bromo-1,6-dihydro-6-oxo-1-phenyl-4-pyridazinyl oxamicacid compound with 2-dimethyl amino-ethanol (1:1)
Oxycarboxin (DCMOD)	5,6-Dihydro-2-methyl-1,4-oxathin-3-carboxamide 4,4-dioxide
Para-dichloro benzene	1,4-Dichloro benzene
Paraquat dimethyl sulfate dichloride	1,1'-Dimethyl-4-4-bipyridyl-diyiium ion salts of
Parathion	(O,O-Diethyl-6-nitrophenyl) phosphorothioate
Paris Green	Copper aceto arsenite
Pebulate	S-Propyl-butyl-ethylthiocarbamate
Pentachloronitrobenzene	Pentachloronitrobenzene
Pentachlorophenol	Pentachlorophenol
Permethrin	3-Phenoxy benzyl (*Cis-trans*-3- (2,2-dichlorovinyl)-2,2-dimethyl-cyclo propane carboxylate
Phenthoate	S-α (-ethoxycarbonyl benzyl-O,O-dimethyl phosphorodithioate
Phenyl mercuric acetate	Phenyl mercuric acetate
Phenyl mercurichloride	Phenyl mercurichloride
Phenyl mercuricurea	Phenyl mercuricurea
Phorate	O,O-Diethyl S-(ethylthiomethyl) phosphorodithioate
Phosalone	S-(6-Chloro-2-oxobenzoxazolin-3-yl) methyl-O,O diethyl-phosphorodithioate
Phosmet	O,O-Dimethyl-S-phthalimid-O-methyl-phosphorodithioate
Phosphamidon	2-Chloro-2-dithylcarbiamoylo 1-methylvinyldimethyl phosphate

APPENDIX B (continued)
List of Pesticides, Included in the Insecticide Act of 1968 (India)

Pesticides	Chemcial name
Phosphorus paste	Phosphorus paste
Phoxim	O-α cyano binzylidene amino O,O-diethyl phosphorothioate
Picloram (Tordon)	4-Amino-3,5,6-trichloropicolinic acid
Pindone	2-Pivaloyl-indane-1,3-dione
Piperonyl butoxide	5-[2-(2-Butoxyethoxy) ethoxymethyl]-6- propyl-1-3-benzodioxole
Pirimiphos methyl	O-(2-Diethylamino)-6-methylpyrimidin-4-O,O-yl-dimethyl phosphorothioate
Potassium cyanide	Potassium cyanide
Propanil	3,4 (Dichloropropionanilide
Propagite	2-(4,t-butyl) Phenoxy-cyclohexyl prop-2-ynyl sulfite
Propineb	Polymer of zinc propylenebisdithio carbamate
Propoxur (Baygon)	2-Isopropoxyphenylmethyl carbamate
Propyzamide	3,5-Dichloro-N-(1,1-dimethyl propynyl) benzamide
Pyrnachlor	2-Chloro-N-(-methyl-2-propynyl) acetanilide
Pyracarbolid	3,4-Dihydro-6-methyl-pyran-5-carboxanilide
Pyrazon (PCA Xpyramin)	5-Amino-4-chloro-2-phenyl-3-(2H)-pyridazinone
Pyrazophos	O-6-Ethoxy carbonyl-5-methylpyrazolo (1,5-a) pyrimidin-2yl-O,O-diethyl phosphorothioate
Pyrethrins	4-Hydroxy-3-methyl-2-(2,4-pentadeenyl)-2-cyclopenten-1-one
Quinalphos	O,O-Diethyl-O-quinoxalin-2-yl phosphorothioate
Quinomethiomate	6-Methyl-2-oxo,1,3-dithiolo (4,5-b) quinoxaline
Rabicide	4,5,6,7-Tetrachloropthalide
Rotenone	1,2,12,12a,α-Tetrahydro-2a-isopropyl-8-9-dimethoxy-1) benzo-pyrano-(3,4-b)-furo-(2-3-H)(1) benzopyran-6(6a H)one
S-421	bis-(2,3,3,3-Tetra chloropropyl) ether
Schradan	Octa methyl diphosphoramide
Sclex	3-(3,5-Dichlorophenyl)-5,5-dimethyl oxazolidinedione-2,4
Simazine	2-Chloro-4,6-bis-(ethylamino)-S-triazine
Sindone A	1,1-Dimethyl-4,6-di-isopropyl-5-indanyl ethyl ketone
Sindone B	1,1,4-Trimethyl-6-isopropyl-5-indanyl ethyl ketone
Sirmate	3,4-or 2,3-dichlorobenzyl N-methyl carbamate
Sodium cyanide	Sodium cyanide
Sodium fluoroacetate	Sodium fluoroacetate
Sodium fluorosilicate	Sodium fluorosilicate
Streptomycin	O-2-Dioxy-2-(methyl amino)-α-L-gluco-pyranosyl-(1)-2-O-5 deoxy-3-C-formyl-α-lyxofuranosyl-(1,4)-N,N-bis (aminoiminomethyl)-D-streptamine
Strychmine	Strychindin-10-one
Sulfoxide	1,2-Methylene-dioxy-4[2-(octylsulphinyl propyl)] benzene
Sulfur	Sulfur
Swep	Methyl 3,4-dichlorocarba-nilate
Tavron G	2,2,2-Trichloroethyl stryrene
2,4,5-TB	4-(2,4,5-Trichlorophenoxy) butyric acid
Tecnazene	1,2,4,5-Tetrachloro-3-nitrobenzene
Temephos	$O,O,O'O'$-Tetramethyl O,O'-thiodi-p-phenylenediphosphorothioate
TEPP	Tetraethyl pyrophosphate
Terbacil	3-$tert$-Butyl-5-chloro-6-methyluracil
Terbutyrn	2-$tert$-Butylamino-4-ethylamino-6-(methylthio)-1,3-5-triazine
Terracur	5-Carboxymethyl-2-methyl-2-H-1,3,5-thiadiazine-2-thione
Tetrachlorpvinphos (Cardona)	2-Chloro-1(2,4,5-trichlorophenyl) vinyl dimethyl phosphate
Tetradifon	2,4,4'5-Tetrachlorodiphenyl sulphone
Tetramethrin	3,4,5,6-Tetrahydro phthalimidomethyl ($\pm$)-cis, trans-chryssanthemate
Thallium sulfate	Thallium sulfate
Thiometon	S-[2-(Ethylthio) ethyl] O,O-dimethyl phosphorodithioate
Thionazin (Nemafos)	O,O-Diethyl-O-pyriazinyl phosphorothioate
Thiophanate-M	1,2-di-(3-Methoxy-carbonyl-2-thioureidobenzene

APPENDIX B (continued)
List of Pesticides, Included in the Insecticide Act of 1968 (India)

Pesticides	Chemcial name
Thiram	*bis*-(Dimethyl thiocarbamoyl) disulfide
Tolyl mercury acetate	Tolyl mercury acetate
Toxaphene	Chlorinated comphene containing 67% to 69% chlorine
Tranid	exo-3-Chloro-endo-6-cyano-2-norbornanone-*O*-methylcarbamoyl oxime
Triadimefon	1-(4-Chlorophenoxy)-3,3-dimethyl-1-(1H-1,2,4-triazol-1-yl)-2-butanone
Triallate	*S*-2,3,3-Trichloroallyl-di-isopropyl thiocarbamate
Trichlorfon	Dimethyl (2,2,2-trichlorol-hydroxy ethyl)phosphate
Trichlorophenoxy acetic acid (2,4,5-T)	Trichlorophenoxy acetic acid
Trichlorphon	Dimethyl-4-tridecyl morpholine
Tridemorph	2,6-Dimethyl-4-tridecylmorpholine
Trifluralin	2,6-Dinitro-*NN*-dipropyl-4- (triflouromethyl) benzamine
Triforine	1,4-di-(2,2,2-Trichloro-1-formamidoethyl piperazine
Triorthocresyl phosphate	Triorthocresyl phosphate
Tunio (Methazole)	2,(3,40Dichlorophenyl)4-methyl-1,2,4-oxadiazalidine-3,5,dione
Udonkor	*N*-(beta-Cyanothyl) monochloroacetamide
Vacor	*N*-3-pyridyl methyl-*N*-*p*-nitrophenyl urea
Vamidothion	*O,O*-Dimethyl-*S*-[2-(1-methyl carbamoyl ethyl thio) ethyl] phosphorothioate
Vegetta	Ethylene thiuram monosulfide
Vernolate (Vernam)	*S*-Propyl (dipropyl thiocarbamate)
Warfarin	3-α-Acetonylbenzyl-4-hydroxy-coumarin)
Zimet	
Zinc phosphide	Zinc phosphide
Zineb	Zinc ethylene *bis*-dithiocarbamate
Ziram	Zinc dimethyl-dithiocarbamate
Zulate	
Dikar	A blend of Dithane M-45 and Tech. Karathane
Dinocap	Mixture of 4 & 5 parts of 2,4-dinitro-6-octo-phemyl crotonatesto 2 parts of the isomer of 2,6-dinitro-4-octylphenyl crotonates
Plictran	Tricyclohexyl tinhydroxide derivatives
Metox	Chorsulficide
Triorphocroesyl phosphate	Triorthocresyl phosphate

REFERENCES

1. **Muller, P.,** *DDT, The Insecticide Dichlorodiphenyl Trichloroethane and its Significance,* Vol. 2, Birkhauser, Verlag, Basel, 1949.
2. **Lorenz, W. and Sasse, K.,** Grehard Schrader and the development of organophosphorous compounds for crop protection, in *Pflanzenschutz-Nachr.,* 21, 5, 1968.
3. **Natarajan, P.,** Introduction of pesticides, *Pesticide Information,* 13, 22, 1987.
4. **Binder, D.,** *New York Times,* June 26, 1989.
5. **Morarity, F.,** *Pollutants and Animals: A Factural Perspective,* Allen and Unwin, London, 1974.
6. **Bogan, J. A. and Bourne, W. R. P.,** Organochlorine levels in Atlantic sea birds, *Nature,* 240, 358, 1972.
7. **Gaskin, D. E., Hodrinet, M., and Frank, R.,** Organochlorine pesticide residues in harbour porpoises from the Bay of Fundy region, *Nature,* 233, 499, 1971.
8. **De Long, R. L., Gilmartin, W. G., and Simpson, J. G.,** Premature births in California sea lions, association with high organochlorine pollutant residue levels, *Science,* 181, 1168, 1973.
9. **Le Boeuf, B. J. and Bonnell, M. L.,** DDT in California sea lions, *Nature,* 234, 108, 1971.
10. **Weaver, L., Gunnerson, C. G., Breidenbach, A. W., and Lichtenberg, J. J.,** Chlorinated hydrocarbon pesticides in major U.S. river basins, *U.S. Public Health Rep.,* 80, 481, 1965.

11. **Dikshith, T. S. S., Kumar, S. N., Raizada, R. B., Srivastava, M. K., and Ray, P. K.,** Residues of 1-naphthol in soil and water samples in and around Bhopal, India, *Bull. Environ. Contam. Toxicol.,* 44, 87, 1990.
12. **Sarkar, A. and Sen Gupta, R.,** DDT residues in sediments from the Bay of Bengal., *Bull. Environ. Contam. Toxicol.,* 41, 664, 1988.
13. **Gardner, A. L. and Iverson, R. E.,** The effect of aerially applied malathion on an urban population, *Arch. Environ. Health,* 16, 823, 1968.
14. **Mc Laughlin, L. A. Jr. and Snyder, C. H.,** Encephalopathy in a child following exposure to malathion, *Ochsner Clin. Rep.,* 2, 37, 1956.
15. **Baker, E. L.,** Epidermic malathion poisoning in Pakistan Malaria workers, *Lancet,* 1, 31, 1978.
16. **Karnik, V. M., Ichaporia, R. N., and Wadia, R. S.,** Cholinesterase levels in diazinon poisoning. I. Relation to severity of poisoning, *J. Assoc. Physicians India,* 18, 337, 1970.
17. **Reich, G. A., Gallaher, G. L., and Wiseman, J. S.,** Characteristics of pesticide poisoning in South Texas, *Texas Med.,* 64, 56, 1968.
18. **Carson, R.,** *Silent spring,* Houghton-Mifflin, New York, 1962.
19. **Henderson, G. L. and Woolley, D. E.,** Tissue concentrations of DDT: correlation with neurotoxicity in young and adult rats, *Proc. West. Pharmacol. Soc.,* 12, 58, 1969.
20. **Harrison, R. D.,** Comparative toxicity of some selected pesticides in neonatal and adult rats, *Toxicit. Appl. Pharmacol.,* 32, 443, 1975.
21. **Walker, A. I. T., Thorpe, E., Robinson, J., and Baldwin, M. K.,** Toxicity studies on the photoisomerization product of dieldrin, *Med. Fac. Landbouwwet. Rijksuniv. Gent.,* 36, 398, 1971.
22. **Donoso, J.,** Review of environmental effects of pollutants: XII. Endrin, U.S. Dept. Commerce, Nat. Tech. Inf. Serv., Washington, D.C., 1979.
23. **Krijnen, C. J. and Boyd, E. M.,** The influence of diets containing from 0 to 81 percent of protein on tolerated doses of pesticides. *Comp. Gen. Pharmacol.,* 2, 373, 1971.
24. **Boyd, E. M., Dubos, I., and Krijnen, C. J.,** Endosulfan toxicity and dietary protein, *Arch. Environ. Health,* 21, 15, 1970.
24a. **Dikshith, T. S. S., Raizada, R. B., Singh, R. P., Kumar, S. N., Gupta, K. P., and Kaushal, R. A.,** Acute toxicity of hexachlorocyclohexane in mice, rats, rabbits, pigeons and fresh water fish, *Vet. Human Toxicol.,* 31, 113, 1989.
25. **O'Brien, R. D.,** *Toxic Phosphorous Esters, Chemistry, Metabolism and Biological Effects,* Academic Press, New York, 1960.
26. **Loshadkin, N. A. and Snirnov, V. V.,** A review of modern literature on the chemistry and toxicology of organophosphorous inhibitors of cholinesterases, New Jersey Assoc. Tech. Services Inc., Glen Ridge, NJ, 1962.
27. **Heath, D. F.,** *Organophosphorous Poison, Anticholinesterases and Related Compounds,* Pergamon Press, New York, 1961.
28. **Frest, C. and Schmidt, K. J.,** *The Chemistry of Organophophorous Pesticides,* 2nd revised edition, Springer-Verlag, New York, 1982.
28a. **Kuhr, R. J. and Dorough, H. W.,** *Carbamate Insecticides: Chemistry, Biochemistry, and Toxicology,* CRC Press, Cleveland, Ohio, 1976.
29. International Agency for Research in Cancer, *Monographs on the Evaluation of Carcinogenic Risks of chemicals to Man,* Vol, 12, IARC, Lyon, France, 1976.
30. **Bainova, A.,** Herbicides in, *Toxicology of Pesticides,* Interium Document No. 9, World Health Organization, Geneva, 1982, 145.

Chapter 2

BIOTRANSFORMATION OF PESTICIDES: THE ROLE OF THE MIXED FUNCTION OXIDASE SYSTEM IN PESTICIDE TOXICITY

T. A. Popov and B. J. Blaauboer

TABLE OF CONTENTS

I. INTRODUCTION

Organisms live in environments containing many chemicals that threaten their survival. This chemical hostility is as old as life itself, although the present environment contains an increasing amount of manmade chemicals such as pesticides, drugs, food additives, and environmental pollutants resulting from industrial activities. Thus, the survival of organisms has been and is dependent on the development of mechanisms to remove foreign substances from the body.

Many xenobiotics (from xenos = foreign and bios = life) that are nonpolar will not be readily excreted from organisms. Especially in terrestrial organisms lipophilic chemicals would tend to be retained and even accumulated in the body if they were to remain unchanged upon uptake. This will result in an indefinite toxic action. The majority of xenobiotics, however, are metabolized to less lipophilic compounds which are excreted more easily. Therefore, the toxicity of many chemicals is largely dependent upon their rate of metabolism. The system of the metabolism of xenobiotics in the organism is referred to as biotransformation. In this system an important role is played by the mixed function oxidases.

Most xenobiotics undergo biotransformation in two phases. In phase I, the molecule is changed in one or more places. Groups such as OH, -COOH, $-NH_2$ are unmasked or introduced into the molecule by oxidation, reduction, or hydrolysis. Some of these products are eliminated from the body without further change. Many others, however, are still not hydrophilic enough to be excreted into urine or bile, and are metabolized in a second phase of biotransformation (Figure 1).

Introduction or unmasking of groups in the phase I reactions provides "*a handle*", which can be used for the attachment of an endogenous compound. In phase II, the metabolic product of phase I or the original compound if it possesses a polar group, is conjugated with glucuronate, sulfate, glycine, or other groups. The resulting metabolites are less lipotropic, more polar i.e., more water-soluble charateristics that facilitate their excretion.

Nonsynthetic reactions in phase I may either increase or decrease the toxicity of the compound. If biotransformation produces a more toxic metabolite the term bioactivation is used. Phase II, also called synthetic biotransforming reactions, are usually detoxifying ones.

Biotransformation has been studied more thoroughly than any other aspect of xenobiotic kinetics. A number of reviews have been published on the general features of the biotransformation of foreign compounds.[1-4] or specific groups of xenobiotics.[5-7] Many tissues are capable of metabolizing xenobiotics. Quantitatively the highest activities of biotransformation reactions are found in the liver. Other organs with relatively high activities in this respect are the lung, the intestine, the skin, and the kidneys. These organs all have in common that they are in contact with the exterior of the body or, as is the case with the liver, can form a "*filter*" for compounds entering the body *via* the intestine wall. Therefore, these organs come into contact with xenobiotics surrounding the organism. Moreover, they can play a role in the excretion of foreign compounds and also in the excretion of endogenous waste products. A special role is played by the adrenals, where the metabolism of steroid hormones takes place. In this metabolism hydroxylation reactions, catalyzed by mixed function oxidases, are very important.

The mixed function oxidase (MFO) system catalyzing the majority of the reactions mentioned is an integral part of the smooth endoplasmic reticulum (SER), attached to, and embedded in the lipid layers of its membranes (Figure 2). In Table 1 the most important phase I reactions are shown. Many oxidations and also some reductions are performed by mixed function oxidases.

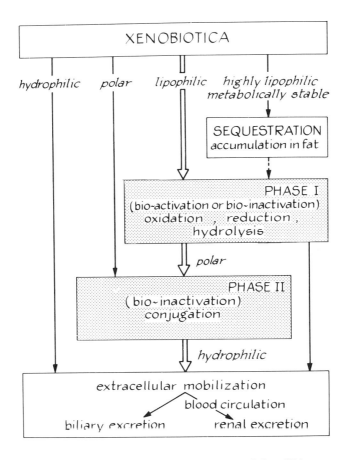

FIGURE 1. General scheme of the role of phase I and phase II biotrans-
formation reactions in the kinetics of xenobiotics. (From Henderson, P.
Th., Metabolism of Drugs in Isolated Hepatocytes and Proliferating Liver
Tissue, Ph.D. thesis, University of Nijmegen, 1971).

II. MIXED FUNCTION OXIDASE

A. GENERAL CHARACTERISTICS

The enzymatic machinery for drug oxidation has been termed as a mixed function
oxidase[8] or monooxygenase[9], since in the course of the reaction, one atom of the oxygen
molecule is reduced to water and the other is incorporated into the compounds undergoing
oxidation. The oxidative reactions include alkyl-, aryl-, and N-hydroxylation, epoxide formation, N- and O-dealkylation, deamination, desulfuration, and dechlorination of a wide
variety of substances (Table 1). Most of these reactions result in hydroxylation of the
compound.[10b]

A schematic representation of the MFO is shown in Figure 3. Arrows indicate the
hypothetical reaction sequence for oxidation of xenobiotics. The substrate (SH) combines
first with the oxidized form of cytochrome p-450 to form a complex which is then reduced
by an electron yielded by the NADPH-flavoprotein (FP_1) chain. In turn, the reduced substrate-
cytochrome p-450 complex reacts with molecular oxygen and the oxygenated complex
accepts a second electron from the NADH-flavoprotein (FP_2)-cytochrome b_5 chain. This
second electron can also be donated by the NADH-FP_1 chain. In Figure 3 this possibility
is shown as the dotted line representing a bridge between the two electron-donating chains.
Donation of the second electron to the cytochrome p-450 substrate-oxygen complex activates

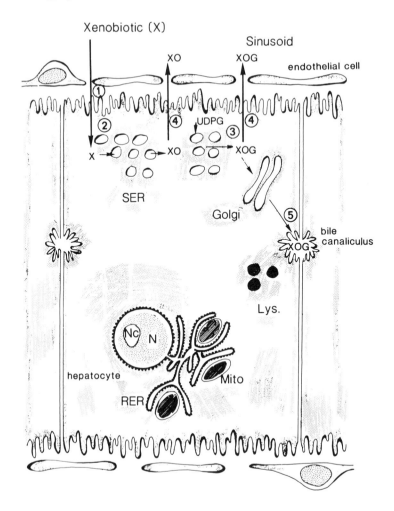

FIGURE 2. Localization of biotransformation reactions in liver parenchymal cells and transport processes involved in the cellular secretion of metabolites. (1) Uptake of a xenobiotic; (2) phase I biotransformation (e.g., oxidation); (3) phase II biotransformation (e.g., glucuronidation); (4) excretion via blood and kidney (if $M \leq$ ca. 300); (5) excretion via bile (if $M \geq$ ca. 300). Abbreviations: N: nucleus; Mito: mitochondria; lys: lysosomes; RER: rough endoplasmic reticulum; SER: smooth endoplasmic reticulum; X: xenobiotic; XO: oxidized xenobiotic metabolized, produced by the MFO system; UDPG: UDP-glucuronic acid; XOG: xenobiotic-glucuronide.

the oxygen. In the next step, one atom of "activated oxygen" is reduced to water, while the other oxidizes the substrate to form an intermediate complex (O-cyt p-450-SH). This complex is labile and promptly breaks up generating oxidized substrate (SOH) releasing cytochrome p-450 for another cycle.

Some authors erroneously refer to oxidation involving MFO as "microsomal oxidation". Such a term is only valid for *in vitro* conditions, that is, following SER disruption after homogenization and centrifugation.

More schematically, the monooxygenase (MFO) reactions can be described by the equation:

$$SH + NAD(P)H + H^+ + O_2 \quad \xrightarrow{MFO} \quad SOH \quad + NAD(P)^+ + H_2O \quad (1)$$

TABLE 1
Most Common Types of Phase I Biotransformation Reactions

	Type of reaction	Example of substrate compound	Metabolite(s)
		A. Oxidation	
I.	Mixed function oxidase dependent		
	Aromatic hydroxylation	R–⟨ ⟩	R–⟨ ⟩–OH
	Aliphatic hyroxylation	R–CH₃	R–CH₂OH
	Epoxidation	R–C–C–R′ (H H)	R–C——C—R′ (O, H)
	N-Hyroxylation	⟨ ⟩–NH₂	⟨ ⟩–NHOH
	O-Dealkylation	R–O–CH₃	ROH + CH₂O
	N-dealkylation	R–NHCH₃	R–NH₂ + CH₂O
	S-dealkylation	R–S–CH₃	R–SH + CH₂O
	Deamination	R–CH–CH₃ (NH₂)	R–C–CH₃ (=O) + NH₃
	Sulfoxidation	R–S–R′	R–S –R′ (→ O)
	Dechlorination	CCl₄	[CCl₃ ·]⟶ CHCl₃
	Oxidative desulfuration	R₁–O (S) P (R₂–O) (O–R₃)	R₁–O (O) P (R₂–O) (O–R₃)
II.	Amine oxidation	R–CH₂–NH₂	R–CHO + NH₃
III.	Dehydrogenation	CH₃–CH₂–OH	CH₃CHO + CH₃COOH

TABLE 1 (continued)
Most Common Types of Phase I Biotransformation Reactions

Type of reaction	Example of substrate compound	Metabolite(s)
	B. Reduction	
Azo reduction	$R\text{-}N{=}N\text{-}R'$	$R\text{-}NH_2 + R'\text{-}NH_2$
Nitro reduction	$R\text{-}NO_2$	$R\text{-}NH_2$
Carbonyl reduction	$R\text{-}C\text{-}R'$, $=O$	$R\text{-}CH\text{-}R'$, $-OH$
	C. Hydrolysis	
Esters	$R\text{-}C\text{-}O\text{-}R'$, $=O$	$R\text{-}C\text{-}OH + R'\text{-}OH$, $=O$
Amides	$R\text{-}CONH_2$	$R\text{-}COOH + NH_3$

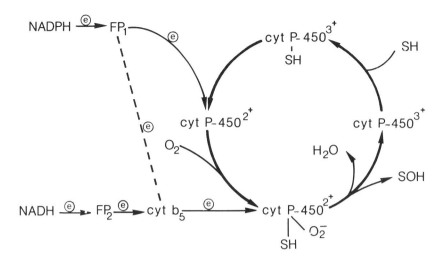

FIGURE 3. Scheme of the oxidation of a xenobiotic (SH) by the mixed function oxidase system. For further details see text.

In the scheme outlined in Figure 3, the compound being metabolized (substrate "SH") may represent any of the wide variety of xenobiotics: pesticides, organic solvents, medicaments, ethanol, and many other substances foreign to the body. It may also be one of a number of endogenous substrates that include saturated and unsaturated fatty acids, cholesterol, steroid hormones, bile acids, and prostaglandins.[11]

Key enzymes in the overall reaction are

1. Cytochrome p-450
2. NADPH-cytochrome p-450 reductase (FP$_1$), the flavine enzyme involved in the oxidation of NADPH
3. NADH-cytochrome b$_5$ reductase (FP$_2$)
4. Cytochrome b$_5$

Incorporation in membranes is essential for enzymic activity. This provides the structural environment necessary for the interaction with lipophilic substrates and the requirements for a well-organized transfer of electrons.[12] The pivotal component, cytochrome p-450, a hemoprotein (or better a group of homoproteins), was first described by Klingenberg[13] as a co-binding pigment. Cytochrome p-450 takes its name from the absorption peak in the difference spectrum at 450 nm of its reduced form combined with carbon monoxide. The hemoprotein is located in the SER of many cell types, but mainly in the hepatocytes, of all vertebrates and also in insects and other arthropods, in bacteria, bacteroids, and in yeast.[14] Plants can perform similar oxidation reactions, but little is known about the properties of the enzyme involved.[15] In these reactions molecular oxygen takes part and the electrons are donated by NADH.[16] Cytochrome p-450 is not identical in all tissues or species. Differences are seen in adrenal and hepatic cytochrome p-450 and also in MFO systems from different species.

During the action of the MFO system some "leakage" of active oxygen may exist in the form of the superoxide anion radical (O_2^{-}·). This is thought to happen *via* the breakdown of the oxygenated cytochrome p-450 substrate complex.[17]

$$[SH\text{-}Fe^{2+}\text{-}O_2 \quad \longleftrightarrow \quad SH\text{-}Fe^{3+}\text{-}O_2^{-}] \quad \longrightarrow \quad SH\text{-}Fe^{3+} + O2^{-}\cdot \qquad (2)$$

This reactive form of oxygen may dismutate to H_2O_2 and also the highly reactive OH radical can be formed. All these types of "active oxygen" may affect cellular structure. In many cell types, e.g., in liver cells, defense mechanisms — superoxide dismutase (SOD), glutathione peroxidase, catalase, etc., are present to scavenge these oxidative radicals in order to minimize the cellular damage.

The leakage of active oxygen species may be due to nonoptimal conditions for the transfer of the second electron into the MFO cycle.[18] Another possibility is that substrates that are poorly metabolized by cytochrome p-450 because they are poor acceptors of the oxygen from the complex, are responsible for elevated amounts of superoxide anion radical production by the system.[18]

On the other hand, the MFO system can act as a peroxidase. In this case, the oxygen atom necessary for the oxidation of substrates can be donated by H_2O_2 or by (lipid) hydroperoxides.[17]

$$SH + H_2O_2 \xrightarrow{\text{MFO}} SOH + H_2O \qquad (3)$$

$$SH + ROOH \xrightarrow{\text{MFO}} SOH + ROH \qquad (4)$$

B. CYTOCHROME P-450 ISOENZYMES, AND BINDING CHARACTERISTICS

Since many different compounds are metabolized by the MFO-system, it has been suggested for a long time that multiple forms of the enzyme system exist.[10] Indeed, experiments with inducing compounds led to the finding that different forms of cytochrome p-450 can be induced. Several groups of inducers could be distinguished, of which phenobarbital, 3-methylcholanthrene and pregnenolone-16-α-carbonitrile were the first compounds to be used. This led to the conclusion that at least three forms of the enzyme exist. One form, induced by 3-methyl-cholanthrene and related compounds has a different CO-binding characteristic with a peak in the difference spectrum at 448 nm and has therefore been named for some time as cytochrome p-448.[19]

In recent years, our knowledge of this multiple enzyme system has greatly increased by using isolation techniques: X-ray crystallography, immunologocal characterization, and amino acid sequencing.[20-23] Thus, in rat liver SER at least 14, and probably 16 isoenzymes of the cytochrome have been characterized.[24,25] In other organs other than the liver and in other species other forms can be found. These isoenzymes have different functional and organizational characteristics. However, it can be shown by comprising the amino acid sequence that even bacterial and eukaryotic cytochrome p-450s all are members of the same protein family and have a common architectural design.[26]

Thus, the wide variety of substrates for the MFO system are metabolized by distinct but related isoenzymes. However, some overlap in substrate specificity and in inducibility can occur and this has led to some confusion over the identity and nomenclature of isoenzymes. These isoenzymes are in some cases named after their respective inducing agent, e.g., cytochrome p-450PB as the isoenzyme(s) found after induction with phenobarbital.[27] The additions commonly used are UT for untreated, PB for phenobarbital, MC for 3-methylcholanthrene, BNF for B-naphthoflavone, and PCN for pregnenolone-16-a-carbonitrile. Other authors use this nomenclature with a modification: p-450 (PB-1), (PB-2), etc. or P-450PB-A, PB-B, etc., indicating that one inducing agent may produce more than one isoenzyme.[28,29] In another system the isoenzymes are named P-450a, p-450b, etc.[24]

While insight into the multiplicity of the cytochrome p-450 system is progressing rapidly, the relationships between each of the forms and the biotransformation of different substrates remain to be defined. At least two types of substrates can be distinguished, based on the location and morphology of the site of interaction between substrate and cytochrome ("binding site"). Differences in binding sites are reflected in the form of the different spectra of cytochrome p-450 with and without substrate. Substrates interacting with the oxidized form of the cytochrome while producing "enzyme substrate complexes" with an absorption maximum at 390 nm are termed "type I" compounds. Another group of substrates will produce complexes with an absorption maximum around 420 nm and are called "type II" compounds. The type I binding site is located at the protein moiety of the cytochrome, while the type II compounds react with the sixth ligand position of the heme-iron. Among the type I substrates are the compounds that can induce increased metabolism by the MFO system: many pesticides, steroid hormones, barbiturates, and many other drugs. Aniline and other amines, as well as isocyanides and certain steroids and alcohols are type II compounds.[30]

These changes in absorption reflect changes in the so-called spin state of the heme-iron. Four out of six ligands of this iron can be attributed to the porphyrin ring, the fifth ligand is a cysteine residue of the protein moiety, while the sixth ligand position may be occupied either by a hydroxyl group in the protein or by water. Binding of a substrate to cytochrome p-450 changes the ligand properties of the 6th ligand position and leads to a rearrangement of the electron pairing pattern of the heme-iron. This iron has five d-electrons. In the low-spin state two pairs of electrons are formed, leaving one electron unpaired. In the high-spin state all five d-electrons are unpaired. Native cytochrome p-450 is either in the high-spin or in the low-spin state. Binding of a type I compound to the active site on the protein moiety leads to a shift from low-spin to high spin cytochrome p-450, which is reflected in the changes in absorbance with a maximum at 390 nm. Type II compounds are binding to the heme-iron resulting in a conversion to the low-spin state and this is observed in a change in absorbance with a through at 390 nm and a maximum around 420 nm.[31]

Some compounds (i.e., nitrogenous bases, thiols, and other toxic chemicals) can form stable complexes with cytochrome p-450 by interacting with the 6th ligand position. Since the change in spin state is an essential characteristic for the mixed function oxidase activity of cytochrome p-450, the formation of these stable complexes inactivates the enzyme and instead may lead to an enhanced production of active oxygen species like superoxide, peroxides, and the hydroxyl anion radical.[18] Many compounds are metabolized by cytochrome p-450 with the formation of carbenes or other reactive intermediates. These metabolites may also form stable complexes with the cytochrome, resulting in inhibition of its normal enzymic activity.

Most data on the biochemistry and biophysics of the cytochrome p-450 system have been derived from studies with mammalian hepatic systems, where the highest activities for phase I biotransformation reactions can be found. In other mammalian tissues and organs and in other species MFO systems are known to occur as well. The fat body and the gut are principal sites for oxidative biotransformation in insects.[32-34] In spite of some differences, all animals appear to utilize a very similar MFO system for oxidation of xenobiotics.

C. INDUCTION AND INHIBITION OF THE MFO SYSTEM

A very distinctive feature of the mixed function oxidase system is its ability to be induced or inhibited by certain xenobiotics. These changes of enzyme activity may result in an increased or diminished toxicity of the compounds to be metabolized by the MFO system.

Over 200 different compounds of very diverse structure have been shown to enhance MFO activity. There are two main groups of inducing agents. One group consists of a wide variety of pesticides (e.g., DDT, dieldrin, lindane), environmental pollutants (e.g. chlorinated biphenyls), drugs (e.g. barbiturates, imipramine), food additives (e.g. butylated hydroxytoluene). These compounds all produce similar changes in the MFO system and the classical example in this group is phenobarbital. A second group of inducing agents consists of polycyclic aromatic hydrocarbons (many of them are known as strong carcinogenic agents), tetrachloro-dibenzo-dioxin (TCDD), polychlorinated biphenyls, and other xenobiotics. The prototype of this group is 3-methylcholanthrene (3-MC).[35,36]

The major requirement for the compounds in the first group of inducers is that these compounds are substrates of the MFO system with a relatively low rate of biotransformation. Therefore, the "enzyme substrate complexes" exist for relatively longer periods. This results in a decreased amount of enzyme available for reaction.[37] This enzyme inhibition in the first 1 to 12 h after administration of the inducers is followed by increased synthesis of the enzyme, resulting in an increased MFO activity. *De novo* synthesis of the enzyme is demonstrated by an increased incorporation of ^{14}C-orotic acid into nuclear RNA and increased RNA/DNA ration and messenger RNA production in the nucleus. The induction can be blocked by inhibitors or protein synthesis, e.g., actinomycin-D, puromycin, and ethionine. The enhancement of MFO activity is accompanied by an enhanced activity of NADPH-cytochrome p-450 reductase, an increase in liver weight, and in the amount of smooth endoplasmaic reticulum (SER) in hepatocytes. This "classical" induction of the MFO system is also known as the "substrate-type" of induction.

Administration to animals of the second group of inducers (e.g., 3-MD) results in a distinctly different type of enzyme induction.[35,36] One major distinction is to be seen in the carbon monoxide difference spectra: the absorption maximum is located at 448 nm. Parke[38] listed these differences as follows:

- Cytochrome p-448 rather than cytochrome p-450 is produced
- There is no simultaneous increase in cytochrome p-450 reductase
- Cytochrome p-448 tends to exist as a stable complex containing the inducing agent
- In the mammalian placenta, cytochrome p-448, but not cytochrome p-480 is inducible

Recent information suggests that 3-MC also induces at least two isoenzymes, one of which is cytochrome p-448.[24] It has been postulated that inducers belonging to this group bind to a receptor in the hepatocyte cytosol and that the inducer-receptor complex interacts with structures in the cell's nucleus. This interaction would regulate the synthesis of the cytochrome p-450 isoenzymes involved.[39,40] The inducers from the second group enhance biotransformation of foreign compounds to a much more limited degree than do the inducers from group one.

The ability of some xenobiotics to enhance MFO activity (phase I reactions) can extend to induction of enzymes involved in conjugation reactions (phase II). Reactions in both phases can be increased *in vivo* following administration of a wide variety of foreign compounds such as polycyclic hydrocarbons, DDT, and polychlorinated biphenyls.[41,42] However, the induction in the hydroxylation step usually precedes that in the glucuronidation step. The interdependence of the induction of MFO and UDP-glucuronosyltransferase (the enzyme catalyzing glucuronidation) and the time sequence of the two phenomena suggest that these induction processes might be coupled.[42] Although being subsequent events in the metabolism of xenobiotics, both processes may have different control mechanisms of their biosynthesis.

The number of known MFO inhibitors is much smaller. Interference can occur with various steps or components of the MFO system. Inhibition may be "competitive" or "noncompetitive". Competitive (reversible inhibition occurs when two or more substrates compete simultaneously for the same active site on the cytochrome. The inhibitory effect of inducers of the first group (e.g. phenobarbital), occurring in the early stage of their action, is an example of competitive inhibition. The best known inhibitor of the MFO system, SKF-525A (β-diethylamino-ethyl diphyenyl propylacetate), is another example of a competitive substrate. Pretreatment with this compound results in an inhibition of the biotransformation of other MFO substrates for several hours. Competitive inhibition of cytochrome p-450 can be highly specific because of the differences in specificity of the active sites in different isoenzymes.

Noncompetitive (irreversible) inhibition of MFO can be the result of covalent binding of the inhibitor to the enzyme. The formation of stable enzyme-substrate complexes blocks the metabolism of other MFO substrates. Many examples exist of the formation of such stable complexes as a result of the bioactivation of substrates by the MFO system itself. This so-called "suicide action" of the cytochrome p-450 system is observed with some methylenedioxyaryl compounds that are in use as insecticide synergists. The best known compound from this group, piperonyl butoxide can act as a noncompetitive inhibitor of MFO after its biotransformation to a carbene and other reactive intermediates.[43]

Nonreversible inhibition of cytochrome p-450 can be observed with many xenobiotics such as nitroso compounds, some amines, etc. Heavy metals of metal-containing compounds (e.g. cadmium and mercury) are MFO-inhibitors as well. Methyl mercury inhibits the MFO system by impairing the structure of SER membranes and interaction with components of the system. Other examples are CCl_4, carbon disulfide, and halothane.[44]

Inhibition of the MFO system can also occur at the site of NADPH-cytochrome p-450 reductase (FP_1 in Figure 3). If the flow of reducing equivalents from NADPH is blocked or diverted, MFO activity will be decreased. The bipyridilium herbicides paraquat and diquat are good electron acceptors of the reductase. The compounds are then reduced to stable free radicals. Reaction with oxygen reconverts the radicals to the original ions. Thus, paraquat and diquat not only inhibit the MFO system in microsomes by competing for the electrons donated by the reductase but also are competing for oxygen.[45,45]

D. OTHER FACTORS INFLUENCING MFO ACTIVITY
1. Species and Strain

Sensitivity to the toxic action of xenobiotics varies among different animal species. It is known that the intrinsic toxicity of a substance and its concetration present in the tissues determine its toxic effects in an organism. Therefore, species differences in toxicokinetics and in biotransformation are very important factors in understanding species differences in toxicity. As far as biotransformation is concerned, these differences may be qualitative (different pathways) or quantitative (different kinetic characteristics).[47] These differences apply to both pahse I and phase II reactions. The implications of a relative change in the metabolism via alternative pathways are sometimes very clear. For example, lindane treatment leads to a significant increase in liver tumor incidence in CF1 mice while in Osborne-Mendel rats it is not carcinogenic.[48] This is correlated with a higher MFO activity in mice, a higher inducibility of MFO by lindane, a larger increase in absolute and relative liver weight after lindane treatment, and with lower epoxide hydrolase activity than in rats. Sensitivity to the toxic action of chemicals may also depend on the animal strain. For example, Oesch et al.[48] reported that lindane is carcinogenic for CF1 mice but no for B6C3F1 mice.

Comparative studies of the biotransformation and toxicokinetics in animals show a relationship between the rate of oxidative xenobiotic metabolism and the body weight of the animal species.[44] The ratio between the log of the oxidative biotransformation and the log of the body weight was shown to be linear for the following species: mouse, hamster, rat, guinea pig, rabbit, cat, dog, minipig, and sheep.[49] Man seems to be an exception, having lower rate of oxidative metabolism of exogenous chemicals than would be predicted from the body weight.[44]

This linear relationship suggests that the rate of MFO-dependent oxidation is depending on tissue oxygen concentration rather than tissue concentrations of the xenobiotic. An important consequence is that detoxication by MFO in the smaller animal species normally used in laboratory experiments is fast in comparison with larger animals, including man. This may cause problems in the extrapolation of toxicity data from rodents to man: the equivalent dose based on body weight may be more toxic to man. On the other hand, in case of bioactivation reactions catalyzed by the MFO system, the small rodents will produce bioactivated metabolites to a higher degree than man. Such activations occur with many mutagens and carcinogens and could be an explanation for the higher incidence of mutagenic and carcinogenic effects in the smaller experimental animals, such as the mouse and the rat. These species differences must be taken into consideration when toxicity data are to be extrapolated from one species to another and to man.

Evidence obtained by a number of investigators indicates that no one species is identical to another, both qualitatively and quantitatively, in the biotransformation of a single exogenous chemical. A striking example is the ability of man and the rat to convert DDT to DDE and the inability of the rhesus monkey to produce more than a trace of metabolite.[7]

2. Age

Age has an important effect on the biotransformation of xenobiotics. A systematic study of pesticides and other xenobiotics shows that newborn animals are generally more susceptible than adults regardless of the route of administration.[50] The same may apply to man: children are normally more susceptible to poisons. Brodeur and Du Bois[51] studied the effects of 15 organophosphorus insecticides and defoliants in weanling male rats and in adults and found toxicity ratios (weanlings/adults) to be between 0.2 to 4.1 with a mean of 1.8. Calves and lambs are much more susceptible than adult cattle or sheep to sprays or dips of chlordane, dieldrin, and lindane.[52] In other cases older animals were less resistant to xenobiotics. Lu et al.[59] showed that newborn rats are over 20 times more resistant to DDT than adults.

Such age differences can be explained by considering the role of the MFO system in the bioactivation (toxification) or bioinactivation (detoxification) of the chemical in question.[53] Accordingly, the neonatal rat, with a poorly functioning MFO system, is resistant to the toxic effect of CCl_4 until the age of at least 7 days, at which time the ability to metabolize the agent has appeared.

Age differences concerning MFO component activity and metabolic potential have been reported.[54,55] MFO activity is almost lacking in rat fetus and newborn, but its activity increases rapidly during the early days or weeks of life. The development of the rat MFO system has been investigated by Mac Donald et al.[56] by analyzing its components in fetuses and young pups of postconceptional age 18-54 days. Cytochrome p-450, cytochrome b_5, and NADPH-cytochrome c reductase were present and increased with age before birth. The major increases were detected in the first 2 days after birth. Again, the cytochrome p-450 concentration increased markedly at puberty, whereas the reductase activity increased before puberty and reached the adult level at puberty. Metabolism of warfarin to specific metabolites indicated that the isoenzyme cytochrome p-450 UT-C began to predominate at 37 days postconception. The dominant position of this isoenzymes in the hepatic cytochrome p-450 pool increased with age.

Senescence also affects drug metabolism and aging animals show differences in reponse to inducing agents.[57,58] These differenes are associated with a decrease in cytochrome p-450 concentrations and enzyme activities and with changes in the inducibility of enzyme components. In juvenile rats (5 to 6 weeks old) significant cytochrome p-450 induction was found after a four-week treatment with 0.05 ppm 8-monohydroxymirex, whereas in adult rats (12 to 14 weeks) induction only occurred with at least 10 ppm of this compound.[59] In the same study 4-hydroxylation of aniline was more readily induced in juvenile than in adult rats, whereas N-demethylation of aminopyrine had a higher inducibility in adults.

Induction of the MFO system is also controlled by the hormonal status of the organism. Administration of o,p'-DDT to newborn rats resulted in elevated levels of cytochrome p-450 in prepubertal animals (day 20). However, in adult rats no effect of this neonatal treatment on the cytochrome p-450 amounts was found.[60]

The very low levels of MFO activity in fetal and neonatal experimental animals are associated with the development of the SER. In these species this development does not occur until after birth, while in man, the SER appears in the first or second trimester of pregnancy and has attained a substantial activity by the time of birth.[61] Therefore, toxicity findings concerning effects on the fetus or the neonate are not easily extrapolated from rodents to man.

In conclusion, on the basis of age differences in MFO activity, it might be predicted that neonatal and immature animals will be less resistant to pesticides that are detoxified by MFO than adults and will be more resistant to chemicals that are bioactivated by these enzyme systems.

3. Sex

Consistent differences between males and females in pesticide toxicity have been shown in the rat and the mouse. Calculations from oral toxicity data of 69 pesticides showed that in rats the ratio (male/female) in oral LD_{50} ranged from 0.21 to 4.62 with an average of 0.94.[7] Sex differences in mice generally are less pronounced, and no significant differences in susceptibility to pesticides or other xenobiotics are found between the sexes of other species.

The sex differences in rat and mouse are to a large degree associated with MFO activity and inducibility in the liver. In the absence of intentional induction, MFO activity is higher in the males of these species.[62,63] However, the inducibility of MFO by foreign compounds is usually greater in the female rat. Since quantitative measurements show equal amounts of microsomal cytochrome p-450 in males and females,[10] it is suggested that the sex differences reflect qualitative differences in the MFO system. Bentley et al.[64] have found that the treatment of rats and mice with the formamidine insecticide chlordimeform enhanced the activity of MFO. However, the extent of induction depended upon the reaction studied, the sex, and species of the animal selected. Microsomal cytochrome p-450 content was elevated in both male and female rats and mice, O-dealkylation of ethoxycoumarin was increased in male and female rats but not in mice, while N-deethylation of ethylmorphine was elevated in mice but not in rats. Hydroxylation of benzo(a) pyrene was increased in female rats and mice, but not in males.

The effects of chlordecone and mirex treatment of the MFO-system was investigated by Ebel[65] in male and female rats. Treatment with both pesticides resulted in higher levels of cytochrome p-450 in a time and dose-dependent manner. The apparent enzyme kinetics (V_{max} and K_m) for the O-demethylation of p-nitroanisole were determined. In male rats the maximum rate of p-nitroanisole metabolism was increased with about 100% with chlordecone and 50% with mirex. The apparent k_m was elevated about 40- and 18-fold after treatment with chlordecon and mirex, respectively. In females, p-nitroanisole metabolism was reduced slightly by treatment with either agent and the apparent K_m was increased about 14-fold by chlordecone treatment and unaffected by mirex.

The validity of sex differences seems to be supported by their disappearance after treatment of females with androgens. Treatment of male rat with estrogens also affects the MFO system.[62] It should be pointed out that the ability of sex steroids to enhance biotransformation of xenobiotics appears to parallel their anabolic rather than their androgenic activity.

4. Nutrition

The activity of mixed function oxidases is profoundly affected by the nutritional status of animals. This may result in changes in the toxicity of pesticides or other xenobiotics exceeding 100%. For this reason knowledge of the nutritional status of animals used in toxicity studies is very important.[44]

The general effects of protein, lipid, vitamins and other dietary constituents on the toxicity of xenobiotics have been known for some time.[66,67] A low-protein diet decreases the amount of cytochrome p-450 and the MFO activity. Accordingly, this increases the toxicity of pesticides that are detoxified by biotransformation and decreases the toxicity of pesticides that exert their adverse effects as toxic metabolites.[68] When protein restriction is severe anb especially when it is complete, susceptibility to some pesticides is increased dramatically.[7] Although an increase in dietary protein does not have a very dramatic impact, high protein levels may give rise to an enhanced toxicity of pesticides that are primarily activated by MFO and to a higher resistance to xenobiotics that are detoxified by MFO.

Complete protein restriction prevents induction of liver MFO in rats by compounds that normally result in an enhancement of enzyme activity. Biotransformation of the organo-thiophosphate malathion to its activated metabolic malaoxon was increased in livers of chickens given different MFO inducers: β-naphthoflavone, 3-methylcholanthrene, butylated hydroxytoluene, and polychlorinated biphenyls. Malaoxon dealkylation — one of the de-toxification reactions of this compound was decreased in birds fed a low-protein diet and this was correlated with decreases in the amount of cytochrome p-450 and p-448.[69]

The biotransformation of xenobiotics is also dependent on dietary lipid. Intake of lipids, especially phospholipids and unsaturated fatty acids, is essential for the normal activity of MFO[70,71] Deficiency of these lipids may lead to a loss of activity with enhanced toxicity of certain pesticides. It is possible that chemical carcinogens given to animals on a high-fat diet especially in the presence of a simultaneous deficiency of lipotropes would give rise to increased levels of lipid peroxidation, resulting in an increased occurrence of mutation and carcinogenesis.[44]

The effects of a high protein diet (59% casein) or a high fat diet (50% saturated fat) on the toxicity of parathion and dichlorvos in growing male rats was studied by Purshottam and Srivastava.[72] Both the high protein and the high fat diet significantly protected against mortality from parathion but not from dichlorvos. Hydroxylation of aniline was increased significantly by both diets, whereas hepatic microsomal cytochrome p-450 and the demeth-ylation of aminopyrine were unchanged.

Vitamins are other essential dietary constituents that may affect the integrity and activity of the hepatic MFO system. Vitamin A (retinol) deficiency has been shown to impair the activity of MFO: retinol-deficient rats exhibit lower levels of liver cytochrome p-450 which results in impairment of the biotransformation of xenobiotics.[73] The effects of vitamin A on the inducibility by xenobiotics seem to be influenced by stress: cold or noise diminished the effects of DDT on cytochrome p-450 levels in the liver.[74] Matkovics et al.[75] studied the effects of vitamin A deficiency on the action of organothiophosphate pesticides. They ob-served an inhibition of protein synthesis by these pesticides in the liver of vitamin A deficient rats. Addition of vitamin A compensated to some extent the cholinesterase-inhibiting action of the pesticides, while vitamin E addition had a more pronounced effect in normal rats.

A requirement for vitamin C (ascorbic acid) for the phase I biotransformation reactions is also known: a severe deficiency (more than 7% depletion results in an impairment of the MFO.[76]

Administration of vitamin E (α-tocopherol) to rats increases hydroxylation reactions in phase I. Vitamin E deficiency has been shown to decrease the activity of MFO.[77]

The effect of dietary essential amino acids and vitamins A, C, and E on the inducibility of the liver MFO system by lindane was studied by Sharmanov et al.[78] Deficiency in these amino acids and vitamins in male rats led to an induction of MFO within the first 2 h after a single dose of lindane (18 mg/kg), but after this period the induction was significantly lower than in animals on a normal diet. This deficiency in essential nutrients also caused a delay in the induction of the MFO system in rats treated daily for 3 months with lindane at a dose of 0.9 mg/kg.

Thus, MFO activity may strongly be affected by the nutritional status of animals. Moreover, extensive or prolonged administration of xenobiotics may lead to significant nutritional demands for ascorbic acid and, in the case of enzyme-inducing agents, for folate.[71]

III. THE ROLE OF MIXED FUNCTION OXIDASE IN CHRONIC PESTICIDE TOXICITY

A. CHANGES IN FMO DURING CHRONIC EXPOSURE TO PESTICIDES

Although animal death resulting from acute effects of exposure to pesticides may be of immediate concern, species survival will be dependent on the ability of animals to adapt to chronic low-level exposure to environmental xenobiotics, including pesticides. The animal's survival in general is related to its capacity to adjust itself to changes in a broad range of environmental factors. These adjustments are associated with deviations in functional and structural parameters, reflecting the animal's adaptative potential.

The ability of animals to survive chronic low levels of environmental pesticides and other xenobiotics is to a large degree dependent on the adaptative potential of the liver. The most consistent responses in vertebrates to the exposure of many pesticides are both structural and functional changes in the liver, including increases in enzyme activities, in size and number of cellular organelles, and in cell and organ size.[59] There is a clear relationship between induction of MFO and liver enlargement, mostly associated with a proliferation of SER.

The increase in liver mass is a compensatory response in which the liver is reacting to an increased functional demand.[79] The enlargement represents "real" growth and in most instances consists of a hyperplastic component (i.e. an increase in cell numbers) and a hypertrophic component (cellular enlargement).[59]

A study with a wide range of xenobiotics indicated that with only a few exceptions, xenobiotics causing liver growth also induced hepatic metabolism of foreign compounds.[80] In this study the insecticides DDT, pyrethrum, and dieldrin appeared to be moderate inducers, whereas mirex was a highly potent inducer. Similar results were obtained in a 1-year experiment described by Yarbrough et al.[81] Male mice were fed comparable dose levels of p,p'-DDT and mirex. NADPH-cytochrome c reductase activity and cytochrome p-450 content was determined periodically in liver microsomes. These parameters showed significantly greater changes in animals exposed to mirex as compared with those exposed to DDT. With mirex, cytochrome p-450 content remained elevated throughout the treatment period with exposure levels of 1.78 mg/kg and 17.80 mg/kg and no significant changes occurred with time. In DDT-treated animals no significant dose or time response of cytochrome p-450 content was found at the same exposure levels.

The induction of the hepatic MFO system after chronic exposure to DDT has been studied in different animal specis.[82-85] Oral administration of p,p'-DDT (5,15, and 50 mg/kg/day) for 21 days to rats and baboons resulted in increased concentrations of hepatic cytochrome p-450. In rats all dose levels gave equivalent increase in the enzyme system whereas in baboons the enhancement was dose related.[86] In squirrel monkeys, lower doses (0.5 and 5 mg/kg/day) for up to 6 months significantly increased MFO activities as measured by the metabolism of p-nitroanisole and O-ethyl-O-4-nitrophenyl phenylphosphothionate (EPN).[87] DDT appeared to be a more potent inducer than toxaphene during a 13-week exposure period in rats.[88] A strong MFO induction was observed in the first 6 weeks with a gradual decline in the next 7-week exposure period.

Chronic dieldrin exposure (2 to 5 mg/kg for 52 days) to female rats resulted in increases in liver weight, microsomal protein, and cytochrome p-450 together with an initial induction of aniline and p-nitrobenzoate metabolism.[89] This was followed by a decrease in metabolism of these substrates to levels lower than those of controls, while liver weight and microsomal levels of protein and cytochrome p-450 remained elevated. This phenomenon, associated with a lack of correlation between activity and content of cytochrome p-450, has been termed hypertrophic, hypoactive endoplasmic reticulum. In an eight-week dieldrin exposure study Stevens et al.[90] found elevated activities of NADPH-cytochrome c reductase, NADPH-oxidase, and cytochrome p-450 levels in both male and female rats, but only a slight reduction in specific substrate metabolism.

The measurement of MFO components and/or MFO activity with a large variety of substrates has been used frequently in evaluating the effects of a wide range of pesticides. It is now clear that many pesticides used as insecticides, herbicides, fungicides, larvicides, etc., having very different chemical structures do affect MFO components and activity. Induction of MFO as a result of chronic exposure has been reported for many organochlorine insecticides: DDT,[59,81] Dieldrin,[91] chlordecone,[92] mirex,[93,94] and 8-monohydroxymirex.[95] Chronic exposure to pyrethrins leads to a moderate induction of MFO with effects of some biotransformation reactions.[96] Slight induction of MFO is reported to occur after chronic exposure to carbamates.[97]

The number of pesticides known to be inhibitors of MFO is much smaller. Inhibitory effects are reported for the exposure to thiophosphate insecticides,[98,99] thiocarbamates[97,98] to amidines,[100] and to bipyridilium compounds.[45]

In conclusion, the study of effects of pesticides on the MFO system can indicate damaging effects of components of the enzyme system and its activity. Moreover, these studies will increase our knowledge of the role of the MFO system in the mechanisms of chronic intoxication with pesticides and in pesticide interaction.[92,101-103] Since so many examples exist of pesticides that alter MFO activity, as well as examples of pesticides of which the toxicity is determined by MFO activity, it is very important to pay attention to the inter-relations between pesticides and this enzyme system in evaluating the risk of the use of pesticides.

B. MFO AND ADAPTATION TO PESTICIDES

Adaptation is an extremely important phenomenon in understanding the relation between the toxic action of a xenobiotic and the response of the organism. It is difficult, however, to assess the nature of this response, in particular since it is not easy to distinguish between the "physiological normal" and "compensated pathology".

The "normal" is a natural state of the organism and its vital activities. This state is relatively steady and at the same time flexible, for it reflects the dynamics of environmental change. Depending on the intensity and duration of exposure as well as on the body's adaptive potential, pesticides may produce varying degrees of change in functional parameters, which may or may not remain within the limits of physiological fluctuations. Detection of early deviations from the physiological normal situation is particularly complicated by the fact that the observed value for any functional parameter integrally reflects two processes: the action of the pesticide and the counteraction of the organism (i.e., adaptation). Hence, determination of the latter is only theoretically possible. Such an approach has been used to explore chemical toxic action in "pure form", i.e. making no allowance for adaptation.[98] Relating the theoretical cummulative effect (TCE) as calculated for a given parameter by way of mathematical modeling, to the experimentally observed value (OV) enables definition of adaptation in relative units:

$$\text{Adaptation (rel. units)} = \frac{\text{TCE} - \text{OV}}{\text{TCE}} \qquad (5)$$

Using Formula 5, curves describing the process of adaptation were shown to assume the shape of fluctuations that gradually faded away (Figure 4). Moreover, this general pattern was found to be maintained with various toxic agents (e.g., the organothiophosphate chlorpyrifos, tetrachloromethane, the organochlorine compound milbex) over the whole range of doses compatible with life.[98,104] These findings lead us to presume that the adaptation processes in an organism follow general rules.

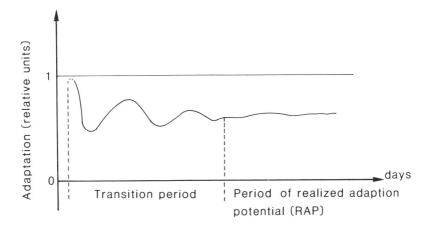

FIGURE 4. Typical curve representing the adaptation of an organism to repeated exposure to a foreign compound with effects on functional parameters.

The oscillatory nature of adaptation dynamics is conceivably related to predominance of different defense and adjustment mechanisms and their synchronization. Depending on the type of exposure, various adaptation mechanisms appear to come into play, both general mechansims (e.g., increased rate of regenerative processes, synchronization of physiological and biochemical processes with environmental challenges, etc.) as well as more or less specific mechanisms (e.g. changes in biotransformation rates).

In the adaptation curve, the first phase showing fluctuations that gradually subside characterizes transitional adaptive processes leading to the attainment of a steady state level (Figure 4). The last phase in the curve illustrates the realization of the organism's adaptive potential to a particular type of exposure. A plot of the exposure rate vs. the realized adaptive potential (RAP) has the shape of a decreasing exponent. Such a curve is valid for exposures that are compatible with life, i.e. do not exceed the adaptive potential of an organism. Thus, adaptation is operative in both maintaining the balance with environmental factors as well as in the process of transition to establishment of a new balance.

The limits of organims's adaptive potential and the dynamics of transition processes determine which type of adaptation to a particular exposure will result, namely:

1. Steady State (Physiological) Adaptation

This type is manifest in the maintenance of steady equilibrium at the expense of structural and functional changes that stay within the range of physiological fluctuations.

2. Compensation or *Compensatory Adaptation*

This is manifest in the recovery from imbalance to attain a qualitatively new steady state at the expense of structural and functional changes that indicate straining of compensatory mechanisms. In the above two types of adaptation, RAP is within the limits of physiological fluctuations. Transition processes, however, remain within these limits only for steady state adaptation, whereas for compensatory adaptation these limits are exceeded.

3. Adaptation to High-Intensity Exposures or Adaptation in Pathology

Such adaptation occurs at the expense of structural and functional changes going beyond the limits of physiological fluctuations. The extent or RAP deviation from the relative unit-adaptation indicator is dependent upon rate, multiplicity, and schedule of exposure to the noxious factor. Any substantial change in the latter characteristics will provoke renewal of transition processes. Prolonged straining of compensatory mechanisms may result in their impairment (adaptation failure or exhaustion). Other possible causes of failure include intercurrent illness, malnutrition, etc.

Establishment of a new equilibrium in an organism as a result of the action of pesticides or other chemical compounds may lead to an increasing tolerance to a noxious agent. For example, rats that had received 2 mg/kg dieldrin for 28 days survived 25 consecutive daily doses of 5 mg/kg, a dosage producing 70% mortality in untreated rats.[89] In terms of the classification above this resistance can be explained as compensation. However, in these experiments the livers of rats pretreated with moderate dosages of dieldrin showed definite indications of damage in response to the higher dosage. Therefore, compensatory adaptation may result in a situation that can be described as a "premorbid state".[98]

Very often tolerance to a compound is a result of an organism's increased ability to metabolize it. It has shown that the enhanced metabolism responsible for tolerance is mediated by an increased MFO activity. In the case of a pesticide that is detoxified via a reaction catalyzed by the MFO, MFO-inducing pesticides will be capable of producing tolerance. Since these inducing compounds never have a specific action, this also explains another adaptive phenomenon known as increased nonspecific tolerance.[105] As an example, mice made tolerant to the organothiophosphate disulfoton were "coss-tolerant" to chlorphyrifos as well as to the carbamate insecticide propoxur.[106] Another example of cross-tolerance not associated with changes in MFO activity is the tolerance to hypoxia of subjects exposed to carbon monoxide.

Resistance is another adaptive phenomenon, characterized by changes in the genetic properties of a species. In this case the species has the ability to develop a genotype that can cope successfully with a toxic agent. This phenomenon is found especially in fast-multiplying species like insects. More than 100 insect species like mosquitos and flies, many of them known to be a vector in disease, are now resistant to one or more pesticides.[107] An example of resistance in a vertebrate species is the Norway rat, which developed a resistance to warfarin.[7]

C. MFO AND PESTICIDE INTERACTIONS

Changes in MFO activity belong to the major biochemical mechanisms of pesticide interaction. Metabolic interactions occur primarily through the ability of one compound (A) to modify the enzyme(s) responsible for the metabolism of another chemical (B). If B is inactivated by a given enzyme system, the ability of A to inhibit or stimulate the enzyme's activity, the combined dosage of A and B will result in synergism (potentiation) or antagonism of the biological activities of B. The opposite effect will be observed if the enzyme system activitates B.[108] Since the MFO system is involved in the primary attack of many lipophilic xenobiotics,[99,109,110] interactions involving the MFO system are likely to have the widest toxicological implications.[108] However, pesticide interactions can occur through modifications of any of the enzymes involved in biotransformation.

An example of the interaction between pesticides and other chemicals is given in the study by Popov and Zadorozhnaya.[111] By using the model of the *in situ* perfused rat liver[112] the metabolism of chlorpyrifos (Dursban) as well as the effects of this organophosphorus compound on cholinesterase (ChE) activity in blood was determined. Livers were perfused with diluted rat blood (4 vol blood + 1 vol Ringer-Lock solution). Rats were pretreated for 4, 8, or 15 days with tetrachloromethane (CCl_4, 200 mg/kg bw, daily oral dosage in sunflower oil) or with the organochlorine pesticide milbex (30 mg/kg bw daily oral dosage calculated on the basis of the active ingredient CPAS). After preparing the liver for *in situ* perfusion, chlorpyrifos (10μg/ml) was added to the perfusate. Samples of perfusate were taken after 5, 15, and 30 min. After this time the livers were prepared for EM morphological examination. Analysis of chlorpyrifos and its major metabolites was achieved by GLC and TLC. Cholineesterase activity was measured by a method modified after Hestrin.[113]

Figure 5 shows the disappearance of chlorpyrifos (A) and the appearance of its PO-analogue (B) in the perfusate during recirculating perfusion of rat livers. In C, the inhibition

% 4 days treatment 8 days treatment 15 days treatment

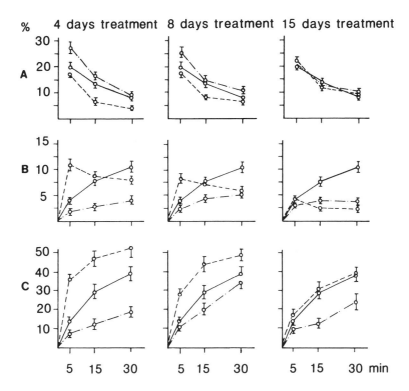

FIGURE 5. Adaptation to prolonged exposure to Milbex and tetrachloromethane. Rats were treated for 4, 8, and 15 days with Milbex or tetrachloromethane (CCl$_4$). Chlorpyrifos bioactivation was determined in the *In situ* perfused rat liver and the cholinesterase activity was measured in the perfusion medium (rat erythrocyte suspension). (A) Chlorpyrifos concentration in perfusion medium; (B) concentration of the PO metabolite of chlorpyrifos in medium; (C) cholinesterase inhibition; (O———O: control; O---O: after Milbex treatment; O-·-·-O: after CCl$_4$ treatment. Data represent means ± s.e.m. of 4 perfusions; results are expressed as percentages of t = 0.

of cholineesterase activity is shown. Data represent means ± SEM of four perfusions as percentages of t = O. Line 1 represents results with livers from control rats, line 2 with livers from milbex-pretreated rats, and line 3 with livers from CCl$_4$-pretreated animals.

The very fast inhibition of ChE in the beginning of the experiments is a reflection of the high velocity of oxidative desulfuration catalyzed by the MFO system in the liver. This metabolite is a 40 times more potent ChE inhibitor as compared with the parent compound. Milbex, a known inducer of MFO activity, causes a faster disappearance of chlorpyrifos from the perfusate after 4 days of pretreatment. Parallel with this faster disappearance, more PO analogue and higher degree of ChE inhibition was found. The dealkylated PO metabolites are also found in high concentrations after milbex pretreatment (the monoethyl metabolite: 3.7 ± 0.2 arbitrary units at 5 min after the start of the chlorpyrifos perfusion and 11.3 ± 1.5 units at 30 min; the completely dealkylated metabolite: 29.5 ± 4.4 arbitrary units at 5 min and 54.5 ± 2.6 units at 30 min), while both metabolites cannot be detected in the control perfusions. The concentration curves of the PO-metabolite (Fig 5B) suggest that these dealkylation products are formed from the PO metabolite. Thus, milbex not only causes an induction of the bioactivation reaction, but there is also an enhancement of the bioin-activation reactions.

Prolonged treatment with milbex for 8 and 15 days, respectively, results in a less pronounced effect on chlorpyrifos uptake from the perfuste. After 15 days treatment no significant difference with nonpretreated livers is seen. This is reflected in the initial velocity of PO analogue formation, while in later stages of the perfusion (i.e., after 15 and 30 min) the dealkylation is more abundant. It seems, however, that the initial rate of desulfuration strongly determines the inhibition of ChE. Ultrastructural findings in the livers show that after an initial hyperplasia and an increase in SER per cell and some necrosis in other areas of the liver, a prolonged treatment of animals with milbex leads to a compensatory adaptation.

Pretreatment of animals with CCl_4 results in an inhibition of chlorpyrifos biotransformation, which is also reflected in a strongly diminished ChE inhibition. Here, no dealkylation is found. Prolonged treatment leads to adaptational changes as well: after 8 days a diminished effect of the pretreatment is seen on chlorpyrifos kinetics. EM morphological examination shows that this functional adaptation is paralleled by ultrastructural changes. After 4 days, dystrophy and micronecrosis in the centrilobular parts of the livers are observed. The same changes are seen after 8 days, however, by then hyperplasia and hypertrophy can be found in other regions of the liver, resulting in a mozaic pattern of morphological changes and this explains the functional adaptation.

After 15 days, CCl_4-treated livers show a normal uptake of chlorpyrifos from the medium. However, there is less PO analogue formation and less ChE inhibition. A possible reason for this finding is that a repeated treatment with CCl_4 leads to a strong detoxification by the production of hydrolyzed metabolites (i.e., thiophosphoric acid and phosphoric acid).

These studies show that there can be dramatic changes in the effects of pesticides in animals when certain other compounds are present and that these interactions can be the result of changes in the metabolism of the compounds by the MFO system. It is also clear that prolonged treatment of animals will lead to adaptational changes. In the case of CCl_4 treatment, three different stages of adaptation can be distinguished:

1.   Dystrophic structural changes reflected in diminished functional activity of MFO system (4 days).
2.   Reparative regeneration with (partial) functional improvement (8 days). This can be followed by a 3rd stage:
3.   Structural and functional recovery.

For milbex treatment the adaptation seems to consist of a change in biotransformation pathways. After an initial stage of stimulated bioactivation of chlorpyrifos the induction of the bioinactivation reaction results in a correction to the normal situation.

The results presented above confirm that changes in the activity of the MFO system and the consequent rearrangement of biotransformation pathways represent a basis for the understanding of mechanisms of adaptation to pesticides. Another conclusion is, that MFO induction by a pesticide can potentiate the toxic action of another pesticide that is bioactivated.

With developments that improve our understanding of the MFO system, some long-known or recently arisen phenomena may now be explained. Thus, catastrophic population depletions among certain avian species following the massive application of DDT was found to be related to disorders in calcium metabolism resulting in egg shell thinning and rapid steroid hormone breakdown resulting from the MFO-inducing action of this pesticide. This mechanism probably underlies the gonadotropic effects demonstrated for a number of organochlorine pesticides such as DDT and dieldrin.

IV. CONCLUSION

It is clear that pesticides can have marked effects on oxidative biotransformation in mammals, and therefore have the potential to cause a variety of toxic interactions in animals. A major question is whether or not a certain level of induction or inhibition of MFO activity is in itself a toxicological hazard, especially if one takes into consideration that many carcinogens are known MFO inducers. Therefore, the appraisal of MFO activity may contribute to solving a wide range of current problems in the theory and practice of pesticide toxicology. Of particular interest are the possibilities to enhance the adaptive capacity to toxic exposures and to control toxicokinetics and the related dynamics. Furthermore, the evaluation of MFO activity in laboratory animals contributes to our increased understanding to distinguish between the "normal" and a compensated pathology particularly in studies related to a health standard setting.

REFERENCES

1. **Williams, R. T.,** *Detoxication Mechanisms,* Chapman and Hall, London, 1959.
2. **Parke, D. V.,** *The Biochemistry of Foreign Compounds,* Pergamon Press, Oxford, 1968.
3. **Gillette, J. R., Conney, A. H., Estabrook, R. W., Fouts, J. R., and Mannering, G. J., Eds.,** *Microsomes and Drug Oxidation,* Academic Press, New York, 1969.
4. **LaDu, B. N., Mandel, H. G., and Way, E. L., Eds.,** *Fundamentals of Drug Metabolism and Drug Disposition,* Williams & Wilkins, Baltimore, 1971.
5. **O'Brien, R. D.,** *Toxic Phosphorus Esters. Chemistry, Metabolism and Biological Effects,* Academic Press, New York, 1960.
6. **Heath, D. F.,** *Organophosphorus Poisons. Anticholinesterases and related Compounds,* Pergamon Press, New York, 1961.
7. **Hayes, W. J. Jr.,** *Toxicology of Pesticides,* Williams & Wilkins, Baltimore, 1975.
8. **Mason, H. S.,** Mechanisms of oxygen metabolism, *Science,* 125, 1185, 1957.
9. **Hayaishi, O.,** *Oxygenases,* Academic Press, New York, 1962.
10. **Gillette, J. R. E., and Jollow, D. J.,** Drug metabolism in liver, in *The Liver,* Becker, F. F., Ed., Marcel Dekker, New York, 1974, 165.
11. **Schenkman, J. B. and Kupfer, D., Eds.** *Hepatic Cytochrome p-450 Mono-Oxygenase System,* Pergamon Press, Oxford, 1982.
12. **Guengerich, F. P.,** Isolation and purification of cytochrome p-450 and the existence of multiple forms, *Pharmacol. Ther.,* 6, 99, 1979.
13. **Klingenberg, M.,** Pigments of rat liver microsomes, *Arch. Biochem. Biophys.,* 75, 376, 1958.
14. **Mannering, G. J.,** Microsomal enzyme system which catalyzes drug metabolism, in *Fundamentals of Drug Metabolism and Drug Disposition,* LaDu, B. N., Mandel, H. G., and Way, E. L., Eds., Williams & Wilkins, Baltimore, 1971, 206.
15. **Casida, J. E. and Lykken, L.,** Metabolism of organic pesticide chemicals in higher plants, *Annu. Rev. Plant Physiol.,* 20, 607, 1969.
16. **Galliard, T. and Stumpf, P. K.,** Fat metabolism in higher plants, *J. Biol. Chem.,* 241, 5806, 1966.
17. **Bast, A.,** Interactions of Drug Metabolites with Hepatic Cytochrome p-450. Some implications for Drug Metabolism, Ph.D. thesis, University of Utrecht, The Netherlands, 1981.
18. **Paine, A. J.,** Excited states of oxygen in biology: their possible involvement in cytochrome P-450 linked oxidations as well as in the inductrion of the P-450 system by many diverse compounds, *Biochem. Pharmacol.,* 27, 1805, 1978.
19. **Alvares, A. P., Schilling, G., Levin, W., and Kuntzman, R.,** Studies on the induction of CO-binding pigments in liver microsomes by phenobarbital and 3-methylcholanthrene, *Biochem. Biophys. Res. Commun.,* 29, 521, 1967.
20. **Ryan, D., Lu, A. Y. H., West, S., and Levin, W.,** Multiple forms of cytochrome P-450 in phenobartial — and 3-methylcholanthrene-treated rats, *J. Biol. Chem.,* 250, 2157, 1976.
21. **Ryan, D., Lu, A. Y. H., Kawalek, J., West, S. B., and Levin, W.,** Highly purified cytochrome P-448 and P-450 from rat liver microsomes, *Biochem. Biophys. Res. Commun.,* 64, 1134, 1979.
22. **Welton, A. F., O'Neal, F. E., Chaney, L. C., and Aust, S. D.,** Multiplicity of cytochrome P-450 hemoproteins in rat liver microsomes, *J. Biol. Chem.,* 250, 5631, 1975.
23. **Coon, M. J. and Black, S. D.,** Comparative structures of P-450 cytochromes, in *Proc. 4th Int. Symp. Comparative Biochemistry, Cytochrome P-450,* Beerse, Belgium, 1985, 26.
24. **Vlasuk, G. P., Ryan, D. E., Thomas, P. E., Levin, W., and Walz, F. G., Jr.,** Polypeptide patterns of hepatic microsomes from Long-Evans rats treated with different xenobiotics, *Biochemistry,* 21, 6288, 1982.

25. **Bandiera, S., Ryan, D. E., Levin, W., and Thomas, P. E.,** Evidence for a family of four immuno-chemically related iozymes of cytochrome p-450 purified from untreated rats, *Arch. Biochem. Biophys.,* 240, 478, 1985.

26. **Dus, K. M.,** P-450$_{LM}$ isozymes — evolution of structure and function, *Proc. 4th Int. Symp. Comparative Biochemistry, Cytochrome P-450,* Beerse, Belgium, 1985, 20.

27. **Newman, S. L. and Guzelian, P. S.,** Identification of the cyanopregnenolone-inducible form of hepatic cytochrome P-450 as a catalyst of aldrin epoxidation, *Biochem. Pharmacol.,* 32, 1529, 1983.

28. **Yoshioka, H., Miyata, T., and Omura, T.,** Induction of phenobarbital-inducible form of cytochrome P-450 in rat liver microsomes by 1,1-di (p-chlorophenyl)-2,2-dichloroethylene, *J. Biochem. (Tokyo),* 95, 937, 1984.

29. **Kaminsky, L. S. and Guengerich, F. P.,** Cytochrome P-450 isozyme/isozyme functional interactions and NADPH-cytochrome P-450 reductase concentrations as factors in microsomal metabolism of warfarin, *Eur. J. Biochem.,* 149, 479, 1985.

30. **Schenkaman, J. B., Remmer, H., and Estabrook, R. W.,** Spectral studies of drug interaction with hepatic microsomal cytochrome, *Mol. Pharmacol.,* 3, 113, 1967.

31. **Boyd, G. S.,** Biological hydroxylation reactions, in *Biological Hydroxylation Mechanisms,* Boyd G. S. and Smellie, R. M. S., Eds., Academic Press, New York, 1972, 1.

32. **Casida, J. E.,** Mixed-function oxidases involvement in the biochemistry of insecticide synergists, *J. Agric. Food. Chem.,* 18, 753, 1970.

33. **Wilkinson, C. F. and Brattsten, L. B.,** Microsomal drug-metabolizing enzymes in insects, *Drug. Metab. Rev.,* 1, 153, 1972.

34. **Naquira, C., White, R. A., and Agostin, M.,** Multiple forms of *Drosophila* cytochrome P-450, in *Biochemistry, Biophysics and Regulation of Cytochrome P-450 Proc. 3rd Eur. Meeting on Cytochrome P-450,* Gustafsson, J. A., Carlstedt-Dure, J., Mode, A., and Rafter, J., Eds., Elsevier, Amsterdam, 1980, 105.

35. **Parkinson, A., Robertson, L. W., Safe, L., and Safe, S.,** Polychlorinated biphenyls as inducers of hepatic microsomal enzymes: effects of di-ortho substitution, *Chem. Biol. Interact.,* 35, 1, 1981.

36. **Robertson, L. W., Parkinson, A., Bandiere, S., and Safe, S.,** Potent induction of rat liver microsomal drug-metabolizing enzymes by 2,3,3',4,4'5-hexabromobiphenyl, a component of Firemaster, *Chem. Biol. Interact.,* 35, 13, 1981.

37. **Parke, D. V.,** Induction of the drug metabolizing enzymes, in *Enzyme Induction,* Parke, D. V., Ed., Plenum Press, New York, 1975, 207.

38. **Parke, D. V.,** Biochemical mechanisms of chemical interactions, in *Combined Exposures to Chemicals,* WHO Interim Document 11, Copenhagen, 1983, 52.

39. **Gielen, J. E., Goujon, F. M., and Nebert, D. W.,** Genetic regulation of aryl hydrocarbon hydroxylase induction. II. Simple Mendelian expressing in mouse tissues in vivo, *J. Biol. Chem.,* 247, 1125, 1972.

40. **Poland, A. and Glover, E.,** Comparison 2,3,7,8,-tetrachloro-dibezno-p-dioxin, a potent inducer of aryl hydrocarbon hydroxylase, with 3-methylcholanthrene, *Mol. Pharmacol.,* 10, 349, 1974.

41. **Vainio, H.,** Enhancement of hepatic microsomal drug oxidation and glucuronidation in rat by 1,1,1-trichloro-2,2-bis(p-chloro-phenyl) ethane (DDT), *Chem. Biol. Interact.,* 9, 7, 1974.

42. **Vainio, H.,** Linkage of microsomal drug oxidation and glucuronidation, in *Proc. 6th Int. Congress of Pharmacology,* Pergamon Press, Oxford, 1976, 53.

43. **Franklin, M. R.,** Methylenedioxyphenyl insecticide synergists as potential human health hazards, *Environ. Health Perspect.,* 14, 29, 1976.

44. **Parke, D. V.,** Biochemical studies in the risk assessment of toxic chemicals, in Risk Assessment, *WHO* Interim document 6, Copenhagen, 1982, 186.

45. **Kreiger, R. I., Lee, P. W., Black, A., and Fukuto, T. R.,** Inhibition of microsomal aldrin epoxidation by diquat and several related bipyridilium compounds, *Bull. Environ. Contam. Toxicol.,* 9, 1, 1980.

46. **Steffen, C. and Netter, K. J.,** On the mechanism of paraquat action on microsomal oxygen reduction and its relation to lipid peroxidation, *Toxicol. Appl. Pharmacol.,* 47, 593, 1979.

47. **Williams, R. T.,** Inter-species variations in the metabolism of xenobiotics, *Biochem. Soc. Transact.,* 2, 359, 1974.

48. **Oesch, F., Frieberg, T., Herbst, M., Paul, W., Wilhelm, N., and Bentley, P.,** Effects of lindane treatment on drug metabolizing enzymes and liver weight of CF$_1$ mice in which it evoked hepatomas and in nin-suseptible rodents, *Chem. Biol. Interact.,* 40, 1, 1982.

49. **Walker, C. H.,** Species differences in microsomal mono-oxygenase activity and their relationship to biological half-lifes, *Drug. Metab. Rev.,* 7, 295, 1978.

50. **Lu, F. C., Jessup, D. C., and Levallee, A.,** Toxicity of pesticides in young rats versus adult rats, *Food Cosmet Toxicol.,* 3, 591, 1965.

51. **Brodeur, J. and Du Bois, K. P.,** Comparison of acute toxicity of anticholinesterase insecticides of weanling and adult male rats, *Proc. Soc. Exp. Biol. Med.,* 114, 509, 1963.

52. **Radeleff, R. D.,** *Veterinary Toxicology,* Lea and Febiger, Philadelphia, 1964.
53. **Durham, W. F.,** Body burden of pesticides in man, *Ann. N.Y. Acad. Sci.,* 160, 183, 1969.
54. **Richey, D. P. and Bender, D. A.,** Pharmacokinetic consequence of aging, *Annu. Rev. Pharmacol. Toxicol.,* 17, 49, 1977.
55. **McMartin, D. N., O'Connor, J. A., Fasco, M. J., and Kaminsky, L. S.,** Influence of aging and induction on rat liver and kidney microsomal mixed function oxidase systems, *Toxicol. Appl. Pharmacol.,* 54, 411, 1980.
56. **Mac Donald, M.G., Fasco, M. J., and Kaminsky, L. S.,** Development of the hepatic mixed function oxidase system and its metabolism warfarin in the perinatal rat, *Dev. Pharmacol. Ther.,* 3, 1, 1981.
57. **Chadwick, R. W., Linko, R. S., Freal, J. J., and Robbins, A. L.,** The effect of age and long-term low-level DDT exposure on the response to enzyme induction in the rat, *Toxicol. Appl. Pharmacol.,* 31, 469, 1975.
58. **Fabacher, D. L. and Hodgson, E.,** Induction of hepatic mixed function oxidase enzymes in adult and neonatal mice by kepone and mirex, *Toxicol. Appl. Pharmacol.,* 39, 71, 1976.
59. **Yarbrough, J. D., Chambers, J. E., and Robinson, K. M.,** Alterations in liver structure and function resulting from chronic insecticide exposure, in *Effects of Chronic Exposures to Pesticides on Animal System,* Chambers, J. E. and Yarbrough, J. D., Eds., Raven Press, New York, 1982, 25.
60. **Lamartiniere, C. A., Luther, M. A., Lucier, G. W., and Illsley, N. P.,** Altered imprinting of rat liver monoamine oxidase by o,p'-DDT and methoxychlor, *Biochem. Pharmacol.,* 31, 647, 1982.
61. **Gillette, J. R. and Stripp, B.,** Pre- and postnatal enzyme capacity for drug metabolite production, *Fed. Proc.,* 34, 172, 1975.
62. **Kato, R.,** Sex related differences in drug metabolism, *Drug. Metab. Rev.,* 3, 1, 1974.
63. **Goble, F. C.,** Sex as a factor in metabolism, toxicity, and efficacy of pharmacodynamic and chemotherapeutic agents, *Adv. Pharmacol. Chemother.,* 13, 173, 1975.
64. **Bentley, P., Staeubli, W., Bieri, F., Muecke, W., and Waechter, F.,** Induction of hepatic drug-metabolizing enzyme following treatment of rats and mice with chlordimeform, *Toxicol. Lett.,* 28, 143, 1985.
65. **Ebel, R. E.,** Hepatic microsomal-p-nitroanisole O-demethylase. Effects of chlordecone or mirex induction in male and female rats, *Biochem. Pharmacol.,* 33, 559, 1984.
66. **Campbell, T. C. and Hayes, J. R.,** Role of nitrition in the drug metabolizing enzyme system, *Pharmacol. Rev.,* 26, 171, 1974.
67. **Wattenberg, L. W., Loub, W. D., Lam, L. K., and Speier, J. L.,** Dietary constituents altering the response to chemical carcinogens, *Fed. Proc.,* 35, 1327, 1976.
68. **Krijnen, C. J. and Boyd, E. M.,** The influence of diets containing 0—81% of protein on tolerated doses of pesticides, *Comp. Gen. Pharmacol.,* 22, 373, 1971.
69. **Ehrich, M., Larsen, C., and Arnold, J.,** Organophosphate detoxification related to induced hepatic microsomal enzymes of chickens, *Am. J. Vet. Res.,* 45, 755, 1984.
70. **Hietanen, E., Laitinen, M., Vainio, H., and Hanninen, O.,** Dietary fats and properties of endoplasmic reticulum. II. Dietary lipid induced changes in activities of drug metabolizing enzymes in liver of rats, *Lipids,* 10, 467, 1975.
71. **Parke, D. V.,** The effects of nutrition and enzyme induction in toxicology, *World Rev. Nutr. Diet.,* 29, 96, 1978.
72. **Purshottam, T. and Srivastava, R. K.,** Effect of high-fat and high-protein diets on toxicity of parathion and dichlorvos, *Arch. Environ. Health,* 39, 425, 1984.
73. **Colby, H. D., Kramer, R. E., Greiner, J. W., Robinson, D. A., Krause, R. F., and Canady, W. J.,** Hepatic drug metabolism in retinol-deficient rats, *Biochem. Pharmacol.,* 21, 1644, 1975.
74. **Truhaut, R., Ferrando, R., and Fourlon, C.,** Interactions entre la vitamine A et le DDT: influence due froid et du bruit, *C.R. Acad. Sci. III,* 299, 759, 1984.
75. **Matkovics, B., Szabo, L., Ivan, J., and Gaal, I.,** Some further data on the effects of two organophosphate pesticides on the oxidative metabolism in the liver, *Gen. Pharmacol.,* 14, 689, 1983.
76. **Zannoni, V. G., Flynn, E. J., and Lynch, M.,** Ascorbic acid and drug metabolism, *Biochem. Pharmacol.,* 22, 2365, 1973.
77. **Horn, L. R., Machlin, L. J., Barker, M. D., and Brin, M.,** Drug metabolism and hepatic heme proteins in the vitamin E-deficient rat, *Arch. Biochem. Biophys.,* 172, 270, 1976.
78. **Sharmanov, T. Sh., Nurmagambetov, T. Zh., Bakanov, S. H. A., and Amirov, B. B.,** Effect of acute and chronic lindane poisoning on the function of the liver microsome mono-oxygenase system in rats maintained on a diet deficient in lysine, methionine, threonine and vitamins A, C and E, *Vopr. Med. Khim.,* 31, 114, 1985.
79. **Schulte-Hermann, R.,** Reactions of the liver to injury, in *Toxic Injury of the Liver,* Farber, E. and Fisher, M., Eds., Marcel Dekker, New York, 1979, 365.
80. **Schulte-Herman, R.,** Induction of liver growth by xenobiotic compounds and other stimuli, *Crit. Rev. Toxicol.,* 3, 97, 1974.

81. **Yarbrough, J. D., Chambers, J. E., Grimley, J. M., Alley, E. G., Fang, M. M., Morrow, J. T., Ward, B. C., and Conroy, J. D.,** Comparative study of 8-monohydroxymirex and mirex toxicity in male rats, *Toxicol. Appl. Pharmacol.,* 58, 105, 1981.
82. **Hart, L. G. and Fouts, J. R.,** Effects of acute and chronic DDT administration on hepatic microsomal drug metabolism in the rat, *Proc. Soc. Exp. Biol. Med.,* 114, 388, 1963.
83. **Platt, D. S. and Cockrill, B. L.,** Liver enlargement and hepatotoxicity: an investigation into the effects of several agents on rat liver enzyme activities, *Biochem. Pharmacol.,* 16, 2257, 1967.
84. **Gillette, J. W.,** Microsomal epoxidation: effect of age and duration of exposure to dietary DDT on induction, *Bull. Environ. Contam. Toxicol.,* 3, 159, 1969.
85. **Copeland, M. F. and Cranmer, M. F.,** Effects of *o,p'*-DDT on the adrenal gland and hepatic microsomal enzyme system in the beagle dog, *Toxicol. Appl. Pharmacol.,* 27, 1, 1974.
86. **Down, W. H. and Chasseaud, L. F.,** The effect of DDT on hepatic microsomal drug-metabolizing enzymes in the baboon: comparison with the rat, *Bull. Environ. Contam. Toxicol.,* 20, 592, 1978.
87. **Cranmer, M., Peoples, A., and Chadwick, R.,** Biochemical effects of repeated administration of *p,p'*-DDT on the squirrel monkey, *Toxicol. Appl. Pharmacol.,* 21, 98, 1972.
88. **Kinoshita, F. K., Frawley, J. P., and Du Bois, K. P.,** Quantitative measurement of induction of hepatic microsomal enzymes by various dietary levels of DDT and toxaphene in rats, *Toxicol. Appl. Pharmacol.,* 9, 505, 1966.
89. **Hutterer, F., Schaffner, F., Klion, F. M., and Popper, H.,** Hypertrophic hypoactive smooth endoplasmic reticulum: a sensitive indicator of hepatotoxicity exemplified by dieldrin, *Science,* 161, 1017, 1968.
90. **Stevens, J. T., Oberholser, K. M., Wagner, S. R., Greene, F. E.,** Content and activities of microsomal electron transport components during the developments of dieldrin-induced hypertrophic hypoactive endoplasmic reticulum, *Toxicol. Appl. Pharmacol.,* 39, 411, 1977.
91. **Walker, A. J. T., Thorpe, E., and Stevenson, D. E.,** The toxicology of dieldrin (HEOD). I. Long-term oral toxicity studies in mice, *Food Cosmet. Toxicol.,* 11, 415, 1972.
92. **Klingensmith, J. S. and Mehendale, H. M.,** Potentiation of CCl_4 lethality by chlordecone, *Toxicol. Lett.,* 11, 149, 1982.
93. **Kaminsky, L. S., Piper, L. J., McMartin, D. M., and Fasco, M. S.,** Induction of hepatic microsomal cytochrome p-450 by mirex and kepone, *Toxicol. Appl. Pharmacol.,* 43, 327, 1978.
94. **Klingensmith, J. S. and Mehendale, H. M.,** Hepatic microsomal metabolism of CCl_4 after pretreatment with chlordecone, mirex, or phenobarbital in male rats, *Drug. Metab. Dispos.,* 11, 329, 1983.
95. **Strik, J. J. T. W. A., Centen, A. H. J., Janssen, M. M. Th., Harmsen, E. G. M., Villeneuve, D. C., Chu, I., and Valli, V. E.,** Toxocity of photomirex with special references to porphyria, hepatic P-450 and glutathione levels, serum enzymes, histology and residues in the quail and rat, *Bull. Environ. Contam. Toxicol.,* 24, 350, 1980.
96. **Springfield, A. C., Carlson, G. P., and Defeo, J. J.,** Liver enlargement and modification of hepatic microsomal drug metabolism in rats by pyrethrum, *Toxicol. Appl. Pharmacol.,* 24, 298, 1973.
97. **Mountie, J., Rivera, F., Goudonnet, H., Escousse, A., and Truchot, R. C.,** Etude de l'influence des pesticides carbamines sur l'induction des enzymes hepatiques du rat et sur les modifications des phospholipides microsomaux, *Arch. Latinoam. Nutr.,* 33, 664, 1983.
98. **Popov, T.,** Biologic and Mathematical Modelling of Intoxication, D.Sc. thesis, University of Kiev, 1977.
99. **Uchiyama, M., Yoshida, T., Homma, K., and Hongo, T.,** Inhibition of hepatic drug-metabolizing enzymes by thiophosphate insecticides and its drug toxicological implications, *Biochem. Pharmacol.,* 24, 1221, 1975.
100. **Budris, D. M., Yim, G. K., and Schnell, R. C.,** Effect of acute and repeated chlordimeform treatment on rat hepatic microsomal drug metabolizing enzymes, *J. Environ. Pathol. Toxicol. Oncol.,* 5, 175, 1984.
101. **Mehendale, H. M.,** Potentiation of halomethane hepatotoxicity: chlordecone and carbon tetrachloride, *Fundam. Appl. Toxicol.,* 4, 295, 1984.
102. **Perucca, E. and Richens, A.,** Drug interactions with phenytoin, *Drugs,* 21, 120, 1981.
103. **Neal, R. A., Sawahata, T., Halpert, J., and Kamataki, T.,** Chemically reactive metabolites as suicide enzyme inhibitors, *Drug. Metab. Rev.,* 14, 49, 1983.
104. **Glushkov, V. M., Sanotskij, I. V., Antomonov, Yu. G., and Kotova, A. B.,** Response to repeated chemical exposures, Institute of Cybernetics, Kiev, 1978.
105. **Lyublina, E. I., Minkina, N. A., and Rylova, M. L.,** Adaptation to industrial poisons as a phase of intoxication, *Leningrad Meditsina,* 1971.
106. **Costa, L. G. and Murphy, S. D.,** Unidirectional cross-tolerance between the carbmate insecticide, Propoxur and the organophosphate disulfoton in mice, *Fundam. Appl. Toxicol.,* 3, 483, 1983.
107. **Brown, A. W. and Pal, R.,** *Insecticide Resistance in Arthropods,* 2nd ed., WHO, Geneva, 1971.
108. **Wilkinson, C. F. and Denison, M. S.,** Pesticide interactions with biotransformation systems, in *Effects of Chronic Exposures to Pesticides on Animal Systems,* Chambers, J. E. and Yarbrough, J. D., Eds., Raven Press, New York, 1982, 1.

109. **Blumberg, W. E.,** Enzymic modification of environmental intoxicants: the role of cytochrome p-450, *Q. Rev. Biophys.,* 11, 481, 1978.
110. **Ullrich, V., Roots, I., Hildebrandt, A., Estabrook, R. W., and Conney, A. H.,** Eds., *Microsomes and Drug Oxidations,* Pergamon Press, New York, 1977.
111. **Popov, T. and Zadorohnaya, T.,** Cadence of hepatocyte structure and function changes in exposure to pesticides, *Bull. Exp. Biol. Med.,* 83, 273, 1977.
112. **Popov, T.,** A unit for perfusion of rat liver in situ, *Bull. Exp. Biol. Med.,* 81, 122, 1975.
113. **Hestrin, S.,** The reaction of acetylcholine and other carboxylic acid derivatives with hydroxylamine and its biological application, *J. Biol. Chem.,* 180, 249, 1949.

Chapter 3

METABOLISM AND TOXICOKINETICS OF PESTICIDES IN ANIMALS

G. Carrera and A. Periquet

TABLE OF CONTENTS

I. INTRODUCTION

When a pesticide enters the animal body through ingestion, inhalation, or dermal absorption it is subjected to body metabolism by a variety of mechanisms. There are several chemical or biochemical transformations that a pesticide may undergo in the animal. The majority of the pesticides are essentially lipophilic in nature and contain certain functional groups which undergo well-recognized biochemical reactions. These reactions lead to compounds that are more polar than the parent molecule and hence more easily excreted from the body. In fact, most metabolic transformations of pesticides are detoxification processes.

The metabolic transformation of pesticides also leads to the formation of more active compounds, for example, as in the case of parathion to paraoxon.

The bioalteration reactions related to pesticides may be categorized as (a) phase I metabolism (biotransformation) and (b) phase II metabolism (conjugation). The phase I metabolism involves a large number of chemical reactions such as hydrolysis, hydroxylation, isomerization, oxidation, epoxidation, dehydrohalogenation, dehalogenation, desulfuration, reduction, and nitrosation. Phase II metabolism or conjugation consists of synthesis reactions in which an endogenous molecule combines with the pesticide or more often with one of its metabolites leading to the formation of a more polar molecular which is easily excreted. Phase II metabolism involves thus, the formation of conjugates through glycoside formation, sulfo conjugation, glutathione conjugation, amino acid conjugation, acetylation, and methylation. The conjugated metabolites are, in fact, the derivatives of the pesticide which have reacted with a natural component of the animal to form a new material. This kind of reaction generally involves the formation of a free metabolite which in the second step converts into a conjugate. Many activities of phase I and phase II enzymes in various organs, tissues, and subcellular fractions are shown in Tables 1 and 2. The ability to metabolize pesticides

TABLE 1

Metabolic Activities of Some Enzymes in Various Rat Organs and Tissues

Organs	Epoxide hydrase[a]	Aromatic hydroxylase[b]	UDPG transferase[c]
Liver	138	2	36
Kidneys	21	0.02	77
Lungs	5	0.02	40
Intestine	5	0.006	—
Skin	5	0.006	—

[a] nmol of styrene glycol/mg microsomal nitrogen/15 min.
[b] pmol of *p*-amino/phenol/mg fresh tissue/min.
[c] nmol of conjugated 4-methylumbelliferone/mg microsomal proteins/h.

TABLE 2

Subcellular Localisation of Some Enzymes Metabolizing Xenobiotics

Subcellular fractions	Epoxide hydrase[1]	Aromatic hydroxylase[b]	UDPG transferase[d]	GSH epoxide transferase[d]
Nucleous + membrane residues	—	5	—	—
Mitochondria	42	8	—	—
Microsomes	392	84	36	—
Cytosol	13	0	—	224

[a] nmol of styrene glycol/mg microsomal nitrogen/5 min.
[b] pmol of *p*-amino phenol/mg fresh tissue/min.
[c] nmol of conjugated 4-methylumbelliferone/mg microsomal proteins/hr.
[d] nmol of conjugated styrene-oxide/mg microsomal proteins/min.

by species of animals differs both quantitatively and qualitatively and is modulated by several factors. We discuss in this chapter the general pathways of pesticide metabolism and the factors that influence the metabolic pathways.

II. GENERAL PATHWAYS OF PESTICIDE METABOLISM

A. METABOLIC REACTIONS IN PHASE I
Many of phase I microsomal reactions involve cytochrome p-450 monooxygenases also called *mixed function oxydases*; they are constituted of three essential elements, the p-450 cytochrome, the NADPH-cytochrome p-450 reductase, and the phosphatidylcholine. The hydroxylation of the substances by these enzymes takes place according to a six-step catalytic cycle which is now quite well known.[1] Studies in recent years particularly in relation to the purification and characterization of the cytochrome P-450 monooxygenases proved that they exist in a number of forms and the system is much more complex than supposed.[2,3]

Other phase I microsomal reactions do not use the p-450 cytochrome as *catalyzer*. Several studies have shown that the enzymatic system, allowing in particular the N-oxygenation of secondary and tertiary amine and the S-oxygenation of thiols, sulfurs, thioamides, and thiocarbmates, is different from the p-450 cytochrome system and leads mainly to flavine use. An FAD monooxygenase which did not contain hemoprotein and metallic ions (except for traces of zinc) has been isolated, purified, and characterized. The catalytic mechanism still remains uncertain and a pathway chain has been proposed.[4] The other phase I reactions such as oxidations, reductions, dehydroxylations, and hydrolysis are, however, not microsomal although their enzymes are present in mitochondria and cytoplasm.

1. Microsomal Reactions
a. Hydroxylations

These are reactions that take place during the metabolism of several pesticides. The reaction involves an aliphatic carbonate bond, for example, carbaryl which on hydroxylation through the hepatic microsomal system requires NADPH and oxygen.[5] The aliphatic hydroxylation reactions generally occur according to an electrophile reaction mechanism. Studies have shown that the K_m and V_{max} of these reactions do not depend, or little depend, on the carbonate bond substitutes. The hydroxylation reaction speed by cytochrome p-450 is relatively fast as compared with other steps in the oxidation process. The stoichiometry of the aliphatic hydroxylation reactions has been studied in the reconstituted system containing highly purified cytochrome p-450.[6] It is now possible to show that the ratio between used NADPH, oxygen consumption, and oxygenate water production as 1:1:1.

Hydroxylation reaction can occur on an aromatic ring as in the case of lindane or carbaryl. The latter is metabolized by the enzymes of the liver microsomes into 1-naphthyl-N-hydroxymethyl carbamate; 4-hydroxy-1-N-methylcarbamate; 5-hydroxy-1-naphthyl-N-methylcarbamate, and in 5,6-dihydro-5,6-dihydroxy-1-naphthyl-N-methylcarbamate which could be the last formed metabolite.[7,8]

It has been generally seen that the primary amines are hydroxylated by MFO with cytochrome p-450, whereas the secondary amines are by oxidase amines, for example, the N-desalkylation of trifluraline in rats and dogs[9] and the O-desalkylation of the dichlorvos.[10]

b. Hydrolysis

Pesticides which have the ester groups are degraded by chemical or enzymatic hydrolysis with the breakdown of the molecule by the addition of water. For instance, carbaryl is quickly hydrolyzed in animals by esterases yielding carbonic acid which is instantaneously decomposed into carbon dioxide and methyl or dimethyl amine.[8] Organophosphorus insecticides are also hydrolyzed but by different enzymatic processes. The general reactions are summarized in Equation 1 which demonstrates the hydrolysis pathways.

$$(RO)_2\overset{S\,(O)}{\overset{\|}{P}}-X \;+\; H_2O \dashrightarrow (RO)_2\overset{S\,(O)}{\overset{\|}{P}}-OH \;+\; HX \tag{1}$$

$$(RO)_2\overset{S\,(O)}{\overset{\|}{P}}-X \;+\; H_2O \dashrightarrow (RO)(HO)\overset{S\,(O)}{\overset{\|}{P}}-X \;+\; ROH$$

Malathion, for example, can be hydrolyzed in five different sites as shown in Equation 2.

$$(MeO)_2-\overset{S}{\overset{\|}{P}}-S-CH-COO-Et \tag{2}$$
$$\qquad\qquad\qquad\quad |$$
$$\qquad\qquad\qquad CH_2COO-Et$$

The hydrolysis reactions are catalyzed by a large variety of enzymes. The esterase polymorphism was noted in many organs (kidney, liver, brain, testes, and intestine). The nonspecific esterases are detected in rat liver microsomes by immunological techniques which allowed the detection of ten different antigens, and these vary in concentrations depending upon the sex of the animal. Some of them are induced by phenobarbital.[11,12] From paraoxon, metabolized by rat hepatic microsome, p-nitrophenol has been detected due to an esterase A activity and β-naphthol, due to an esterase B activity.[13]

c. Epoxidation

The microsomal enzymes are responsible for the epoxidation of the double bonds present in many cyclodiene insecticides such as heptachlor, aldrin or dieldrin[14] and for example, the *in vivo* epoxidation has been shown in dogs and in rats.[15,16] It was clearly shown that epoxide formation catalyzed by cytochrome p-450 monooxygenase is stereospecific with the intervention of different isoenzymes working with different forms of cytochrome p-450.[17] Even though epoxides are stable compounds, they can undergo hydration reactions as in the case of heptachlor giving a dihydrodiol which later metabolizes and excretes out.[18] These epoxides are very reactive to biological macromolecules (proteins and nucleic acids) and are often more toxic than the parent compounds. For instance, heptachlor, aldrin, and isodrin are respectively epoxidized into dieldrin and endrin.[19]

d. Desulfuration

The desulfuration is a classic metabolic pathway of organophosphorus pesticide containing a phosphorothioic moiety. This reaction in animals often leads to a more reactive and toxic compound than the initial substance. The desulfuration of malathion into malaoxon and of parathion into paraoxon are good examples of these types of reactions.[20—22] In fact, the *in vitro* studies with reconstituted system revealed the important steps of parathion metabolism by hepatic microsomes. The parathion cytochrome p-450 bond (sulfur atom) may be due to cystein residue and the presence of cytochrome p-450 antibody can prevent this bond.[23]

e. Dehydrohalogenation and Deshalogenation

The most common example of this type of reaction in animals is the enzymatic conversion of DDT into DDE. DDT can also undergo a reductive dechlorination and yield DDD.[24] The metabolic conversion of DDT in animals can follow two pathways. One of them goes through the conversion of *p,p'*-DDT to *p,p'*-DDE, the other consists in an oxidation of the aliphatic part of *p,p'*-DDT to form *p,p'*-DDA, which is the major excretion product in many animals. Generally, vertebrates produce both *p,p'*-DDE and *p,p'*-DDD from *p,p'*-DDT.[25] Another example of the removal of a halogen from a pesticide molecule is the reductive debromination of the 3,4,5-tribromo-N-N-α-trimethyl 1-H-pyrazole-1-acetamide which is the major metabolic pathway in rats.[26]

f. Oxidoreductions

Several oxidation reactions such as the epoxidation and hydroxylation have already been mentioned. A particular example of oxidation dealing in the metabolism of pesticides containing an R-S-R group has been reported by March et al.[27] For example, compounds like demeton are oxidized to sulfoxide and then sulfone, and these metabolites can significantly contribute to the biological activity of the compound. The sulfoxidation is an important metabolic pathway of a carbamate insecticide like aldicarb.[8]

g. Isomerizations

This type of reaction in relation to pesticides, though seldom seen in animals, has shown in rats, an isomerization reaction during the metabolism of methomyl *in vivo*.[28] Methomyl exists in two geometrical configurations, though one of them is more stable than the other. In fact, the transformation to the labile isomer is necessary before the metabolism into acetonitrile and carbon dioxide.

h. Nitrosations

Certain pesticides which contain a nitrogen group react with nitrites to form N-nitrosocompounds, many of which have mutagenic properties.[29] This reaction is a purely chemical synthesis (nonenzymatic), strongly dependent on pH and strong acidity conditions. For example, herbicides such as atrazine or triazines can be transformed into nitrosaminated compounds in such conditions.[30] Nitrosamines can also be formed from the dithiocarbamate fungicides such as ziram, ferbam, and thiram.[31] Similarly the carbamates and substituted ureas more easily react with the nitrites to yield nitrosamines. For instance, many N-methyl-carbamate pesticides are nitrosed and the resulting compounds have mutagenic and carcinogenic potentialities in experimental animals.[32-35]

2. Nonmicrosomal Reactions

Several oxidases and dehydrogenases present in mitochondria and cytoplasm catalyze the oxidation of xenobiotics but examples concerning pesticides are rare in literature. Oxidation of tyramine which is a degradation product of tyrosine is generally mentioned as an example. Nonmicrosomal hydrolases are relevant to the metabolism of ester and amide xenobiotics and of certain phosphorodithioate pesticides such as parathion and dimethoate.[36]

B. PHASE II METABOLIC REACTIONS

Metabolic conjugations involving pesticides have been studied in detail.[37-40] It has been shown that pesticides which after having undergone phase I reactions possess -OH, COOH, -NH$_2$, NHOH, or SH groups can be conjugated with endogen compounds.[41,42] In animals, the most important endogen compounds are glucuronic acid, sulfate, glutathione, and amino acids. During phase II reactions, the xenobiotics or more frequently its metabolites are transferred to coenzymes of the intermediate metabolism but the enzymes which catalyze this transfer are specific. These coenzymes may be classified into four groups:

1. Uridine diphosphate coenzymes (conjugation with glucuronic acid)
2. Adenosine coenzymes (sulfoconjugation, phosphoric acid ester formation, methylation)
3. Coenzyme A (acetylation, glycine conjugation)
4. Glutathione

1. Glucuronic Acid Conjugations

This is the most frequent conjugation mechanism. It concerns the compounds having alcohol, phenol, carboxylic, thiol, and amine functions. The formation of glucuronoconjugated compound is carried out in two steps:

Step 1. Biosynthesis of coenzyme UDPGA:

$$GIP + UTP \xrightarrow{\text{uridyltransferase}} UDPG + P^2O_7^4$$

$$UDPG + 2NAD \xrightarrow{\text{UDP deshydrogenase}} UDPGA + 2\ NADH_2$$

(3)

Step 2. Transfer by a UDP glucuronyl transferase of the glucuronyl radical to the aglycone.

$$UDPGA + ROH \xrightarrow{\hspace{3cm}} R-OC_6H_9O_6 + UDP \qquad (4)$$

Glucuroconjugation can occur on O- or N-atoms. O-glucuronidation occurs for example in the metabolism of carbaryl, DDT, propham, and ferbam[43-45] while N-glucuronidation occurs in the metabolism of carbofuran, mobam, and meobal.[46]

2. Sulfoconjugation

Several pesticides (with alcohol, phenol, or amine functions) can be transformed into the corresponding sulfates under the action of sulfotransferase. These reactions are fairly common in animals and take place in two steps. The endogenous donor of the group is 3'-phosphoadenosine-5' phosphosulfate (PAPS), which is an activated form of sulfate.

Step 1. PAPS synthesis:

$$ATP + SO_4^{2-} \xrightarrow[\substack{ATP\ Sulfate \\ Adenylytransferase}]{} APS + P_2O_7^{4-}$$

$$APS + ATP \xrightarrow[\substack{ATP-Adenylyl\ Sulfate \\ -3'\ phosphotransferase}]{} PAPS + ADP$$

(5)

Step 2. Transfer by a sulfotransferase of the hydroxylated xenobiotics on the active sulfate.

$$PAPS + R - OH \longrightarrow R - OSO_3H + PAP \quad (6)$$

3. Methylation

Methylation is a relatively minor pathway in the metabolism of a xenobiotic. However, organophosphate insecticides containing a thiolate ester bond can be biochemically disrupted and this may yield S-methylated metabolites. For example, methidalthion quickly disrupts in rats giving 4-methylsulfinylmethyl and 4-methylsulfonylmethyl derivatives.[47] Phosalone as well as menazon also gives the same metabolites in rats where the degradation route was obvious.[48,49] The methylated metabolites have no anticholinesterasic activity and are 15 to 50 times less toxic than original insecticides.[50]

Fonofos (Dyfonate) used for soil treatment also undergoes similar biotransformation: the thiophenol moiety released by the oxidative P-S cleavage of fonofos or by the hydrolysis of the oxon, is rapidly methylated and subsequently oxidized to sulfoxide and sulfone in rats.[51-53]

4. Acetylation

The aromatic amines and the sulfonamides are acetylated in the presence of acetyl coenzyme A according to Equation 7:

$$CH_3CO - S - CoA + R - NH_2 \xrightarrow{Acylase} RNHCOCH_3 + CoASH \quad (7)$$

Acetylation is mainly a reaction against foreign amines and is a simple modification of normal reaction processes, for example, conversion of choline to acetylcholine and acetylation of the -SH group of coenzyme A. Acetylation of foreign amines is usually regarded as a general reaction of aromatic amines and some unnatural aromatic acids such as α-amino-α-phenylbutyric acid and phenylcysteine. There are isolated examples of acetylation of other amino groups. It has been reported that the possible existence of additional forms of metabolic acetylation of foreign compounds should be considered since *active formyl* groups and acyl esters of coenzyme A other than acetyl have been detected in the tissues.[54] In fact, Asulam (methyl-4-aminobenzenesulfonyl carbamate) an herbicide, has been identified in the urine of rats as N-acetylasulam and N-acetylsulfanilamide.[35]

5. Amino Acid Conjugation

Those pesticides which contain an aromatic carboxylic acid group can be conjugated after activation by the coenzyme A with certain amino acids and in particular glycine (Equation 8):

$$CoA - SH + RCO - S - CoA + H_2O \longrightarrow RCO - S - CoA +$$
$$H_2NCH_2COOH \longrightarrow RCONHCH_2COOH + CoA - SH$$

(8)

Isoxathion (karphos) an organophosphorus insecticide has been shown to conjugate with glycine to form hippuric acid.[56] Similarly, taurine conjugation occurs in the metabolism of cypermethrin which is the cyano analog of permethrin. This α-cyano-3-phenoxybenzyl ester is metabolized *in vivo* to 3-phenoxybenzoic acid. The major urinary metabolite of both cypermethrin and 3-phenoxybenzoic acid in mice has been identified as 3-phenoxyben-zoyltaurine.

6. Glutathione Conjugation

Glutathione is closely involved in the metabolism of xenobiotics. In fact, aliphatic or aromatic pesticides can be conjugated with glutathione yielding S-alkyl and S-aryl cysteine and then mercapturic acids. These reactions are catalyzed by glutathione transferases which are localized in the soluble fraction of the cell.

The general scheme of the reaction is represented in Equations 9 to 12; more information regarding conjugations with glutathione is discussed by Hutson.[57]

$$RX + GSH \xrightarrow{GSH-S-transferase} RSG + HX \tag{9}$$

$$RSG \xrightarrow{\gamma-glutamyltransferase} R-CyS-Gly + Glutamate \tag{10}$$

$$R-CyS-Gly \xrightarrow{Peptidase} R-SCH_2CHCOOH + Glycine \atop NH_2 \tag{11}$$

$$R-SCH_2CHCOOH + acetyl-CoA \xrightarrow{Transferase} R-SCH_2CHCOOH + CoA \atop NH_2 \quad NHCOCH_3 \tag{12}$$

The organophosphate triester insecticides, the S-triazine herbicides, the thiocarbamate fungicides, as well as the diphenyl ethers and the organothiocyanates are good substrates for glutathione-S-transferases.[58] Diazinon is degraded in rat into diethyl phosphorothioic acid and S-(2-isopropyl-4-methyl-6-pyrimidinyl) glutathione.[59,60]

C. FACTORS INFLUENCING THE METABOLIC REACTIONS

Many factors are known to influence the activity of phase I and phase II enzyme reactions in animals. These could be due to intrinsic factors such as species, sex, age, pathological and hormonal state, pregnancy, circadian rhythms which are independent of pesticide exposure, or due to extrinsic factors which depend on exposure to the pesticide.[61] In fact, these factors play a significant role and modulate the toxicity of pesticides in animals. In other words they influence on every level of toxicokinetics: absorption, distribution, metabolism, and elimination (ADME) of the pesticide. Information on the interaction of pesticides is inadequate.[62]

1. Intrinsic Factors
a. Species and Strain

It has been demonstrated in the previous pages how enzymes of phase I and phase II have different activities in species of animals. The basal values of hepatic microsomal activities and their response to induction suggest differences in species and strains of animals.[63-65] Furthermore, the ethnic differences in man have shown differential storage of pesticides.[66,67]

b. Age

Age and size of an animal apparently are the most important factors which influence susceptibility. For example, a comparison of the toxicity of 16 anticholinergic insecticides in young and adult rats demonstrated susceptibility of the young rat over the adult one.[68] Carbophenothion is five times more toxic for young than for the adult rat while mevinphos, trichlorfon, and carbaryl are twice as toxic. However, the toxicity of malathion, DDT, and dieldrin is more for the adult rat followed by the 2-week-old rat and the newborn one respectively.[69] The variation in the metabolic activities of the enzymes before and after birth, as well as the glucoroconjugation and the sulfoconjugation activities[70,71] seems to explain the susceptibility of animals to pesticide-induced toxicity.

c. Sex
The activities of hepatic microsomal enzymes are highly dependent on sex; they are generally higher in the male than in the female of the immature animal.[72] *In vivo* and *in vitro* studies have shown increased metabolism of azinphospmethyl in the male than in the female animal.[73] Another example is parathion which causes greater toxicity to female rat as compared to male. The decreased susceptibility of the male rat to parathion is related to the increased activity of the hepatic cytochrome p-450 monooxygenase enzyme system which metabolizes parathion to nontoxic metabolites. This enzyme system in male rat seems to be androgen dependent.

d. Nutrition
Information is now available to show that state of nutrition alters the toxicity of xenobiotics in animals.[74-77] It has been shown that altered levels of protein, lipid, and vitamins in the diet significantly influence the toxicity of a pesticide.[78,79] Ascorbic acid-deficient diet, for example, impaired both the induction of O-demethylase and the stimulation of the glucuronic acid system by DDT.[80]

2. Extrinsic Factors
The extrinsic factors associated with the pesticide toxicity can be listed as follows: the physico-chemical properties of the pesticide, route of exposure, vehicle used, concentration of the pesticide, and environmental conditions like temperature and humidity etc. which normally alter the rate of absorption of the compound. For instance, parathion causes greater toxicity at 38°C than at 25°C to experimental animals, while sarin and DDT become more toxic under hypothermic conditions.[81,82]

Several pesticides are more toxic by oral administration than by dermal route, for example, lindane, mirex, malathion, phosphamidon. These pesticides have a lower LD_{50} value by the oral route than through the dermal route.[83] Different solvents are used as vehicles to deliver the pesticide either in the form of a spray or emulsion concentrate. Dipterex, for instance, is more toxic with sesame oil as a vehicle than either with water or dimethyl sulfoxide or with water plus emulsifier.[84]

Toxicity of a pesticide is significantly modulated by interaction between pesticides and other chemical compounds. For example, combinations of organophosphorus compounds like malathion + EPN, or malathion + TOCP show a varied degree of potentiation.[85,86] The mechanism seems to lie in the interference of one compound with the process of detoxification of the other.

III. METABOLISM OF SELECTED PESTICIDES

A. ORGANOCHLORINE INSECTICIDES
The organochlorine insecticides are lipid soluble compounds, generally highly chlorinated, with a slow rate of metabolism which frequently leads to bioaccumulation.

1. DDT

In spite of extensive literature on the metabolism of DDT many aspects of phase I and II metabolism remain unknown. It was argued whether or not the conversion of DDT to DDD is due to intestinal flora or due to the enzymatic system localized in the animal tissues. Ottoboni and Ferguson[87] have shown that rats exposed to DDT accumulated DDD in liver lipids at concentrations greater than those in the general body fat. Further they showed that axenic and normal rats feeding on DDT accumulate the same levels of TDE,[88] which indicates that the contribution of intestinal microflora is negligible.

The capacity of transforming DDT to DDD seems to be variable for different species.[89] In this way, the metabolism of DDT in rats would lead first to DDD and after dechlorination to DDMU (1-chloro-2,2-*bis*(p-chlorophenyl)ethylene) which is then transformed into DDMS (1-chloro-2,2-*bis*(p-chlorophenyl)ethane). DDMS yields excreted DDA (*bis*(p-chlorophenyl)acetic acid) via DDOH (2,2 *bis*(p-chlorophenyl) — ethanol). However, Datta et al. suggest that DDT is metabolized into DDD and DDE and then to DDMU in rat and finally is excreted in the form of DDA.[90,91] Liver, kidney, and brain of female rat dosed chronically with DDT has been shown to contain the same level of DDT. Liver is the only tissue which stores more DDD than DDT and the concentration of DDD in this organ is higher than that of DDE while the opposite is observed in all other tissues.[92,93] Similarly, it has been shown that in newborns of a mother dosed with ^{14}C-DDT, the DDT concentration in the liver decreased by 60% in 28 days while that of DDD and DDE simultaneously increased by 36 and 22% respectively which corresponds to the hepatic metabolism of DDT.[94] In rats dosed for 4 months with DDT, the level of DDT and its metabolites in liver, kidney, brain, and blood decreased in the following order: DDA>DDT>DDD>DDE. In fat tissue, the level of DDD decreased more rapidly than that of DDT and DDE.[95]

The reductive systems which dechlorinate DDT into DDD were studied extensively in rat liver.[96] Two independent systems, one requiring cytochrome p-450 and the other FAD are postulated. In the first system, DDT seems to bind directly with the reduced cytochrome p-450. The electron is transferred from NADPH to the reduced p-450-substrate complex *via* NADPH reductase. Because of the rapid turnover of the system it has been indicated that the last electron transfer to the substrate releases the reduced cytochrome which can react again with the substrate. This system does not involve any form of oxidized p-450 because sesamex and piperonyl butoxide have no inhibitory effects. The second system requiring FAD, is identical to the flavoprotein-flavin cofactor system.[97] It is heat stable and affected by pH changes. It has been shown that ^{14}C-DDT, incubated with rat hepatic microsomes and NADPH produces reactive intermediates which covalently bind to microsomal proteins and lipids.[98] DDD is rapidly formed from DDT under anaerobic conditions, but when DDD is used as a substrate, binding to microsomal proteins occurs only in the presence of oxygen. Sodium dithionate, added to microsomes produced ^{14}C-DDT phospholipid and protein binding and DDD formation, but failed to support DDD metabolism or binding. In fact, the reductive formation of a DDT free-radical intermediate leads to the formation of DDD which binds preferentially to microsomal lipids.

Earlier studies have shown metabolites of DDT in the feces, bile and urine of rats as amino acid conjugated compounds.[99-101] These conjugated DDA compounds, in feces, could represent about 30% of the initial administered dose of DDT.[102] DDT and DDD could be hydroxylated in rats with a hydroxylation preferentially on the 3 and 4 carbon on the ring.[103,104]

Rat feces shows the presence of DDD, DDE, and a form of DDA conjugated with aspartic acid. In rat feces dosed with *p,p'*-DDE, 1,1-dichloro-2-(4-chloro-3-hydroxyphenyl)-2-(4-chlorophenyl)-ethylene (I) and three other metabolites in smaller quantities: the 1,1-dichloro-2-(3-chloro-4-hydroxyphenyl)-2-(4-chlorophenyl)-ethylene (II), and 1,1-dichloro-2-(4-chloro-2-hydroxyphenyl)-2-(4 chlorophenyl)-ethylene (III) and the 1,1-dichloro-2-(4-

hydroxyphenyl-2-(4-chlorophenyl)-ethylene (IV) have been detected. The structure of metabolites I, III, and IV suggests the initial formation of an arene oxide in the metabolic process.[105] Kujawa et al. have shown that, in rats, DDT is transformed into DDD by reductive dechlorination in the liver 30 min after oral administration and that 6 h after administration of 10 mg of DDT to a rat, 60 mg of DDD/kg body weight is found in the liver.[106] After the administration of DDD to rats the dechlorination product DDMU is detected in organs only after short exposures, but permanently in the feces.[107]

Depending upon the compound administered either as DDT or DDD, the urine of female mouse shows different metabolites. For example, after DDT the metabolites identified are DDD, DDMU, DDE, DDA, α-OH-DDA (2-hydroxy-2,2,bis (*p*-chlorophenyl) acetic acid) and DDOH, while after the DDD administration the metabolites are DDMU, DDE, DDA, alpha OH-DDA and DDOH. According to these results, hydroxylation of DDD would give 2,2-*bis*(*p*-chlorophenyl) acetyl chloride which in turn is hydrolyzed to give DDA. The excretion of α-OH-DDA may arise from the initial expoxidation of DDMU to yield 1,2-epoxy-1-chloro-2,2-*bis* (*p*-chlorophenyl)ethane. This chloroepoxide is then hydrolyzed and oxidized to produce the α-OH-DDA.[108]

In mice and hamsters given DDT, 80% of the urinary metabolites detected is recovered as DDA glucuronic acid. Conjugates of DDA with glycine, alanine, and serine are also detected. In mice dosed with DDT, the following compounds, expressed in percent of the administered dose are found in urine: DDT unchanged (0.5%), DDE (0.8%), DDD (0.3%), DBP(*bis*(*p*-chlorophenyl)-benzophenone), (0.1%), DDOH (0.3%) and DDA (0.1%). In hamsters, the metabolites are identical to those of mice but DDE is not detected in urine.[109,110]

Metabolism of DDT, DDD, and DDMU has been studied in female hamsters. The principal metabolites of both DDT and DDD is DDA. DDT and DDD treated animals also excreted small amounts of DDD, DDMU, and DDOH. DDMU is metabolized to significant amounts of DDA, DDOH, α-OH-DDA (2-hydroxy-2,2-*bis*-(*p*-chlorophenyl)acetic acid), 2,2-*bis*-(*p*-chlorophenyl)acetaldehyde and 1,1-*bis*-(chlorophenyl)ethan-1,2-diol. These results have indicated that the metabolic disposition of DDT in the hamster is very similar to that observed in the mouse except that the hamster is not as efficient as the mouse in converting DDT to DDE.[111]

Comparative studies have shown that the rat excretes DDT, DDD and DDE faster than the Japanese quail; DDMU is excreted relatively rapidly and at the same rate in these two species. This suggests that the apparent differences in the rate of excretion of DDT by birds and mammals arise from differences in the conversion of DDT to DDD and DDE or, in the degradation of DDD and DDE to DDMU. The Japanese quails excrete more unchanged DDT, DDD, and DDE than rats. These results reflect the inability of the Japanese quail to metabolize these compounds.[112] The slow degradation of DDE may be responsible for the high amount of DDT recovered as DDE in tissue of Japanese quail and other birds.

In pig, the metabolic conversion of *p,p'*-DDT seems to follow two routes. The first involves the oxidation of the aliphatic part of the molecule to *p,p'*-DDA which is excreted free or conjugated without further modifications. The second is the conversion of *p,p'*-DDT to *p,p'*-DDE which is then excreted in the urine as such or as 3-hydroxy-*p,p'*-DDE.[113]

DDT is essentially observed in the intestine even though a certain absorption takes place in the stomach.[114] It is transported in the organism bound to serum protein in the form of a relatively stable complex.[115] DDT accumulates in body fat in variable quantities depending on the degree of exposure and age.[116,117] Its biological halflife is about 1 month in dog,[118] 2 months in poultry[119] and rat,[120] 3 months in monkey,[121] and 26 months in man.[122]

2. Methoxychlor

Methoxychlor is a structural analog of DDT and is not accumulated in fatty tissue or excreted in milk. The accumulation and elimination of methoxychlor and DDT are significantly different in sheep and in mice. The biological halflife of methoxychlor in sheep is about 10 days, while it is 90 days for DDT, 26 days for DDD, and 223 days for DDE. In mice, after administration of a single dose, 1% of administered DDT is eliminated in 24 h while 98% of methoxychlor is eliminated during the same period of time. In mice, five metabolites of methoxychlor have been isolated in urine and feces.[123,124]

In goats, 17 metabolites of methoxychlor have been isolated from urine and feces.[125] Of these, seven of the metabolites are identified as glucuronide compounds. In contrast, no methoxychlor is detected in the urine of rat because it is preferentially excreted in feces. In fact, in rat, methoxychlor undergoes a hepatic microsomal monoxygenase-mediated activation and the resulting reactive metabolite binds covalently to microsomal components.[126]

3. Aldrin and Dieldrin

Several studies have shown that aldrin is metabolized into its epoxide, the dieldrin in animals and man. This oxidative biotransformation has been used as an assay for hepatic monooxygenase.[127-129] When ^{14}C-aldrin is administered to rats aldrin, dieldrin, and a mixture of metabolites are detected in the feces and in the urine.[130] Rats dosed with ^{14}C-dieldrin, show the presence of dieldrin, syn-12-hydroxy-dieldrin, and trans-4,5-dihydroxy-dihydroaldrin in free and conjugated form in the urine and the feces. In rats, a fraction of dieldrin, as aldrin, is metabolized to dihydrochlordene dicarboxylic acid which is further metabolized to the dimethyl ester and possibly conjugated to amino acids. In rabbits, studies have shown that this animal does not form the acid compounds but can directly excrete the thiol derivative in free or conjugated form.[131] In mice even though the metabolic rate is lower than in rats, the metabolites formed are qualitatively identical. Quantitatively, rat excretes higher amounts of pentachloroketone while larger quantities of more polar metabolites, possibly conjugated, are excreted in urine by the mouse.[132]

In rabbit, on the contrary, six different metabolites are identified in urine, the 6,7-trans-dihydroxydihydroaldrin being the main one.[133]

The toxicokinetics of dieldrin in rat has been studied by Robinson et al.[134] Empirical relationships containing one exponential term in the case of adipose tissue and brain and two exponential terms in the case of blood and liver have been fitted to the results. The halflives of dieldrin in liver were estimated to be 1.3 days for the rapid elimination period and 10.2 days for the slower elimination period. Similar values were estimated for blood. The stimulated halflife for adipose tissue and brain were 10.3 and 3 days, respectively. Storage of dieldrin is more important in adipose tissue than in liver, brain, and blood. The authors observed that elimination of dieldrin from rat may be simulated by a two compartment model.

Sunlight influences aldrin and dieldrin to undergo decomposition into photodieldrin. In rats, photodieldrin is metabolized into pentachloroketone as dieldrin.[135] In Rhesus male monkey, after i.v. administration of ^{14}C-photodieldrin, 45% of the compound is excreted by the animal in 21 days and about two thirds of the excreted radioactivity is detected in urine. The body distribution of the compound shows the highest concentration of photodieldrin and/or metabolites in adipose tissue, liver, and bone marrow. The major metabolite is trans-photoaldrindiol which appears in the urine as glucuronic conjugate and as a free metabolite. Chlorohydroxy-substituted derivative of photodieldrin appears in feces and urine.[136]

4. Isodrin and Endrin

Isodrin is oxidized metabolically to endrin.[137] In rats, the major metabolites of endrin are 12 hydroxyendrin and 12-ketoendrin. The former (hydroxyendrin) is excreted as glucuronide in bile and as 12-hydroxyendrin sulfate in urine.[138] In cows, the metabolic pathways of endrin are similar to those in rats and rabbits. The major metabolite is 12-hydroxyendrin which is found in urine in nonconjugated form. The minor metabolites are 12-hydroxyendrin, 3-hydroxyendrin, and 12-ketoendrin.[139] In rabbit, 12-hydroxyendrin is the major metabolite excreted as sulfate conjugate in urine.[140]

5. Toxaphene

Toxaphene is a very complex mixture of more than 100 polychlorobornane compounds containing 5 to 11 chlorine atoms. In rats, toxaphene components are metabolized via dechlorination and excreted in urine and feces in almost identical proportions. Toxicants A and B are also metabolized to several dechlorination and/or dehydrochlorination products by rats, with reduced cytochrome p-450 acting as the reducing agents.[141-143] In vitro metabolism of toxicants B (2,2,5-endo, 6-exo, 8,9,10-heptachlorobornane) and toxicant C (2-endo, 3,3,5,6-exo, 8,9,10,10-monochlorobornane) by rat liver fraction has shown that no hydroxy metabolite of toxicant B is formed and that toxicant C is metabolized in a dechlorinated product and five hydroxy compounds.[144] The urinary, fecal, and total excretions of ^{14}C toxaphene and two isolated toxaphene fractions (polar fraction 7 and nonpolar fraction 2) are respectively 22.5, 35.7, and 58.2% of the administered dose. The total excretion of fraction 2 is 69.4% while that of the fraction 7 is 65%. In rats, fat seems to contain maximum amount of toxaphene.[145,146]

The distribution of toxaphene has been studied in female mice intravenously injected with ^{14}C-toxaphene. Autoradiographic studies show the compound is initially accumulated in the liver, fat, brain, and kidney, and later a gradual redistribution of the radioactivity occurs in the white fat within 4 h after injection. The depletion in the radioactivity was rapid and only low amounts of the labeled product were present in the adipose tissue after 32 days. In the fetus, in contrast, only liver and adrenals show a distinct labeling. A specific and persistent accumulation of the radioactivity is detected in the adrenal cortex suggesting a possible interference of toxaphene with adrenal steroid hormone synthesis.[146,147]

In dairy cows and buffalo, excretion of toxaphene is rapid through milk and liver; in fact, the residues are logarithmically different after an oral administration of the compound.[149,150]

6. Mirex-Kepone

Mirex is not metabolized in rats. About 58% of the administered dose is recovered as parent compound in the feces, 27.8% in the fat, 3.2% in the muscle, and 1.75% in the liver. Excretion of mirex occurs following a biphasic process with half lives of 38 h and 100 days respectively. Even though mirex is quickly absorbed by liver cell, it is not metabolized by subcellular fractions of rat, mouse, and rabbit liver.[151,152] In fish, the halflife of mirex was greater than 28 days and no degradation products were detected. In the Rhesus monkey, Wiener et al. have shown that 338 days after a single dose of ^{14}C-mirex, less than 0.6% is present in the urine and 7% in the fat itself.[153,154] Similar accumulation of mirex in the fat of the squirrel monkeys has been observed after the administration of photomirex.[155]

Although the conversion of mirex to kepone occurs in soil medium, it has not been reported in animals.[156] In rat, receiving a single dose of ^{14}C-kepone, the highest level of radioactivity declined in all tissues, but increased considerably in liver. The halflives in blood were 8.5 days for the first 4 weeks, 24 days for the next 8 weeks, and 45 days for the final 14 weeks. By 84 days, 65.5% of the administered dose of mirex is excreted in the feces and only 1.6% in urine. This indicates that kepone is well-absorbed and distributed throughout the body; it has a long halflife and disappears more slowly from the liver than from other tissues.[157] The preferential binding of kepone with albumin and HDL seems to explain this unusual tissue distribution. This is in contrast to aldrin which binds preferentially to VLDL and LDL and distributes preferentially to fat tissue.[158,159]

Biotransformation of kepone does not occur in rats, guinea pigs, and hamsters. In pigs, an i.p. injection of kepone resulted in the formation of kepone-alcohol in bile and feces. The reduction and conjugation of kepone in pig are similar to these in man.[160]

7. Endosulfan

In rats, 5 days after a single dose of ^{14}C-endosulfan, 75% of the compound is excreted in feces and 13% in the urine. However, when endosulfan is administered in the diet, 56% of the compound is excreted in the feces and 8% in the urine. Furthermore, after a single oral dose, 47% of the endosulfan is eliminated from the liver via the bile but no enterohepatic circulation is demonstrated. In the excreta and/or tissues, the apolar metabolites identified are sulfate, diol, alpha-hydroxyether, lactone and ether derivatives of endosulfan.[161] In rats, orally exposed to endosulfan for 60 days, the concentration of alpha isomer was the highest in kidney, followed by lung, spleen, testes, and brain; the concentration of beta isomer was more than that of the alpha isomer.[162,163]

8. Chlordane

Administration of [14]C *trans*-chlordane intravenously to rats showed excretion of the compound (29% of the total radioactivity) in the feces and in the urine.[164] The major pathway of the metabolism of *cis*- and *trans*-chlordane is its conversion into oxychlordane probably via the 1,2-dichlorochlordene oxychlordane. Oxychlordane is later metabolized into 1-hydroxy-2-chlorochlordene and into its epoxide: 1-hydroxy-2-chloro-2,3-epoxychlordene. The two other minor products of the metabolism of chlordane are identified as heptachlor the product of loss of HCl from *cis*- and *trans*-chlordane and the chlordane chlorohydrin which can give the 1-2-dihydroxydihydrochlordene.[166,167]

The toxicokinetics of chlordane showed differences in species of animals, for instance, the absorption and distribution of ^{14}C chlordane in mice appeared slower than those in rats. A lower peak radioactivity in tissues and a higher rate of fecal elimination of the compound was seen in mice as compared to those in rats.[168]

9. Heptachlor

In rats, heptachlor is metabolized into 1-exo-hydroxychlordene, which gives 1-2-dihydroxydihydrochlordene via an intermediate: 1-exo-hydroxy-2,2,-exo-epoxychlordene. Another pathway is the formation of heptachlor epoxide which is metabolized into a dehydrogenated derivative of 1-hydroxy-2,3-exo-epoxychlordene.[169] The metabolism of heptachlor, however, is drastically modified by certain compounds which induce phase II enzymes reaction.[170,171]

10. Hexachlorocyclohexane (HCH)

Hexachlorocyclohexane is a mixture of seven chemically distinct isomers; and lindane (gamma isomer) is the potent insecticide.

The metabolism of HCH in animals has shown several possibilities. The traditional group observes that gamma HCH first forms gamma-PCCH which undergoes different changes. In contrast, the other group observe that gamma PCCH is not an intermediate and gamma HCH is immediately hydroxylated to yield various chlorophenols such as 2,4,5-trichlorophenol and 2,3,4,6-tetrachlorophenol. The third pathway is the formation of pentachlorocyclohexanols which are excreted as such or further transformed into various chlorophenols via dechlorination, dehydrochlorination, and dehydrogenation.[172-175] The fourth pathway of lindane metabolism is its aromatization into chlorobenzene and benzene.[176,177]

Different metabolites of lindane are excreted in the form of conjugate. Chlorophenols are seen as sulfates or glucuronide conjugates, and chlorocyclohexane (HCH, PCCH, TCCH) are conjugated to glutathione to give mercapturic acids.[178] Several studies have been carreied out on the metabolism of HCH in experimental animals.[179-182] The tissue distribution pattern

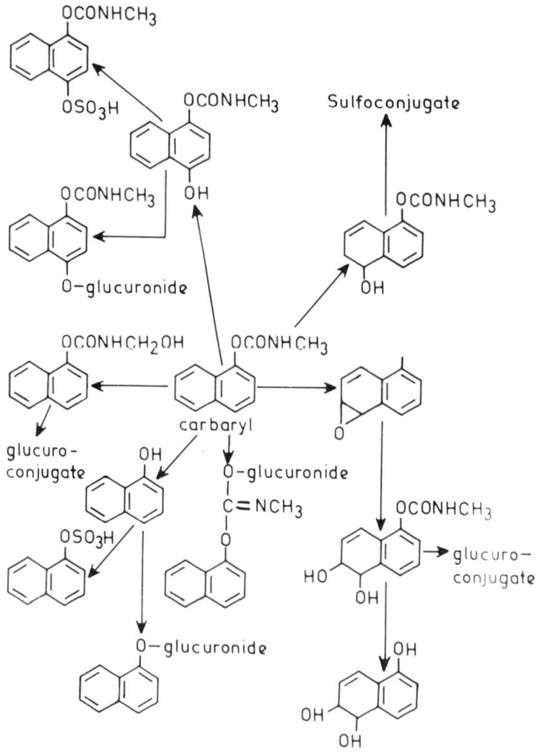

FIGURE 1. Metabolic pathways of carbaryl.[8,191]

of beta and gamma isomers in rats showed significant difference indicating a different metabolic pathway of the two isomers.[183]

B. CARBAMATES

Oxidative degradation through MFO systems appears to be the major metabolic pathway of carbamate pesticides. Ester hydrolysis of carbamate compounds occurs to produce an alcohol or phenolic moiety and a carbamic acid group. The carbamic acid group in the case of methyl-carbamate, is decomposed into carbon dioxide and methylamine while the alcohol or the phenol is conjugated before excretion. Urine is the major medium of excretion of the conjugated metabolites of carbamates in rats and excretion in feces is negligible. Besides, reactions of ester hydrolysis, and alkyl and aryl-hydroxylations are also very common reactions as sulfur oxidations in compounds which contain sulfhydryl groups. The conjugates excreted in animals are often in the form of glucuronide sulfates or glutathione conjugates.

1. Carbaryl

Carbaryl metabolism has been widely studied in different animal species with ^{14}C carbaryl labeled in the ring, or in the methyl or the carbonyl.[184-19] According to these studies, carbaryl is metabolized in two main pathways. The first route, a hydrolytic one, gives 1-naphthol which is quickly eliminated as sulfo- and glucuro-conjugate in urine.[191] The second route, by oxidation on the ring and on the methyl radical leads to the formation of metabolites such as 1-naphthyl-N-hydroxymethylcarbamate, 4-hydroxy-1-naphthyl-*N*-methylcarbamate, 5-hydroxy-1-naphthyl-N-methylcarbamate, and 5,6-dihydro-5,6-dihydroxyl-1-naphthyl-N-methylcarbamate. These compounds are then eliminated in urine in the form of sulfo and glucuro-conjugates. A general scheme of carbaryl metabolism is shown in Figure 1. In addition to glucuronide and sulfate conjugates, glutathione conjugation has been shown in rat and mouse liver preparation although the mercapturic acid was not isolated.[192] The nature of the metabolites in different species such as sheep, guinea pig, monkey, and man are identical to that in rat.[186,193]

Many studies have shown that carbaryl accumulates in tissues of pregnant rats and mice[194-196] and is excreted in milk.[197] A comparison of excretion and distribution of carbaryl in pregnant, nonpregnant, and fetal tissues has been made with ring ^{14}C-carbaryl or carbonyl ^{14}C carbaryl. The results have shown that pregnancy alters the disposition and excretion of carbaryl, which is rapidly distributed in all fetal tissues with highest concentrations in fetal kidney. In fact, 8 h after administration, fetal brain, heart, and lung showed more ^{14}C on a weight basis than the maternal organ. Elimination from the fetus was biphasic. The tissue distribution of radioactivity (carbaryl + metabolites) was biphasic in pregnant and non-pregnant rats. Ring ^{14}C-carbaryl concentrations rapidly declined during the second hour after administration, and after 2 h, the ^{14}C levels declined more slowly. Levels of radioactivity increased in the tissues of treated animal with carbonyl ^{14}C-carbaryl in contrast with animals dosed with ring ^{14}C-carbaryl.[198]

Blood kinetics of carbaryl and the inhibition of plasma acetylcholinesterase have been followed in rats for 24 h after administration of radioactive carbaryl. The kinetics of the radioactivity attributed to unaltered carbaryl is bi-exponential while that of the total ^{14}C activity is tri-exponential. The kinetics are compared with open 2- and 3-compartment models respectively. The exchange rate constant between the various compartments as well as the elimination constant (expressed in h^{-1}) were found to be $K_{12} = 1.93$; $K_{21} = 1.18$, $K_{10} = 2.46$ (2nd compartment model) and $K'_{12} = 18.65$; $K_{21} = 13.9$; and $K'_{13} = 1.14$; $K'_{31} = 0.125$, and $K'_{10} = 0.672$ (3rd compartment model). The 3rd compartment model demonstrated the persistence of radioactivity in the blood which correlated with plasma acetyl-cholinesterase inhibition.

The kinetics of carbaryl is modified by several factors, for example, the nature of the vehicle which alters the digestive absorption of the compound. Blood kinetics of 1-naphthyl-N-methyl (^{14}C) carbamate were determined after an intravenous injection with DMSO and after an intragastric and intraduodenal administration with DMSO, oil, gum tragacanth, and milk. The acetylcholinesterase inhibition and the level of ^{14}C activity were both determined in blood at different intervals of time. The value of the absorption rate constant after intragastric and intraduodenal administration was found to be $0.5 \ h^{-1}$ and $7 \ h^{-1}$ with DMSO, $0.6 \ h^{-1}$ and $0.42 \ h^{-1}$ with oil; $0.13 \ h^{-1}$ and $0.22 \ h^{-1}$ with gum tragacanth, and $0.10 \ h^{-1}$ with milk. The inhibition of acetylcholinesterase was closely related to the absorption rate constants which themselves depended upon the nature of the vehicle employed.[200]

The kinetics of carbaryl are also modified for example, by the experimental hepatic impairment. The blood kinetics of carbaryl were followed after 24 h of oral administration of ^{14}C-carbaryl in control animals and in animals with an altered liver function due to 70% hepatectomy or tranylcypromine treatment. The radioactivity in the blood and, in parallel, cholinesterase inhibition were maintained at a higher level in animals with an altered hepatic function. Tranylcypromine appeared to have a greater effect on blood kinetics and cholin-esterase inhibition than 70% hepatectomy.[201]

2. Tsumacide

Tsumacide (3-methylphenyl-N-methylcarbamate) is metabolized and eliminated essentially in the urine (97% of the dose) and in very small quantities in feces (0.1%) after 24 h in male rats. In females, 70% is excreted in the urine and 4% in the feces. In urine, 3-carboxyphenyl N-methylcarbamate (the major metabolite), 3-hydroxymethylphenyl N-methylcarbamate, and 4-hydroxy-3-methylphenyl N-methylcarbamate are identified in a free or glucuroconjugated form and also 3-methylphenol as a sulfoconjugate. Less than 5% of the tsumacide is metabolized via hydrolysis of the carbamate ester. *In vitro* studies with liver preparations from rabbits, rats, and mice showed metabolism of tsumacide into 3-hydroxymethylphenyl *N*-methylcarbamate and 4-hydroxy-3-methylphenyl N-methylcarbamate.[202,203]

3. Meobal

The metabolism of meobal in rats shows that 92% of the administered dose is recovered in 48 h and 5% in feces, and the untransformed meobal represents less than 3% of the dose. Among metabolites, 3,4-dimethylphenol free, sulfo-, and glucuroconjugates, 3-hydroxymethyl-4-methylphenyl N-methylcarbamate as glucuroconjugate and mainly 4-carboxy meobal have been identified. Other identified metabolites include N-hydroxymethyl analog of 4-carboxymeobal, glucuronide conjugates of 4-hydroxymethyl meobal, and glucuronides of its phenol.[204-206]

4. Banol

Banol is metabolized by rat liver microsomes to 2-chloro-4,5-dimethyl phenyl N-hydroxymethylcarbamate. In vivo studies have shown that rats hydrolyze 52% of banol as indicated by expired ^{14}C carbon dioxide and 35% of the dose is eliminated in urine and 10% in feces. Several studies have shown that urine contained the intact carbamate ester, N-glucuronide of banol and metabolites as sulfate conjugates. Carboxylic acids resulting from oxidation of one or other of the 2-methyl group attached to the phenyl ring and the phenolic acids formed by subsequent cleavage are the major metabolic products with the N-hydroxymethyl-carbamate.[184,207]

5. Propoxur (Baygon, Blattanex)

Propoxur is hydrolyzed in rats by 30% on the basis of the quantity of ^{14}C-carbon dioxide liberated after treatment with radioactive propoxur and 60% of the dose is eliminated in urine.[184] *In vitro* studies show that propoxur is first metabolized to 2-isopropoxyphenyl N-hydroxymethylcarbamate, 2-hydroxyphenyl N-methylcarbamate, and 2-isopropoxy-5-hydroxyphenyl N-methylcarbamate. Distribution, biotransformation, and elimination of propoxur showed that the highest propoxur level was found in the kidney, followed by liver, blood, and brain. A proportional part of 2-isopropoxyphenol (metabolite) in comparison with propoxur was the highest in blood and the lowest in brain. Following an increase of propoxur dosing level, concentrations in kidney and urine elimination of the mother compound is obviously increased.[208]

6. Zectran (Mexacarbamate)

Zectran is essentially metabolized by hydrolysis as shown by 75% of the dose being expired as ^{14}C-carbon dioxide, 17% in urine, and 7% in feces.[184,209] In dog, the only free metabolite identified is 4-dimethylamino-3,5-dimethylphenol, sulfo-, and glucuro-conjugates of the free phenol and conjugates of 2,6-dimethylhydroquinone have also been identified.[210] In vitro studies with the rat liver and human liver enzyme system showed the formation of nine metabolites which contained the carbamate moiety. The major metabolites were 4-dimethylamino-3,5-dimethylphenyl N-hydroxymethylcarbamate and 4-methylamino-3,5-dimethylphenyl N-methylcarbamate. Other metabolites include 4-methylformamido-3,5-dimethyl N-methylcarbamate and 4-amino-3,5-dimethylphenyl N-methylcarbamate.[211-213]

7. Aminocarb (Metacil)

Aminocarb is mainly hydrolyzed in animals. Studies with radiolabeled aminocarb have shown that 70% of the dose is expired as ^{14}C-carbon dioxide, 25% in urine, and only 4% in feces.[184] Studies with rat liver microsome show that aminocarb is metabolized into six products containing the carbamate moiety. The major metabolites are 4-methylamino-3-

methylphenyl N-methylcarbamate, 4-dimethylamino-3-methylphenyl N-hydroxymethylcar-bamate, and 4-amino-3-methylphenyl-N-methylcarbamate.[211-213]

8. Carbofuran (Furadan)

In rats, 45% of carbofuran is hydrolyzed within 48 h as shown by the amount of ^{14}C-carbon dioxide that expires while 38% is eliminated in urine and 4% in feces. The metabolites identified in urine are 2,3-dihydro-2,2-dimethyl-3-hydroxybenzofuranyl-7 N-methylcarba-mate, 2,3,-dihydro-2,2-dimethyl-3-hydroxybenzofuranyl-7 N-hydroxy-methylcarbamate in small quantities, and traces of 2,3-dihydro-2,2-dimethyl-3-ketobenzofuranyl-7 N-methyl car-bamate. Fifty percent of the radioactivity of the urine is as 3-ketophenol, product of the hydrolysis of 2,3-dihydro-2,2-dimethyl-3-ketobenzofuranyl-7 N-methylcarbamate, 21% as carbofuran phenol, 1.5% as 3-hydroxyphenol resulting from the hydrolysis of 2,3-dihydro-2,2-dimethyl-3-hydroxybenzofuranyl-7 N-methylcarbamate, 15% as 3-hydroxycarbofuran, and 4% as the 3-hydroxy-N-hydroxymethyl derivative.[214]

The N-demethylation of carbofuran has been found to be a minor degradative pathway in mice. The major primary metabolites are derived essentially from hydrolytic products such as 3-ketophenol and carbofuran phenol but 3-hydroxycarbofuran is also present as a conjugate.[215] *In vitro* studies with liver microsomes show that carbofuran is metabolized into 3-hydroxycarbofuran, N-hydroxymethyl derivative, 3-hydroxy N-hydroxymethylcar-bofuran, and 3-ketophenol.[214-216] A single intravenous or oral dose of carbofuran caused acetylcholinesterase inhibition in RBC which is correlated with carbofuran plasma concen-trations. Carbofuran showed quick absorption (peak plasma 7 min), distribution and elim-ination ($t_{1/2}$ = 29 min) with 3-hydroxycarbofuran rapidly formed, and is subject to enterohepatic circulation (plasma $t_{1/2}$ = 64 min).[217]

In lactating cows, carbofuran metabolites were detected in milk after an oral treatment of animals. The 3-hydroxycarbofuran, 3-hydroxy N-hydroxymethylcarbofuran, 3-ketocar-bofuran, and nonmetabolized carbofuran were identified as free and/or conjugated metab-olites. Radioactive natural milk components indicated the assimilation of the ^{14}C-carbon dioxide from the hydrolysis of ^{14}C-carbonyl labeled carbofuran.[218]

Biotransformation of N-(2-toluenesulfenyl)carbofuran (2,3-dihydro-2,2-dimethyl-7-ben-zofuranyl N-methyl-N-(2-toluenesulfenyl) carbamate) in mice gives various metabolites dif-ferent from carbofuran (Figure 2). Metabolites II and IV were found in feces, while in urine the phenol VIII, IX, and X were found as conjugates. The major pathway in mice involves the metabolite III as intermediate. Although this metabolite was not excreted, the presence of metabolite IV is indicating the existence of the 3-hydroxy precursor.[219] There is some evidence that N-(2-toluenesulfenyl)carbofuran can form carbofuran via metabolite II inter-mediate.[214]

9. Mobam

Mobam is rapidly metabolized and excreted from the body of rats, goats, and cows. Two major metabolites have been identified in rat urine: the 4-benzothienyl sulfate (65% of the administered dose) and the 4-benzothienyl glucuronide (20% of the dose). A minor metabolite, the 4-hydroxybenzothiofene has also been identified as a free phenol. A dose increase of mobam provokes a decrease in the excretion of glucuronides and an increase in that of sulfoconjugates. In goats and cows 4-benzothieneglucuronide is not excreted but there is an increase of the quantity of excreted 4-benzothienyl sulfate and 4-benzothienyl sulfate-1-oxide. Most metabolites are excreted in the form of phenol conjugates. It is therefore likely that the hydrolysis of the carbamate function is the main metabolic pathway of mobam.[220,221]

10. Aldicarb (Temik), Metomyl (Lannate), Thiocarboxime

Aldicarb, metomyl and thiocarboxine are oximes; patterns of excretion of these com-

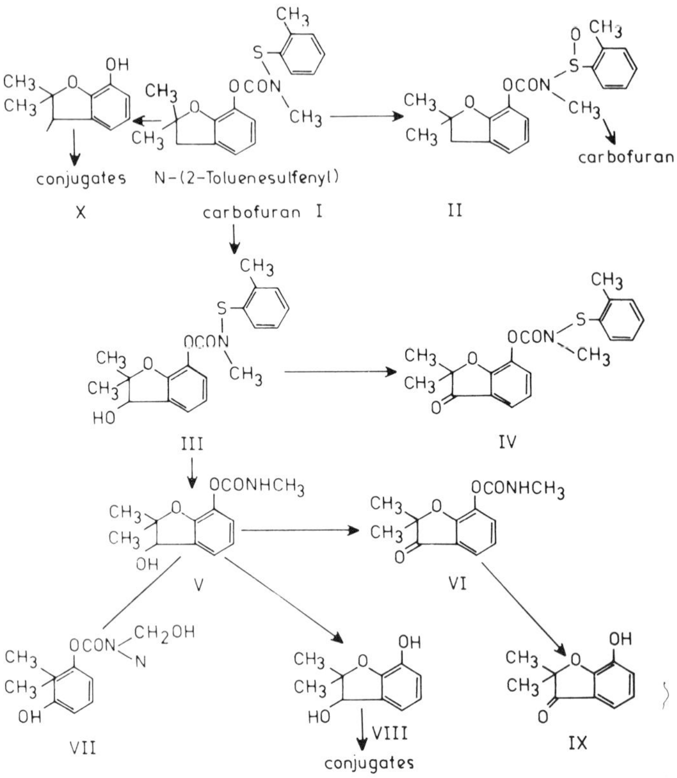

FIGURE 2.   Metabolic pathways of N-(2-toluenesulfenyl) carbofuran.[8,191]

pounds are different from the phenolic carbamate. A general metabolic pathway of aldicarb is shown in Figure 3. Aldicarb is metabolized by rat liver preparations into its sulfoxide, into water soluble metabolites, and into aldicarb sulfone in small amounts. Rats treated with ^{14}C-carbonyl aldicarb excreted 62% of the dose as ^{14}C-carbon dioxide and 30% in urine while with S-methyl ^{14}C-aldicarb, 80% of the radioactivity is excreted in urine and none in expired air.[222] In lactating cows, 80% of the administered radioactivity was present in urine, 0.5% in feces, and 3% in collected milk. Metabolites in urine and milk were the same as those isolated from rats.[223]

[14]C-methomyl is metabolized in rats into carbon dioxide (25%) and acetonitrile (50%). About 12% of the radioactivity was present in urine, 10% in body tissues, and only traces are found in feces.[224] Methomyl is found to be isomerized to the anti-isomer but not the opposite. After hydrolysis, the syn-oxime is essentially converted into CO_2 while the anti-oxime is metabolized into acetonitrile.[225]

[14]C-thiocarboxime is essentially metabolized in rats into CO_2 and acetonitrile in expired air. Urine contained 35% of the administered dose of radioactivity, about 4% in the form of initial compounds, 1.5% as its hydrolysis products as free derivatives, and 30% as O-glucuronides and O-sulfates of the hydrolytic product.[226]

11. Bendiocarb (Ficam)

Bendiocarb metabolism has been investigated in male and female rats treated with ^{14}C-bendiocarb. Excretion was rapid in both sexes and more than 97% of the administered radioactivity was recovered within 72 h. The major routes of excretion are urine (with 90% of the administered dose) and feces (3 to 8%). Breakdown of the molecule to ^{14}C-carbon dioxide represents only to 1 to 3% of the dose. Tissue residue level was very low and there

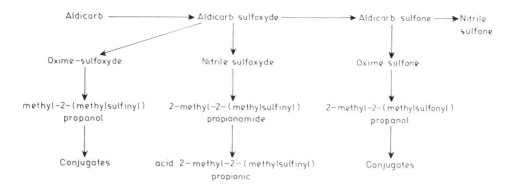

FIGURE 3. Metabolic pathways of aldicarb.[8,191]

was no selective storage of the compound. The major metabolic pathway involved cleavage of the carbamate ester group to yield the 2,2-dimethylbenzo-1,3-dioxol-4-ol which was excreted as a sulfate and glucuronide conjugate. Small amounts of 2,2-dimethylbenzo-1,3-dioxol-4-yl N-(hydroxymethyl)carbamate excreted as conjugate were also found with several minor metabolites which could be ring-hydroxylated derivatives of bendiocarb and 2,2-dimethylbenzo-1,3-dioxol-4-ol.[227].

C. ORGANOPHOSPHORUS INSECTICIDES

The metabolism of organophosphorus insecticides involves a variety of reactions, for instance, oxidative changes through the action of mixed function oxidase and isomerization. Among the biochemical systems which degrade organophosphates, two different groups of enzyme systems are important: namely the oxidative systems and the hydrolytic systems. In the following pages, the metabolic patterns of some organophosphorus insecticides will be discussed.

1. Dichlorvos (DDVP, Vapona)

Dichlorvos undergoes degradation in mammals by vinyl ester linkage giving dichloroacetaldehyde and dimethyl phosphate. It is excreted in urine by O-demethylation to demethyl dichlorvos which is mediated by S-alkyl-glutathione transferase and liver mixed-function oxidase. The O-demethylation of dichlorvos to demethyl dichlorvos also gives formaldehyde and methylmercapturic acid which leads to S-methylcysteine and its S-oxide. The latter is excreted in small quantities in rat urine.[228-230]

Dimethyl phosphate is a major metabolite of dichlorvos because after administration of methyl ^{14}C-dichlorvos, 50% of the radioactivity is excreted in the form of dimethyl phosphate in rat urine and 40% in mouse urine.[231] Demethyl dichlorvos is partially excreted in small quantities (about 2% in rat; 15% in mouse) because it is metabolized thereafter into monomethyl phosphate and dichloroacetaldehyde. Studies carried out with ^{14}C-dichlorvos have shown that dichloroacetaldehyde is further metabolized into glycine and serine, probably via the glyoxal intermediate.[228] The half-life of dichlorvos in blood is extremely short, for example, it is 20 min for rats, 2 min for rabbits, and 25 min for pigs and humans.[228,231] Interestingly, dichlorvos, dichloroacetaldehyde, or dichloroethanol are not found in the tissues of piglets after administration of [14]C- or [36]Cl-dichlorvos to sow.[232] The demethylation of dichlorvos is mediated by glutathione transferase as shown by the decrease of 20% of glutathione in mouse liver.

2. Chlorfenvinphos (Birlane, Supona)

Chlorfenvinphos de-ethylated into phosphate diester 2-chloro-1(2′,4′-dichlorophenyl)vinyl ethyl hydrogenphosphate which is excreted either directly or metabolized later into 2,4-dichlorphenacylchloride, which then metabolizes into 2,4-dichloroacetophenone and then 1-(2′,4-dichlorophenyl) ethanol. The latter is excreted in the form of glucuronide. The reductive dechlorination of the 2,4-dichlorophenacylchloride into the 2,4-dichloroaceto-phenone is mediated by a cytosolic enzyme requiring glutathione as co-factor in rat liver. This process occurs in two steps. In the first step, 2,4-dichlorophenacylchloride reacts with glutathione to yield 2,4-dichloroacetophenone glutathione conjugate. The glutathione conjugate so formed then acts as a substrate for a cytosolic enzyme which catalyzes the nucleophilic attack of the glutathione to yield (2′,4′-dichlorphenyl)ethanol plus GSSG.[235]

Another compound, 2,4-dichlorophenylethanediol has been identified in the form of glucuronide and it could come from either 1 (2′,4′-dichlorophenyl) ethanol or phenacyl alcohol. In mammals, 2-4-dichloromandelic acid has been detected. In rats, it is decarboxylated to give 2,4-dichlorobenzoic acid which is excreted as its glycine conjugate. The selective toxicity of chlorfenvinphos to rats has been attributed to the poor degradation by liver microsomal enzymes and in particular to the low capacity in O-desalkylation reactions in rat liver. For example, rats excrete in urine 32% of desethyl chlorfenvinphos while dogs excrete 70% of the same product. Another difference is in the amount of 1(2′4′-dichlorophenyl) ethanol glucuronide excreted in the urine of rat (41% of the dose) and the dog (40%).[236] In the correlation between theoretical and experimental biotransformation of chlorfenvinphos 13 possible metabolites are obtained from theoretical biotransformation, while experimentally, rat and dog showed only five and four metabolites respectively.[237]

The methyl homolog of chlorfenvinphos, dimethylvinphos (2-chloro-(1-2,4-dichlorphenyl) vinyl dimethylphosphate) is metabolized via glutathione transferase to 2-chloro-1(2′,4′-dichlorophenyl)vinyl methylhydrogenphosphate which is the main metabolite in urine of dogs (44%) and is only excreted in small quantities in rats (3%) probably due to the action of a phosphodiesterase which hydrolyzes this metabolite into 2,4-dichlorophenacyl-chloride. The latter is then metabolized either into 2,4-dichloroacetophenone and then into 1(2′,4′-dichlorophenyl) ethanol, or into 1(2′,4′-dichlorophenyl) ethane diol and thereafter into 2,4-dichloromandelic acid.[238]

3. Tetrachlorvinphos (Gardona, Rabon)

The metabolism of tetrachlorvinphos in rats and dogs is somewhat different. For example, 4 days after a single dose of ^{14}C-(vinyl)-tetrachlorvinphos, 78% of the radioactivity is detected in the urine of rats, 16% in feces, 0.5% in exhaled air, and only 1% in tissue. The metabolites found in urine are desmethyltetrachlorvinphos (4%), 1(2,4,5-trichlorophenyl)ethanol as free (2%) and glucuronide (35%) 2,4,5-trichlorophenylethandiol as free (2.5%), and glucuronide (8%) and 2,4,5-trichloromandelic acid (24%). In dogs on the contrary, 92% of the radioactivity is found in urine. The metabolites in urine are desmethyl tetrachlorvinphos (46%), 2,4,5-trichlorophenylethandiol as free (4%), glucuronide (12%), and 2,4,5-trichloromandelic acid (12%).[239]

The desmethylation of tetrachlorvinphos is catalyzed by the monooxygenase of the liver microsome with liberation of formaldehyde and desmethyl tetrachlorvinphos.[240] However, it is shown that desmethylation of tetrachlorvinphos also occurs in the soluble fraction of the liver which is found to be glutathione dependent. Tetrachlorvinphos in the presence of the soluble enzyme and glutathione, is desmethylated and the methyl radical is transferred into glutathione to yield S-methyl glutathione.[241] A phosphodiesterase catalyzing the formation of methylphosphate and 2,4,5-trichlorophenacyl chloride from the desmethyl tetrachlorvinphos has been found in the soluble fraction of rat and pig liver.[242]

4. Mevinphos (Phosdrin)

Mevinphos is a mixture of *cis* (60%) and *trans* (40%) isomers. Mevinphos is hydrolyzed by cow, calf, and human plasma to yield dimethyl phosphate.[243] *trans*-Mevinphos is degraded faster than the *cis*-isomer by mouse liver homogenates. *cis*-Mevinphos is degraded by the mouse liver glutathione S-alkyltransferase while *trans*-isomer is not demethylated but degraded by hydrolysis at the P-O-vinyl bond by an esterase which requires no glutathione as co-factor. The products of this hydrolysis give methyl acetoacetate and dimethyl phosphate.[241,244] In the detoxification of mevinphos, carboxy esterases do not play any role since carboxyester hydrolyzed metabolites were not found in incubated liver preparations.[245]

5. Dicrotophos (Bidrin, Carbicron)

Dicrotophos is rapidly metabolized in rats, mice, rabbits, and dogs.[246] Three possible metabolic pathways have been shown for dicrotophos. The first which is of minor importance is the O-desmethylation of dicrotophos into demethyldicrotophos. The second is through the hydrolysis of dicrotophos into dimethyl phosphate which is detected in the excreta and to N,N-dimethylacetoacetamide. The third pathway is the N-dealkylation of dicrotophos which yields another insecticide, the monocrotophos (3(dimethoxyphosphinyloxy)-N,N-methyl-6-crotonamide).[246,247]

Studies using ^{32}P and N-^{14}C-methyl-dicrotophos have shown that dicrotophos is first metabolized into monocrotophos via the N-hydroxymethyl intermediate. Monocrotophos is desmethylated via its N-hydroxymethyl derivative to yield the unsubstituted amide, the dimethyl-(1-methyl-2-carbamoyl) vinyl phosphate which is found in very low levels in urine (less than 0.1% of the administered dicrotophos). On the other hand, monocrotophos can be hydrolysated to form the dimethyl phosphoric acid and the N-methylacetoacetamide which is excreted rapidly in urine.[246-248] In the case of dicrotophos, N-dealkylation does not appear to be really a detoxification reaction. In rat, dicrotophos is less toxic than its N-demethylated metabolite monocrotophos which is also less toxic than the unsubstituted amide.[246] It has been shown that 24 h after an i.p. injection of ^{32}P-monocrotophos to rats, 58% of the radioactivity is localized in urine and 5% in the feces. In urine, monocrotophos (34% of the administered dose), dimethyl phosphate (34%), O-demethyl monocrotophos (10%), N-methylol derivative (20%), and phosphoric acid (2%) have been detected.[249]

6. Phosphamidon (Dimecron)

Phosphamidon is rapidly metabolized in rats. About 70% of an oral dose is eliminated in 10 h.[250] The metabolic pathway of phosphamidon is presented in Figure 4.

Four possible metabolic pathways have been proposed from the different identified metabolites in excreta of mammal. The major pathway (I) is a P-O-vinyl hydrolysis resulting in the formation of dimethyl phosphate and α-chloro-acetoacetic acid diethylamine. This compound is probably dehalogenated and then cleaved by deamination and decarboxylation. The hydrolysis of the P-O-methyl bond of phosphamidon (II) which also occurs in animals is a minor pathway of metabolism and yields O-demethyl phosphamidon which is a nontoxic metabolite. The third route leads to the formation of N-desethyl-phosphamidon and phosphamidon amide. The N-ethyl group of phosphamidon is oxidatively eliminated as acetaldehyde through a hydroxylation of the alpha carbon atom. The oxidative N-dealkylation occurs faster with 6-phosphamidon than with the *trans*-isomer. The metabolites N-desethyl-phosphamidon and the phosphamidon amide are more toxic than the parent compounds. Reductive dechlorination (IV) would be another route of metabolism as it suggests excretion of small quantities of dechlorophosphamidon amide in rat urine and goat milk.[248,250,251]

7. Parathion, Methyl Parathion, and Fenitrothion

The metabolic pathways of parathion, methyl parathion, and fenitrothion are the same in animals. A scheme of the metabolism of parathion is shown in Figure 5.

Parathion is the first product which showed that thiophosphates must first be metabolized *in vivo* to become toxic.[252] The conversion of parathion into paraoxon is low compared to

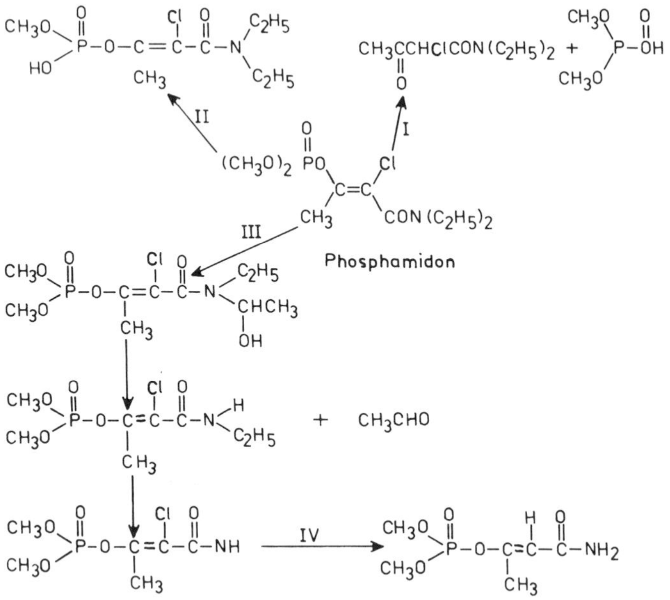

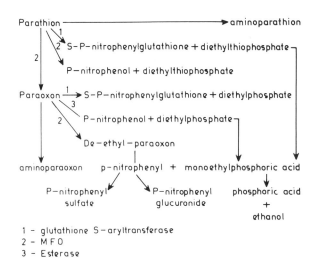

FIGURE 4.   Metabolic pathways of phosphamidon.

Parathion ————————————————→ aminoparathion

FIGURE 5.   Metabolic pathways of parathion. 1 = Glutathione-S-
aryltransferase; 2 = MFO; 3 = esterase.

other metabolic product; it is this conversion that is responsible for the intoxication by
phosphorothionate esters. About 4.5% of the LD_{50} dose administered to rats is converted
into paraoxon in 1 h. This conversion occurs mainly in liver (64%) but also in the gut (21%),
the lungs (13%), and the kidney (1.5%).[253]

In vivo studies have shown that amino paraoxon is not found in appreciable quantities
in the urine of rat but *in vitro* studies suggest that rat tissues have high nitroreductase
activities and the respective amines of parathion and paraoxon are well formed.[254] Paraoxon
and methyl paraoxon are converted into S-P-nitrophenyl glutathione and the corresponding
dialkyl phosphate by soluble liver enzymes in the presence of glutathione. This enzyme,
phosphoric acid triester S-aryl transferase, also metabolizes parathion into S-P-nitrophenyl

glutathione and diethyl thiophosphoric acid.[255-257] A study with several rat strains has shown that de-ethyl paraoxon is the major urinary metabolite of parathion.[257]

The pattern of metabolic transformation of methyl parathion and fenitrothion are quite different from that of parathion, for example, these two compounds are largely demethylated in the first instance.

A study with isolated perfused mouse liver has shown that p-nitrophenol, p-nitrophenol phosphate and p-nitrophenol glucuronide were the metabolic products of paraoxon after a single pass perfusion.[258]

Rat liver homogenates metabolize methyl parathion into methyl paraoxon, and fenitrothion into desmethyl parathion desmethyl fenitrothion and desmethyl paraoxon.[259,260] GSH-alkyltransferase enzyme is found to be responsible for this demethylation. This enzyme in the presence of glutathione catalyzes the transfer of the methyl group of the insecticide on the glutathione, yielding the corresponding demethyl insecticide and the S-methyl glutathione.[261,262] Since phosphoric, thiophosphoric, dimethylthio phosphoric and dimethyl phosphoric acids have been detected in animals exposed to fenitrothion, the main metabolic pathways of fenitrothion are essentially the same as those of methyl parathion and parathion.[263]

Although the molecular alterations and the structure of parathion, methylparathion, and fenitrothion are minor, the toxicity of each product is very different. The insecticide activity of parathion and methylparathion is similar but the mammalian toxicity is somewhat higher. This has been due to the great activity of the mammalian liver enzymes which catalyze the glutathione S-methyl transfer reactions.[262,264] Similarly, the rate of demethylation in mammals is greater with fenitrothion than with methyl parathion.[265] The high degree of selective toxicity of fenitrothion between insects and mammals has been attributed to the difference in rates of activation, and the detoxification and transfer to the target and in the sensitivity of the target enzyme.[263,265-267]

8. Cyanophos

Cyanophos is biodegraded in mammals by aryl ester bond cleavage. The liberated cyanophenol is conjugated with sulfate and the p-cyanophenyl sulfate is excreted in the urine as the main metabolite.[268]

9. Ronnel

The metabolism of ronnel in the rat and cow has shown rapid elimination in urine. The degradation proceeds through the cleavage of both the P-O-phenyl bond giving 2,4,5-trichlorophenol dimethyl thiophosphate and thereafter dimethyl phosphate, and the P-O-methyl bond giving the O-demethylated ronnel.[269,270]

10. Fenthion

A general scheme of the metabolic pathway of fenthion is given in Figure 6. Fenthion sulfoxide and sulfone and fenthion phosphate sulfoxide or sulfone have been identified.[271] The metabolic conversion of the thioether group to the sulfoxide occurs more rapidly than the conversion of sulfoxide to the sulfone and the desulfuration to the phosphate sulfoxide and sulfone.[272,273] Emteres et al. have shown that the kinetics of fenthion in rabbit are not influenced by the route of administration.[274]

11. Chlorpyrifos (Dursban)

Chlorpyrifos is rapidly metabolized in rats and about 90% is excreted in urine. The degradation appears to be due to dealkylation. The metabolites in urine consists of 3,5,6-3,5,6-trichloro-2-pyridinol and its glucuronide; a glucose conjugate of the 3,5,6-trichloro-2-pyridinol has also been detected.[275] Mouse liver perfusion studies *in situ* have shown that

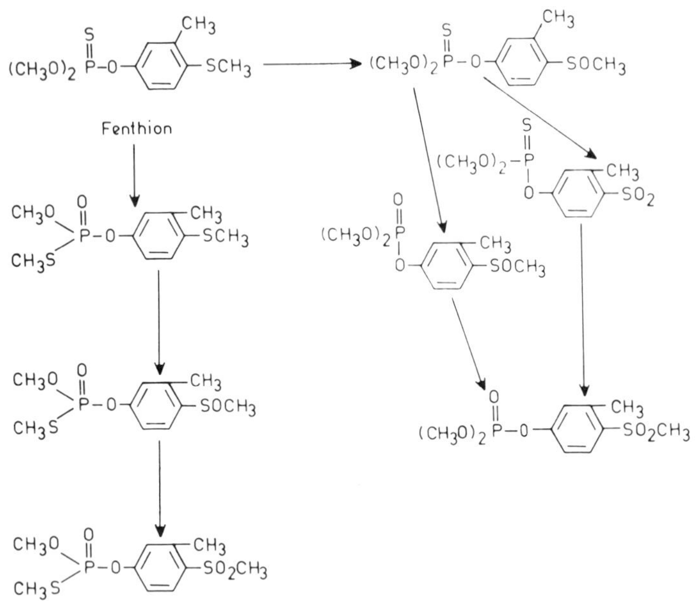

FIGURE 6. Metabolic pathways of fenthion.

chlorpyrifos oxon produced by liver from chlorpyrifos is quickly metabolized within the liver to 3,5,6-trichloro-2-pyridinol and diethyl phosphoric acid.[276,277] Formation of both chlorpyrifos oxon and 3,5,6-trichloro 2-pyridinol requires NDPH and is inhibited by carbon monoxide. The apparent K_m and V_{max} for mouse hepatic microsomal oxidative detoxification of chlorpyrifos to 3,5,6-trichloro 2-pyridinol are 16.1 μM and 263.3 nM/liver/min respectively. The apparent K_m and V_{max} for the oxidative activation of chlorpyrifos to chlorpyrifos oxon are 20 μM and 126.1 nM/liver/min respectively, whereas the apparent K_m and V_m for hepatic microsomal hydrolysis of chlorpyrifos oxon to 3,5,6-trichloro-2-pyridinol are 1.87 mM and 89450.7 mM/liver/min. It has been found that under first order conditions, the capacity of hepatic microsomes to detoxify chlorpyrifos oxon exceeds their capacity to generate chlorpyrifos oxon from chlorpyrifos.[278]

12. Diazinon (Basudrin)

Diazinon undergoes metabolic degradation by the same pathways as parathion and paraoxon (Figure 7). Diazinon and diazoxon are conjugated with glutathione by glutathione S-aryltransferase enzyme of the soluble fraction of rat liver and the products of the reactions give S-2-isopropyl-4-methyl-6-pyrimidinyl glutathione and diethyl thiophosphoric acid.[279] Urinary diethyl thiophosphoric acid is used as an indicator of diazinon exposure.[280]

The metabolism of diazoxon can occur in two pathways. The first and more important is the esterastic pathway conducting to pyrimidinol and diethyl phosphoric acid. The second, of minor importance, is the formation of de-ethyldiazoxon which is not detected on incubation with rat liver microsomes.[256,281] Several studies using ^{32}P-1-ethyl-^{14}C and ring ^{14}C-labeled diazinon and diazoxon have shown different pathways of diazinon metabolism.[256,279,281,282] The side chain is hydroxylated by MFO and this hydroxylation occurs on the tertiary atom carbon of diazinon and diazoxon. Hydroxydiazinon has been found in various organs of sheep dosed with diazinon.[283] In addition to hydroxydiazinon, hydroxydiazoxon, isohydroxydiazinon (6-methylol derivative of diazinon) and the alkene corresponding to the dehydration product of hydroxydiazinon are found as metabolites of diazinon in mice and sheep.[284,285] In rats exposed to diazinon, the diazinon residue is much greater in kidney than in other organs, for instance, liver and brain.[286]

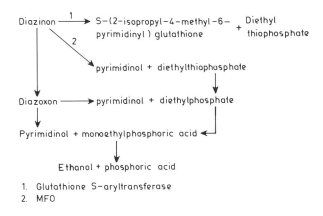

FIGURE 7.   Metabolic pathways of diazinon. 1 = Glutathione-S-aryltransferase; 2 = MFO.

13. Demeton

Demeton exists in two isomer forms: the demeton-S (O,O-diethyl S-2-ethylthioethyl phosphorothioate) and the demeton-O (O,O-diethyl O-2-ethylthioethyl phosphorothioate). Each demeton isomer is first converted into the sulfoxide and then the corresponding sulfone.[287] Demeton-S and demeton-O are rapidly excreted in the mouse within 24 h and about 90% of the metabolites excreted are in the form of hydrolyzed nontoxic products. The remaining products are in the form of demeton-O, its sulfoxide and sulfone, demeton P and its sulfoxide, and the O,O-diethyl O-2-ethylthioethyl phosphate.[250] The methyl analog of demeton-O and demeton-S are demeton-O-methyl and demeton-S-methyl which are metabolized into the corresponding sulfoxide and sulfone. In the presence of traces of water, the intermolecular transmethylation results in the formation of much more toxic sulfonium compounds.[288]

14. Malathion (Cythion, Karbofos)

Malathion appears to degrade rapidly through hydrolytic pathways. *In vitro* and *in vivo* studies have shown that malathion is rapidly activated to malaoxon by P=S to P=O conversion.[289,290] A general scheme of the metabolic pathway of malathion is presented in Figure 8. A study with rats has shown that malathion dicarboxylic acid is the main metabolite in urine. In urine, dimethyl phosphorus diesters, namely O,O-dimethyl phosphate, O,O-dimethyl thiophosphate, and O,O-dimethyl thiophosphonate have been detected.[291] A more recent study in rats has shown that malathion gives rise to α-malathion monocarboxylic acid and β-malathion carboxylic acid. Malathion diacid the most important metabolite has also been detected. The α-malaoxon- or β-malaoxon-monocarboxylic acid represents only 1% of the applied dose whereas demethyl malaoxon is excreted in higher quantity than demethyl malathion.[292]

Several studies have shown that toxicity of malathion is increased or decreased by compounds which act either on the activity of the cytochrome p-450 monooxygenase enzyme or on the activity of the carboxyl esterases.[289,292-294] These compounds appear to modify the toxicokinetics of malathion in the animal. It has been shown that the malathion impurities have a stronger effect in inhibiting carboxylesterase which hydrolyzes the β-carboethoxy moiety of malathion.[295] Malik and Summer have proposed the possible role of glutathione in the detoxication process of malathion.[296]

15. Dimethoate (Rogor, Cygon)

Dimethoate is a carboxyamide instead of a carboxyl ester. In mammals, N-demethylation of dimethoate predominates over both O-demethylation and oxon formation.[297] The impor-

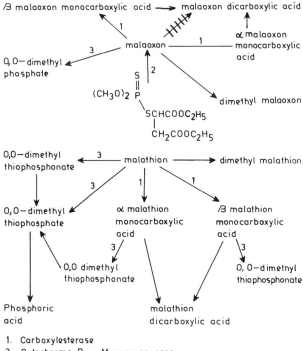

FIGURE 8.   Metabolic pathways of malathion. 1 = Carboxylesterases; 2 = cytochrome p_{450}-monooxygenases; 3 = phosphatases.

tance of the cleavage of the amide bond of dimethioate is responsible for its selective toxicity.[298] The enzymic carboxyamide cleavage of dimethoate in vertebrates occurs almost exclusively in liver. With whole liver homogenates of liver microsomes, dimethoate is degrated to dimethyl phosphorodithioic acid or carboxymethyl dithioate.[299] Guinea pig liver gave only dimethyl phosphorodithioic acid while the degradation of dimethoate in sheep liver homogenate is almost completely due to the amidase yielding the carboxymethyl dithioate.[300]

Dimethoate is rapidly degraded in mammals and eliminated in the urine. In cattle, 90% of the oral dose is found in urine after 24 hr.[301] The main metabolite in urine of cow and sheep is the carboxymethyl dithioate.[302,303] Dimethoate oxygen analog is present in minor amounts and is not hydrolyzed by the amidase. Other metabolites identified are dimethyl phosphorodithioic acid, dimethyl phosphorothioic acid, monomethyl phosphoric acid, and desmethyl dimethoate. The enzymatic ractions which take place in the metabolism of dimethoate are activation of P=S to P=O by desulfuration yielding the oxygen analog of dimethoate, deamidation of amidase yielding the carboxymethyl dithioate, hydrolysis of P-O and P-S bonds by phosphate action, and N-dealkylation by oxidases giving the N-desmethyl dimethoate.

16. Thiometon and Related Compounds

Thiometon, tetrathion, isothioate, disulfoton, and phorate have very similar metabolic pathways in mammals. These compounds are metabolized by oxidation of the thio ether moiety to the corresponding sulfoxide and sulfone and desulfuration of the P-S moiety to P-O producing a phosphorothiolate ester. Phorate incubated with rat liver slices is metabolized into phorate sulfoxide and sulfone and P-O-phorate sulfoxide and sulfone, the oxidation of

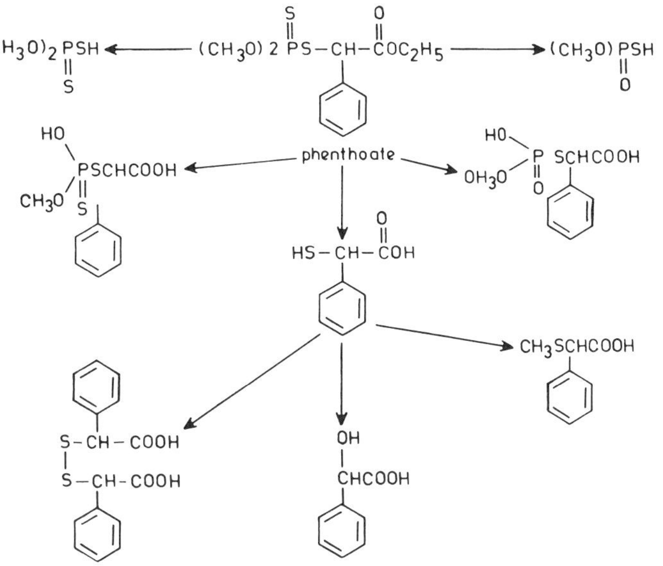

FIGURE 9. Metabolic pathways of phenthoate.

P=S to P=O taking place after the initial state of oxidation is formation of the sulfoxide analog which can be either desulfurated or oxidized to the sulfone. The principal hydrolytic products detected are diethyl phosphoric and diethyl phosphorothioic acids. Phosphorodithioic acid is not found indicating that hydrolysis occurs through cleavage of the P-S bond.[305]

17. Phenthoate
Phenthoate is rapidly metabolized in mouse by P-S and C-S cleavage, O-demethylation, oxon formation, and esterastic cleavage of the carboxy ethyl group. Esterastic cleavage is the major pathway because only 16% of the metabolites identified are the O-demethylated acid, the O-demethylated oxon acid, the dimethyl phosphorodithionate, the dimethyl phosphorothionate and the corresponding product resulting from the cleavage of the P-S bond[306] (Figure 9).

18. Carbophenothion (Trithion, Garrathion)
Carbophenothion is rapidly metabolized by rat and the metabolites detected in urine are the glucuronide, the sulfate of the 4-chlorothiophenol, the 4-chlorophenyl methyl sulfone, the 3-hydroxy-4-chlorophenyl methyl sulfone and its conjugated form, and p-chlorobenzenesulfinic acid. Another S-oxidized compound derived from the p-chlorophenylsulfenylmethyl mercaptan, resulting from the P-S cleavage of carbophenothion has also been identified in small quantities.[307,308]

19. Dioxathion (Delnav)
Dioxathion exists in two forms, the cis- and the trans-isomers. Studies with (^{14}C-ethyl)- or (^{14}C-ring)-labeled cis- and trans-dioxathion have shown that they are rapidly metabolized yielding products of ring fragmentation, O,O-diethyl thiophosphate, O,O-diethyl phosphate, and O,O-diethyl thiophosphonate. Diethylthiophosphate and diethylphosphate are probably the breakdown products of the oxon and the dioxon of dioxathion but diethylthiophosphonate is probably derived from the open ring of dioxathion after its hydroxylation.[309]

20. Phosmet (Imidan)
Phosmet is rapidly degraded and excreted in rats, for instance, about 79% of an oral

dose is eliminated via the urine and 19% via feces.[310] In rats, phosmet is disrupted at the S-C bond giving N-hydroxymethylphthalimide which is rapidly decomposed into phthalamic acid, the major metabolite, and further into phthalic acid.[311] Induction of inhibition of the hydroxylating enzymic systems of the liver affects toxicokinetics of phosmet in large proportion.[312]

21. Phosalone (Zolone)

Phosalone is metabolized in rat by cleavage of the C-S or P-S bond. The P-S bond cleavage of phosalone gives the chlorobenzoxalone-3-yl-methanethiol which is then methylated and oxidized, finally giving the sulfone and the O,O-diethylthiophosphate. The cleavage of the C-S bond gives the chlorobenzoxazolone which is transformed into phenoxazinone via the chloroaminohydroxybenzene.[49]

22. Methidathion (Supracide)

Methidathion is rapidly degraded in mammals. A study on the *in vitro* metabolism of methidathion in rat and mouse liver subcellular fractions shows that the major route of metabolism is via the glutathione S-transferases and the predominant metabolite is desmethyl methidathion. The mixed function oxidases are also involved in the metabolism of methidathion. Four metabolites have been characterized, for example, the desmethyl methidathion, the glutathione conjugate of the heterocyclic moeity of methidathion, the cysteinyl glycine conjugate, and the cysteine conjugate. The other metabolites identified are the oxygen analog of methidathion and methoxythiadiazolin. However, oxidation of the sulfoxide to the sulfone, mediated by the MFO system, appears to be a minor pathway.[313]

23. Azinphosmethyl (Guthion, Gusathion)

Administration of ^{32}P-azinphosmethyl orally to a cow has shown that the compound is metabolized and excreted in urine. ^{14}C-azinphosmethyl, 4-phosphorus free metabolites have been detected in milk, one of which accounts for 90% of the total radioactivity detected.[314] *In vitro* studies with mouse liver microsomes show that in the presence of NADPH and oxygen, azinphosmethyl is metabolized into its corresponding oxon, dimethyl phosphorothionate and dimethyl phosphate. The S-alkyl transferase of the soluble fraction from mouse liver demethylates the azinphosmethyl but not its oxon.[315]

24. Crufomate

Crufomate is rapidly metabolized in animals, for instance, in sheep dosed with ^{32}P-crufomate, 85% of the radioactivity is eliminated in 24 h in urine. Crufomate is disrupted at the P-N bond and the main metabolite excreted is the 4-tert-butyl-2-chlorophenyl methyl phosphoric acid.[316] In sheep dosed with a single oral dose, crufomate is metabolized extensively to yield 27 metabolites, 17 of which have been detected in the blood, the feces, and the urine. Unchanged crufomate is however not detected, probably due to the rapidity of the oxidation of the t-butyl group. However, the product of this hydroxylation, the 4-t-butanolphenyl N-methylphosphoroamidate, represents only 7% of the radioactivity in urine because it is further metabolized into N-formyl derivatives, N-formyl-N-methyl derivatives, and N-demethyl derivatives. The products of the P-O bond cleavage are the 4-t-butyl-2-chlorophenol and its alcohol and acid derivatives.[317]

25. Trichlorfon (Dipterex, Neguvan, Tugon, Dylox)

Trichlorfon is nonenzymatically transformed into dichlorvos at physiological conditions.[318,319] The capacity to transform trichlorfon into dichlorvos seems to vary within the species. In dog dosed with trichlorfon intravenously, the urine contains 63% of the original compounds in the form of glucuronide of trichloroethanol indicating a cleavage of the P-C bond which gives trichloroethanol and O,O-dimethyl phosphoric acid.[320] In the urine of rabbit administered trichlorfon, the desmethyl dichlorvos glucuronide was detected but not the trichloroethanol glucuronide which indicates that the formation of dichlorvos in rabbit is easier than in dog.[321] Thus, trichlorfon has two metabolic pathways which vary with the species. The first pathway is the transformation to dichlorvos desmethyl dichlorvos excreted as glucuronide, O,O-dimethyl phosphate and methylphosphoric acid, as in rabbit. The second pathway is the cleavage of the P-C bond yielding trichloroethanol excreted as glucuronide O,O-dimethyl phosphate and O-methyl phosphoric acid as in dog.

26. Leptophos (Phosvel, Abar)

The metabolism of leptophos has been studied in rats with ^{14}C-phenyl- and ^{14}C methyl-labeled leptophos. Following the administration of a single oral dose of ^{14}C-phenyl leptophos, 46 to 75% of the ^{14}C radioactivity was recovered in the urine after 9 days. Radioactivity was not detected in the expired air. The urinary metabolites identified with O-methyl phenylphosphonic, O-methyl phenylphosphonothioic and phenylphosphonic acids and two other metabolites of unknown structure. Demethylation of leptophos and/or its oxygen analog occurred *in vivo* as confirmed by the elimination of ^{14}C$_2$ in the expired air, from ^{14}C-methyl leptophos. The leptophos seemed to accumulate in subcutaneous fat because 12 weeks after administration traces were still present in the fat; while the degradation products are generally weak inhibitors of the acetylcholinesterase, oxon is a more potent inhibitor than leptophos itself.[321]

In mice, the transformation of leptophos is rapid and only small amounts of the parent compound are present in feces and in urine. The major metabolite is 4-bromo-2,5-dichlorophenol which is mostly excreted as conjugate. The oxon of O-demethyl leptophos is only a minor urinary metabolite and 90% of the radioactivity corresponds as in rats to methyl phenyl phosphonothioic acid, methyl phenyl phosphonic acid, and phenyl phosphonic acid which is the product of phosphodiesterase action on the oxon of the O-demethyl leptophos. The demethylation of leptophos oxon could occur via microsomal oxidation or by S-methyl glutathione transferase action. The absence of O-demethyl-leptophos and phenylphosphonotioic acid in the urine reveals that glutathione mediated-O-demethylation of leptophos is of less importance in relation to the production of 4-bromo-2,5-dichlorophenol.[322]

27. EPN

EPN is the first phosphonate insecticide which was commercialized. An *in vitro* study with rat liver microsomes had shown that EPN induced inhibition of rat liver microsomal carboxylesterase and formation of the EPN oxon (O-ethyl-O-P-nitrophenol phenyl-phosphate) by the cytochrome p-450 monooxygenase stimulated by addition of NAD.[323]

In cat, following a single dermal administration of EPN, the EPN oxon is not identified. After a single dermal dose of ^{14}C-EPN, the radioactivity disappeared exponentially from the administration site at a constant rate of 0.46 day^{-1} corresponding to a half-life of 1.5 days. Most of the absorbed radioactivity was excreted in urine (30%). Only 3% of the ^{14}C was recovered in feces. Only traces of EPN were detected in urine and feces. The metabolites identified were O-ethyl phenylphosphonothioic acid (EPPTA), O-ethyl phenylphosphonic acid (EPPA), and phenylphosphonic acid (PPA). EPN was the major compound identified in the brain, adipose tissue, plasma, liver, and kidney. EPN is eliminated from tissues and plasma according to exponential kinetics. The halflife of the elimination of EPN from plasma was 9.1 days.[324] The metabolism and distribution of EPN in hen are similar to those in cat. After a single oral dose of ^{14}C-EPN, most of the radioactivity was found in excreta (74%) and the metabolites identified were PPA, EPPA, and EPPTA as in cat. In liver, EPPA was the most important metabolite followed by a EPPTA and PPA. EPN disappeared exponentially from the tissue with an elimination plasma halflife of 16.5 days.[325]

D. SYNTHETIC PYRETHROIDS

Synthetic pyrethroids include such important compounds, for example, as permethrin, cypermethrin, fenvalerate, and deltamethrin (Decamethrin). The pyrethroids have (1) a stable alcohol moiety where the alkane side-chain is replaced by aromatic substituents and (2) unstable dimethyl vinyl group on the acid side chain which is modified by either an aromatic substituent as in fenvalerate or by halogen atoms as in the case of permethrin and deltamethrin. This results in hydrolytic degradation rather than oxidative degradation.

1. Permethrin

In the case of permethrin metabolism there are two important degradative forces interacting. The relative ratio of these two forces is determined by the chemical nature of the isomer and the respective biological system. The *trans*-permethrin is more susceptible to esteric attack than *cis*-permethrin. For example, in rats this tendency is very pronounced. The esterase products for *trans*-permethrin constitute about 89% while the oxidase products consitute about 95%. The corresponding figures for *cis*-permethrin are 6 and 20.7% respectively. In contrast, the values for mouse are 91% vs. 74.3% respectively, which suggest the relative importance of oxidative systems.

2. Cypermethrin

The metabolism of *cis, trans*-cypermethrin in rat has been studied by Rhodes et al.[326] The major pathway of metabolism involved cleavage of the ester bond with subsequent hydroxylation and glucuronidation of the cyclopropyl acid moieties, together with hydroxylation and sulfation of the 3-phenoxybenzyl moiety. Elimination of the compound was rapid after the cessation of the exposure, although less rapid from the fat and skin. In fat, *cis*-isomers were eliminated with a halflife of 18.2 days while the average halflife of trans-isomers was 3.4 days. In man, about 78% of the trans cypermethrin is excreted during the same period. In man, as in other animals, ester cleavage and elimination of the *cis*- and *trans*-cyclopropanecarboxylic acid moieties in the free and conjugated form are the major routes of cypermethrin metabolism.[327]

3. Deltamethrin (Decamethrin, Decis)

In rat, deltamethrin is quickly metabolized *in vivo* by liver and blood enzymes. After an intravenous administration, 50% of the dose is cleared from the blood within 0.7 to 0.8 min, and then the rate of clearance is decreased. The major metabolite identified in blood *in vivo* and when deltamethrin is incubated with blood *in vitro* is the 3-phenoxybenzoic acid. Deltamethrin levels in liver peaked at 7 to 10 nmol/g at 5 min and then decreased to 1 nmol/g by 30 min. Peak levels were achieved in the central nervous system within 1 min (0.5 nmol/g), decreasing to 0.2 nmol/g at 15 min. Opposite to the studies with *cis*-methrin, the toxicity did not correlate well with the total amount of radiolabeled or parent deltamethrin in the central nervous system. In contrast, deltamethrin is metabolized less quickly then *cis*-methrin and bioresmethrin.[327,328]

4. Fenvalerate (Sumicidin)

Fenvalerate administered to rats is eliminated rapidly and completely from the body. More than 15 metabolites are found to form the acid portion of the molecule and 4-chloro-α(1-methylethyl)-benzene acetic acid is the main isolated product. Nonmetabolized fenvalerate is the major product in feces but only trace amounts are found in urine.[330] Similar results are found with cows fed fenvalerate.[331]

E. MISCELLANEOUS PESTICIDES
1. Pentachlorophenol (PCP)

Rats dosed with ^{14}C-PCP excreted unchanged PCP (48% of the dose), tetrahydroquinone

(10% of the dose), and glucuronide of PCP (6%). The elimination halflives were 23.9 h for PCP, 24.8 h for PCP-glucuronide and 31.5 h for tetrahydroquinone. In plasma, most of the radioactivity was found to be due to unchanged PCP and only a small fraction was present at PCP glucuronide and TCH was not detectable. The metabolites of PCP are rapidly excreted via urine and are not retained in the body. However, for females given 100 mg/kg, the monophasic elimination had a halflife of 27 h. The highest concentrations were found in liver and kidney and the lowest in brain and fat. About 90% of the PCP in plasma was bound to proteins which probably is responsible for low tissue to plasma ratios and a low rate of renal clearance.[332]

In rhesus monkey there are apparent sex-related differences in the first order clearance of PCP from plasma and excretion in urine. The halflife of PCP in plasma was 83.5 h for females and 72 h for males while the values for urine (excretion) are 92 and 41 hr for females and males respectively. Unlike rat, monkey excretes free unchanged PCP in the urine, and biliary excretion and enterohepatic circulation are the probable explanations for this long halflife of PCP in the body of monkeys.[333]

2. Benomyl

After a single oral dose of ^{14}C-benomyl, 79% of the radioactivity is eliminated in the urine of the rat and 9% in feces within 72 h. During the same period, in dog 16% of the dose was excreted in urine and 83.4% in feces.[334] In mice, 55% of the dose is excreted in urine and 37% in feces. Sheep and rabbits excreted 58 and 67% of the dose in urine and 28 and 24% in feces respectively.[335] In rabbit, sheep, and mouse benomyl is rapidly metabolized and the major metabolites in these three species are the methyl benzimidazol-2-yl carbamate, obtained from benomyl by hydrolytic cleavage of the butylcarbamoyl side chain and the 2-aminobenzimidazole resulting from the cleavage of the carbamate moiety of methyl benzimidazol-2-yl carbamate. In sheep the latter product is the major metabolite excreted in urine and feces and represents about 35% of the administered dose. In urine and feces of these three species of animals, the hydroxylated products of methyl benzimidazol-2-yl carbamate and of 2-aminobenzimidazole which are methyl 5-hydroxybenzimidazol-2-yl carbamate and 5-hydroxy-2-aminobenzimidazole respectively are also found in minor amounts (10%) as sulfate and glucuronide conjugates. *In vitro* studies have shown that the rumen fluid of sheep could hydrolyze the carbamate ester bond of benomyl yielding the 1-butyl-carbamoyl-2-aminobenzimidazole and further the 2-aminobenzimidazole before its absorption.

In rats, dogs, and cows benomyl and methyl benzimidazol-2-yl carbamate are not accumulated in the tissues. In rat and cow, methyl benzimidazol-2-yl carbamate is hydroxylated yielding the methyl-5-hydroxybenzimidazol-2-yl carbamate the major metabolite excreted as glucuronide and sulfate conjugate. In cow, rat, and dog, the hydroxylation in the 4 position of the benzimidazole nucleus of methyl benzimidazol-2-yl carbamate also occurs giving the methyl-4-hydroxybenzimidazol-2-yl carbamate.[334,335]

3. Fuberidazole

Fuberidazole is rapidly absorbed from the gastrointestinal tract of rabbits, rats, dogs, horses, and goats. Fuberidazole is metabolized in these species by two different pathways. In all the species, the furan ring of fuberidazole is hydrolyzed yielding the 4-(2-benzimidazolyl)-4-hydroxybutyric acid. The 4-(2-benzimidazolyl)-4-hydroxybutyric acid represents 90% of the detected metabolite in dogs but only 48% in rats, 45% in horses, 38% in goats, and 35% in rabbits. The second metabolic pathway via the hydroxylation of benzimidazole nucleus leads to the 2-(2-furyl)-5-hydroxybenzimidazole which is detected in the urine of all the species studied except rabbit and dog. The 2-(2-furyl)-5-hydroxybenzimidazole is excreted further in the same proportion as glucuronide and sulfate conjugates in dog, more likely as glucuronide conjugate in horse and goat and as sulfate conjugate in rat and rabbit.[336]

4. Thiabendazole

Thiabendazole is rapidly absorbed by various species such as cattle, goat, pig, rat, and dog. The plasma level shows a climax after 1 to 2 h in dog, 2 to 4 h in rat, and 4 to 7 h in goat and cattle. In all these species, the benzimidazole ring of thiabendazole is hydroxylated yielding hydroxythiabendazole which is found in urine either in a free or conjugated form. The proportion of 5-hydroxythiabendazole glucuronide or sulfate varies according to the species. In rat, unchanged thiabendazole represents 3% of the product detected in urine, 4% is free 5-hydroxythiabendazole, 39% is 5-hydroxythiabendazole sulfate, and 28% is in the form of 5-hydroxythiabendazole glucuronide. In cow, unchanged thiabendazole is not detected in urine. Free 5-hydroxythiabendazole represents 42% of the detected metabolites, 21% is 5-hydroxythiabendazole glucuronide, and 3% is 5-hydroxythiabendazole sulfate. In goat and pig, unchanged thiabendazole represents about 2% of the products excreted in urine while 70 to 94% is 5-hydroxythiabendazole glucuronide.[337,338]

5. Thiophanate

Thiophanate and thiophanate-methyl are metabolized in sheep and mice by cyclization into benzimidazole derivative yielding the methyl benzimidazol-2-yl carbamate. The methyl benzimidazol-2-yl carbamate is then metabolized into methyl 5-hydroxybenzimidazol-2-yl carbamate or into 2-aminobenzimidazole; these 2 latter products further lead to the formation of 5-hydroxy-2-aminobenzimidazole.[339,340]

6. Dimethirimol (Milcurb)

Dimethirimol is metabolized by three pathways in dogs and rats. In rat, the most important metabolic pathway is the formation of 4-(2-hydroxy-4-amino-6-methylpyrimidinyl) butan-2-ol (I) which represents about 20% of the metabolite excreted in urine and 1% in bile. The formation of this product takes places via two intermediates, the 4-(2-hydroxy-4-dimethylamino-6-methylpyrimidinyl) butan-2-ol (III) and the 4-(2-hydroxy-4-methylamino 6-methylpyrimidinyl) butan-2-ol (II). Metabolite II represents 16% in urine and 4% in bile while metabolite III is only found in urine (24% of the dose). A second metabolic pathway is the formation of dimethirimol glucuronide (IV) which represents 2% in the urine and 11% in the bile. The third pathway is the formation of the 2-amino-4-hydroxy-5-n-butyl-6-methylpyrimidine (VI) via the intermediate 2-methylamino-4-hydroxy-5-n-butyl-6-methylpyrimidine (V). Metabolite VI represents 13% of the dose in urine and 3% in bile while metabolite V represents 2% in bile and urine. In dog, unchanged dimethirimol is found in urine (1%) and bile (2%); metabolite I represents 6% in urine and 6% in feces; metabolite II 11 and 3%; metabolite III 21 and 4%; metabolite IV is found only in bile and represents 4% of the administered dose; metabolite V represents 6% in the urine and 2% in bile, and metabolite VI represents 7 and 8% respectively. In dog, another metabolite is formed from metabolite IV, the 4-(2-oxo-3-N-methyl-4-amino-6-methylpyrimidinyl) butan-2-ol which represents 3% of the excreted dose in urine.[341]

In rat, 8 days after an oral dose of (2-^{14}C)-dimethirimol, 87.2% of the radioactivity was found in urine and 10.9% in feces. In dogs, 4 days after an oral dose of (2-^{14}C) dimethirimol, 88.6% was found in urine and 9% in feces. In rats unchanged dimethirimol was not detected in urine but represented only 1% of the dose in bile.

7. Carboxin (Vitavax)

Carboxin is absorbed almost completely in rabbits but poorly so in rat. After an oral dose of ^{14}C-carboxin, 90% of the radioactivity is detected in urine of rabbits in 24 h. Unchanged carboxin represents 10% of the dose in feces and 2% in urine. In rats, during the same period, 40% of the dose is excreted as unchanged carboxin in feces and 15% in urine and only traces of radioactivity are found in tissues after 48 h. The major metabolic

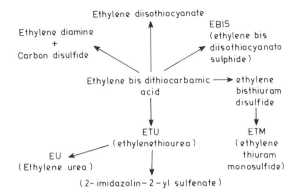

FIGURE 10.   General metabolic pathways of ethylene-*bis*-(dithiocarbamates).

pathway in rat and rabbit is found to be hydroxylation of phenyl ring of the carboxin. Rabbits
hydroxylate 88% of the dose while rats hydroxylate 39% only. The P- and O-hydroxycar-
boxins are excreted in urine as glucuronide in rabbits (62 and 10% of the dose) and rats (26
and 6%). Only traces of the m-isomer conjugate are detected in urine. Free p-isomer is also
detected in feces of rats but not of rabbits.[342] The sulfoxide of the carboxin or of its
hydroxylated derivative is detected in urine of rats and dogs.[343]

8. Pencycuron

Pencycuron is a fungicide used to control plant diseases caused by *Rhizoctoniasolani*.
Eight urinary metabolites and 3 metabolites in both feces and urine are detected in rabbit
exposed to pencycuron. The major urinary metabolites are 1-(*p*-chlorobenzyl)-1-cyclopentyl-
3-(*p*-hydroxyphenyl) urea as free and glucuronide conjugate. In addition, decyclopentylation,
hydroxylation on the 3 position of the cyclopentyl moiety as well as tiol formation and
thiomethylation of the phenyl ring. Glucuronides of these products have also been detected.
Furthermore, a significant amount of pencycuron was also found in feces of the treated
animal.[344]

9. Quinomethionate (Chinomethionat, Morestan)

Quinomethionate is metabolized into 6-methyl-2,3-quinoxalinedithiol plus traces of its
hydroxylated analog.[345] Quinomethionate forms a complex with plasma proteins and particularly with albumins. Studies have shown that absorption and toxicokinetics of quinomethionate in rats are modified by nutrition, particularly by the protein and lipid content of
the diet.[346-348]

10. Ethylene-*bis*-dithiocarbamates

Ethylene-*bis*-dithiocarbamates constitute one of the most important classes of fungicides.
In this group, the most important compounds are maneb, zineb, nabam, mancozeb, and
metiram. The metabolic pathways of these fungicides have been described in several studies.[349]
A general scheme of the metabolism of these products is presented in Figure 10.

Nabam is metabolized *in vivo* and *in vitro* yielding ETU, EBIS, ethylene diamine carbon
hydrogen disulfide, and ethylene diisothiocyanate.[351,352] When ^{14}C-maneb is administered
to rats, 55% of the radioactivity is excreted in feces and urine within 5 days.[353] ^{14}C-maneb
is metabolized in rats into ETU, EBIS, ethylenediamine, and some other unidentified products. ^{14}C-zineb in rat is metabolized into CS_2, sulfur, ETU, and EBIS.[354] Only a small
percentage of an orally administered dose of ^{14}C-maneb and ^{14}C-zineb is excreted in urine
of mice. The major metabolites are ETU and EU which represent both 15% of the radioactivity

and some other more polar products than EU.[355] In animals, mancozeb is metabolized into EBIS, ETU, ethylenediamine, EU, *N*-formyl-ethylene diamine, and *N*-acetyl ethylenediamine.[356]

In rats 73% of the radioactivity from ^{14}C-ETU is excreted in urine during the first 24 h following an oral administration.[357] While 47% is excreted during the same period in guinea pig and mouse[358,359] *in vivo* studies in rats have shown that ETU represents 95% of the urinary metabolites in rats. ETU is metabolized into EU in mice and represents 40% of the metabolites in mouse urine. In mice, ETU is metabolized into EU and 2-imidazolin-2-yl-sulfonate after oxidation of the sulfur atom.[360]

In Rhesus monkey, the major route of ^{14}C-ETU excretion is through urine with an average of 55% of radioactivity.[361]

Dithiocarbamates essentially include Ferbam and Thiram. Ziram is retained for longer periods in rats; 6 days after administration, only a part of the ingested Ziram had been excreted through exhalation or in urine. The largest concentrations of Ziram metabolites are observed in spleen except for carbon disulfide and dimethyldithiocarbamic acid which were found in lung.[362] Approximately 40 to 70% of an oral dose of ^{35}S-Ferbam or ^{14}C-Ferbam is absorbed from the intestinal tract of the rat 24 h after dosing. Most of the absorbed ^{14}C is excreted into urine (42.9%) and bile (1.4%).[363]

11. 2,4-D and 2,4,5-T

The metabolism of phenoxy herbicides has been discussed by Leng.[364] The phenoxy acids, salts, and esters are rapidly absorbed from the gut and widely distributed in tissues. Phenoxy esters are rapidly hydrolyzed in animals, into the corresponding acids which are reversibly bound to plasma protein. Phenoxy acids are rapidly excreted in urine as unchanged or conjugated with glucuronic acid. Metabolism may also occur at high dosage and the rate of clearance from the organism is dependent on the dose level. Rate of formation and elimination of the phenol metabolites from the body depends on dosage levels and on chemical structure of phenoxy compounds administered to the animals.

About 96% of an oral dose of ^{14}C-2,4-D is eliminated as unchanged 2,4-D from sheep within 72 h and nearly 100% from rats within 144 h. After oral administration of ^{14}C-2,4-D to sheep, the level in blood was found to be highest 75 min later and no radioactivity was detected after 24 hr. Urine was the main route of excretion. About 5% of 2,4-D was found 8 h after administration while 90 and 96% were seen 28 and 72 h after, respectively. Only 1% of the radioactivity was found to be present in feces.[365] In goat, a low plasma level of 2,4-D (less than 20 μg/ml) was bound to plasma proteins.[366]

The metabolism of 2,4,5-T in animals has been studied by different workers.[367-369] In dairy cows unchanged 2,4,5-T was detected in urine.[368] Rats and dogs showed different halflives which has been partly due to the differences in the rate of renal excretion of the compound.[369] In rat after i.v. injection, 15.7% of 2,4,5-T is excreted in bile and 4% in urine.[370] Studies of pregnant mice have shown that 2,4,5-T crosses the transplacental barriers with rapid elimination, largely in urine.[371,372] A two-compartment pharmacokinetic model demonstrated saturate renal transport and extensive enterohepatic circulation operating in the distribution and elimination of 2,4,5-T.[373]

12. Trifluralin and Related Compounds

In rats given a single oral dose of ^{14}C-trifluralin 80% of the radioactivity is excreted in the feces while the remaining portion appeared in urine. Trifluralin and N,N'-dipropyl-3-nitro-5-trifluoromethyl-O-phenylenediamine, the amino derivative of fluralin were identified in the feces. Three urinary products isolated and identified are the α,α,α-trifluoro-2,6-dinitro-*p*-toluidine, the α,α,α-trifluoro-5-nitrotoluene-3,4-diamine, and the α,α,α-trifluoro-5-nitro-N-propyl-toluene-3,4-diamine. Another possible metabolite is the α,α,α—trifluoro-2,6-dinitro-N-propyl-*p*-toluidine.[374]

Studies using rat liver microsomes show that trifluralin is extensively metabolized by hydroxylation of the propyl residues and/or N-dealkylation. The most important metabolite is the benzimidazole which is formed via oxidation and reduction processes of the α,α,α-trifluoro-2,6-dinitro-N-ethyl-p-toluidine. Traces of the α,α,α-trifluoro-5-nitrotoluene-3,4-diamine are detected that put in evidence the reductive processes.[375]

Rats show that 72 h after administration of ^{14}C-nitralin, 99.8% of the radioactivity is recovered in excreta. Most of the radioactivity is equally distributed between urine and feces and about 1.5% is found in carcass, skin, and intestine. Analysis of urinary metabolites showed that metabolism proceeds via a complex series of biotransformation involving nitro group reduction, side chain oxidation with the formation of a variety of heterocyclic ring structures. Twenty nine metabolites have been identified in urine but the major metabolite is 7-amino-2-ethyl-5-methyl-sulphonyl-1-propylbenzimidazole which accounts for only 3% of the administered dose.[376]

13. Asulam (Asulox)

Asulam is rapidly excreted in urine and feces of the rat after oral or intravenous administration. In both cases, 75 to 100% of the radioactivity of (ring ^{14}C)-asulam is excreted in urine in 24 h as unchanged asulam (61 to 74%), N^4-acetylsulfanilamide (0.1 to 2.6%).[377]

14. Propham

In rats and goats the urinary metabolites of propham include the sulfate ester of isopropyl 4-hydroxycarbanilate, the glucuronide acid conjugate of isopropyl 4-hydroxycarbanilate, the sulfate ester of 4-hydroxyacetanilide, and other minor unidentified metabolites.[378] The biological halflife of propham in some tissues was short, ranging between 3 and 8 h.[379]

15. Chlorpropham

In rats, the major metabolic pathway of chlorpropham is via p-hydroxylation. After administration of an oral dose of (chain) or (ring ^{14}C)-chlorpropham to rats, 55 and 82.6% of the dose are respectively excreted in urine. p-Hydroxylation is the major metabolic reaction of chlorpropham giving rise to 4 hydroxychlorpropham which is excreted as sulfo- and glucuro-conjugate. The inhibition of sulfoconjugation activity is compensated by an increase of the glucuroconjugation activity whereas the selective inhibition of the glucuroconjugation is not balanced by an increase of the sulfoconjugated derivatives excretion.[380] About 35% of the administered chlorpropham undergoes a hydrolysis of the carbamate group with liberation of m-chloroaniline of isopropanol and CO_2. The formed m-chloraniline would be hydroxylated in o- or p- before being excreted as conjugated derivatives. An hydroxylation of the lateral chain, leading to the formation of 1-hydroxy-2-propyl chlorpropham and then to 1,3-hydroxy-chlorpropham or 1-carboxy-1-ethyl chlorpropham, is also considered as a minor pathway of metabolism.[381]

16. Benthiocarb

Benthiocarb is rapidly absorbed in mice and excreted in 48 h mainly as acidic metabolites in urine (80%), feces (5%), and expired air (1%). The major urinary metabolites are p-chlorohippuric acid (49%), p-chlorobenzoic acid (9%), and traces of p-chlorobenzyl alcohol.[382]

17. Molinate

The major metabolic pathways of molinate involve sulfoxidation and conjugation with glutathione, yielding a mercapturic acid which represents 35.4% of the urinary radioactivity. Ring hydroxylation gives the 3- and 4-hydroxymolinate derivatives which are excreted as free (0.8%) and conjugated (26.1%) compounds. Hydroxylation in the 2-position of the ring and subsequent ring cleavage represents a minor pathway. Hexamethyleneimine (14.6%) and 3- and 4-hydroxyhexamethyleneimine (10.3%) are the major metabolites formed on hydrolysis of sulfoxidized molinate and its hydroxy derivatives. Molinate is degraded by rats and metabolites are excreted in urine.[54]

18. Triazine

The metabolic studies on the s-triazines have been investigated in rats and rabbits and several metabolites are isolated and identified, all retaining the triazine ring intact. Oxidative N-dealkylation is the common metabolic pathway, while simazine yields three metabolites and atrazine yields seven metabolites. Propazine and prometone form three metabolites each, and prometryn has given two metabolites.[383]

19. Terbutryne (Terbutryn, Prebane, Clarosan)

The metabolism of terbutryne in rat and goat is by one or more of the following reactions: S-demethylation, conversion of the methylthio group to a hydroxy group, N-deethylation, oxidation of the terminal carbon of the ethyl group to a carboxylic acid, oxidation of a terminal carbon of the t-butyl group to either an alcohol or a carboxylic acid, and conjugation with glucuronic acid. Animals treated with ^{14}C-terbutryn showed 16 metabolites in their urine and feces.[384]

20. Cyanazine (Bladex, Fortrol)

The major metabolites of cyanazine in rat urine are N-acetyl-S-(4-amino-6-(1-methyl-1-cyanoethylamino)-S-triazinyl)-L-cysteine and 2-chloro-4-amino-6-(1-methyl-1-cyanoethylamino)-S-triazine. Mercapturic acid formation and N-dealkylation are the most important metabolic pathways for cyanazine in rats. Rat urine contains small amounts of the non-dealkylated mercapturic acid and two products of biotransformation of the cyano group, the amine and the 2-hydroxy derivative of the carboxylic acid, which is the major fecal metabolite. In bile two metabolites conjugated with glutathione; the reactive products of glutathione with cyanazine and with its N-deethyl derivative have also been detected.[385]

21. Substituted ureas

Monuron, monolinuron, diuron, and linuron are the substituted ureas. The major metabolites are the completely demethylated compounds and to a minor extent the monomethylated or the methoxylated derivatives. Dealkylation is more important with the dimethyl compounds monuron and diuron than with their methylmethoxy analogs. Monuron and monolinuron are found to be hydroxylated in o- and to a smaller extent in the m-position. Diuron and linuron are hydroxylated in o-position and to a minor extent in the C adjacent to the m-chlorine. All these phenolic metabolites are excreted in urine as glucuro- or sulfoconjugate derivative.[386,387] The metabolism of diuron in rats and dogs shows that tissue residue levels are proportional to the dietary intake but without tissue storage. Excretion is both through feces and urine.[388,389]

The major metabolic pathway of monolinuron is the hydroxylation at the N-methyl group, yielding the N-methylol and then N-demethylated derivatives. p-Chlorophenylurea and its hydroxylated analog are also detected.[390] In pig, monolinuron and its metabolites are mainly excreted in urine. A significant difference has been found in the products of biotransformation formed *in vivo* and *in vitro*. Although the metabolites generated from the aliphatic moiety of monolinuron are found to be identical both in intact and in perfused livers, no aryl hydroxylated products in the o- and m-position could be identified in any of the perfusion experiments with liver of rats.[391]

22. Paraquat and Diquat

Paraquat and diquat show differences in tissue distribution and excretion.[392,393] It has been shown that the labeled paraquat is rapidly distributed throughout the tissue of rats and guinea pig fetuses within 30 min after the administration.[394] Low doses of paraquat (30 to 50 µg/kg) by i.v. injection to dog caused rapid excretion in urine, while larger doses (20 mg/kg) produced renal function impairment and renal failure. The plasma concentration curve and paraquat elimination followed a three-compartment model.[395,396] Several *in vivo* and *in vitro* studies have shown that the uptake and retention of paraquat in the lungs of animals is an energy dependent process[397,398] and is also mediated through the formation of the superoxide ion eventually leading to lipid peroxidation.[399-401]

REFERENCES

1. **Jakoby, W. B.,** *Enzymatic Basis of Detoxication,* Vol. 1, Academic Press, London, 1980.
2. **Ullrich, V., Roots, A., Hildebrandt, A., Estabrook, R. W., and Conney, A. H.,** *Microsomes and Drug Oxydations,* Pergamon Press, Oxford, 1971.
3. **Parke, D. V. and Smith, R. L., Eds.,** *Drug Metabolism,* Taylor and Francis, London, 1976.
4. **Ziegler, D. M.,** Microsomal flavin containing monooxygenation of nucleophilic nitrogen and sulfur compounds, in *Enzymatic Basis of Detoxification,* Vol. 1, Jacoby, W. B., Academic Press, London, 1980, 201.
5. **Leeling, N. C. and Casida, J. E.,** Metabolites of carbaryl (1-naphthyl methyl carbamate) in mammals and enzymatic systems for their formation, *J. Agric. Food Chem.,* 14, 281, 1966.
6. **Nordblom, G. D. and Coon, M. J.,** Hydrogen peroxide formation and stoichiometry of hydroxylation reactions catalyzed by highly purified level microsomal cytochrome p-450, *Arch. Biochem. Biophys.,* 180, 343, 1977.
7. **Stein, K., Portig, G., and Koransky, W.,** Oxidative transformation of hexachlorocyclohexane in rats and with rat liver microsomes, *Arch. Pharmacol.,* 298, 115, 1977.
8. **Khuhr, R. J. and Dorough, H. W.,** *Carbamate Insecticides, Chemistry, Biochemistry and Toxicology,* CRC Press, Boca Raton, FL., 1976.
9. **Emmerson, J. L. and Anderson, R. C.,** Metabolism of trifluralin in the rat and dog, *Toxicol. Appl. Pharmacol.,* 9, 84, 1986.
10. **Bull, D. L.,** Metabolism of organophosphorus insecticides, Natl. Meet. Entomol. Soc. Am., Miami, FL, 1970.
11. **Berzins, F., Blomberg, F., Kjellgren, M., Smyth, C., and Wadstrom, T.,** Crossed immunoelectron-focusing in combination with a zimozan method: studies on esterase active antigens solubilized from rat liver microsomes, *FEBS Lett.,* 61, 77, 1976.
12. **Raffeld, M. and Berzins, K.,** Sex differences in the pattern of esterase active antigens in microsomes from various rat strains, *Biochem. Biophys. Acta,* 499, 24, 1977.
13. **Hinderer, R. K. and Menzer, R. E.,** Comparative enzyme activities and cytochrome p-450 levels of some rat tissue with respect to their metabolism of several pesticides, *Pestic. Biochem. Physiol.,* 6, 148, 1976.
14. **Brooks, G. T. and Harrison, A.,** Hydrolation of HEOD (dieldrin) and the heptachlor epoxides by microsomes from the livers of pigs and rabbits, *Bull. Environ. Contam. Toxicol.,* 4, 352, 1969.
15. **Davidow, B. and Radomski, J. L.,** Isolation of an epoxide metabolite from fat tissues of dogs fed heptachlor, *J. Pharmacol. Exp. Ther.,* 107, 259, 1953.
16. **Tashiro, S. and Matsumura, F.,** Metabolism of trans-nonachlor and related chlordane components in rat and man, *Arch. Environ. Contam. Toxicol.,* 7, 113, 1978.
17. **Bentley, P. and Oesch, F.,** Enzymic mechanisms of oxidation, reduction and hydrolysis in *Foreign Compounds Metabolism in Mammals. Special Periodical Report of the Chemical Society,* 1979, 1989, chap. 2 and 5.
18. **O'Brien, R. D.,** *Insecticides Action and Metabolism,* Academic Press, New York, 1967.
19. **Melnikov, N. N.,** *Chemistry of Pesticides:* Springer-Verlag, New York, 1971, 59.
20. **Eto, M.,** *Organophosphorus Pesticides: Organic and Biological Chemistry,* CRC Press, Cleveland, Ohio, 1974.
21. **Nakatsugawa, T., Tolman, N. M., and Dalam, P. A.,** Degradation of parathion in the rat, *Biochem. Pharmacol.,* 18, 1103, 1969.
22. **Kamataki, T., Belcher, D. H., and Neal, R. A.,** Studies of the metabolism of diethyl p-nitrophenyl phosphorothionate (parathion) and benzphetamine using an apparently homogenous preparation of rat liver, cytochrome p-450: effect of a cytochrome p-450 antibody preparation, *Mol. Pharmacol.,* 12, 921, 1976.

23. **Davis, J. E. and Mende, T. J.,** A study of the binding of sulfur to rat liver chromosomes which occurs concurrently with the metabolism of o,o-diethyl o-p-nitrophenyl phosphorothioate (parathion), o,o,o-diethyl o-p nitrophenylphosphate (paraoxon), *J. Pharmacol.,* 201, 409, 1977.

24. **Sundroik, G., Hutzinger, O., Safe, S., and Platonow, N.,** The metabolism of p,p′-DDT and p,p′-DDE in the pig, in *Fate of Pesticides in Large Animals,* Ivie, G. and Dorough, H., Eds., Academic Press, New York, 1977, 175.

25. **Addison, R. F. and Willis, D. E.,** The metabolism by rainbow trout *(Salmo gairdnerii)* of p,p′-(^{14}C) DDT and some of its possible degradation products labeled with ^{14}C, *Toxicol. Appl. Pharmacol.,* 43, 303, 1978.

26. **Hornish, R. E. and Nappier, J. L.,** Excretion and metabolism of 3,4,5-tribromo N,N-α-trimethyl-1H-pyrazole-1-acetamide in the rat, *J. Agric. Food Chem.,* 26, 1083, 1978.

27. **March, R. B., Metcalf, R. L., Fukuru, T. R., and Maxon, M. G.,** Metabolism of Systox in the white mouse and American cockroach, *J. Econ. Entomol.,* 48, 355, 1955.

28. **Huhtanen, K. and Dorough, H. W.,** Isomerization and Beckman rearrangement reactions in the metabolism of methomyl in rats, *Pest Biochem. Phys.,* 6, 571, 1976.

29. **Elespuru, R. K. and Lijinsky, W.,** The formation of carcinogenic nitroso compounds from nitrite and some types of agricultural chemicals, *Food Cosmet. Toxicol.,* 11, 807, 1973.

30. **Wolfe, N. L., Fepp, R. D., Gordon, J. A., and Fincher, R. C.,** N-Nitrosamine formation from atrazine, *Bull. Environ. Contam. Toxicol.,* 15, 342, 1976.

31. **Eisenbrand, G., Ungerer, O., and Preussman, R.,** Rapid formation of carcinogenic N-nitrosamine by interaction of nitrite with fungicides derived from dithiocarbamic acid *in vitro* under simulated gastric conditions and *in vivo* in the rat stomach, *Food Cosmet. Toxicol.,* 12, 229, 1974.

32. **Lijinsky, W. and Schmahl, D.,** Carcinogenesis by nitroso derivatives of methylcarbamate insecticides and other nitrosamides in rats and mice, *Int. Agency Res. Cancer Sci. Publ.,* 19, 495, 1978.

33. **Seiler, J. P.,** Nitrosation *in vitro* and *in vivo* by sodium nitrite, and mutagenicity of nitrogenous pesticides, *Mutat. Res.,* 48, 225, 1977.

34. **Uchiyama, M., Takeda, M., Suzuki, T., and Yoshikawa, K.,** Mutagenicity of nitroso derivatives of N-methylcarbamate insecticides in microbiological methods, *Bull. Environ. Contam. Toxicol.,* 14, 389, 1975.

35. **Rickard, R. and Dorough, H. W.,** *In vivo* synthesis of 1-naphthyl N-methyl-nitrosocarbamate (nitroso-carbaryl) in the rat and guinea pig, *Pharmacologist,* 20, 146, 1978.

36. **Clayson, D. B.,** Nutrition and experimental carcinogenis. A review, *Cancer Res.,* 35, 3292, 1975.

37. **Dorough, H. W.,** Biological activity of pesticide conjugates, in *Bound and Conjugated Pesticide Residues,* Kaufman, D., Still, G., Paulson, G., and Bandal, S., Eds., American Chemical Society, Washington, D.C., Symposium Series, 29, 1976, 11.

38. **Dorough, H.W.,** Metabolism of insecticides by conjugation mechanisms, *Pharmacol. Ther.,* 4, 433, 1979.

39. **Dorough, H. W.,** Conjugation reactions of pesticides and their metabolites with sugars, in *Advances in Pesticide Science,* Part 3, Geissbuhler, H., Ed., Pergamon Press, New York, 1979, 526.

40. **Mulder, G. J.,** Sulfatation of Drug and Related Compounds, CRC Press, Boca Raton, FL., 1981.

41. **Smith, J. N.,** The comparative metabolism of xenobiotics, *Adv. Comp. Physiol. Biochem.,* 3, 173, 1968.

42. **Jenner, P. and Testa, B.,** Novel pathways in drug metabolism, *Xenobiotica,* 8, 1, 1978.

43. **Dorough, H. W.,** Metabolism of insecticidal methylcarbamates in animals, *J. Agric. Food Chem.,* 18, 1015, 1970.

44. **Miettinen, T. A. and Leskinen, E.,** Glucuronic acid pathway in, *Metabolic Conjugation and Metabolic Hydrolysis,* Vol. 1, Fishman, W., Ed., Academic Press, New York, 1970, 157.

45. **Williams, R. T.,** The biogenesis of conjugation and detoxification products, in *Biogenesis of Natural Compounds,* Bernfelf, P., Ed., Pergamon Press, Oxford, 1967, 427.

46. **Menzer, R. E.,** Biological oxidation and conjugation of pesticidal chemical, *Residue Rev.,* 48, 79, 1973.

47. **Miller, E. C. and Miller, J. A.,** *Progress in Liver Diseases,* Popper, H. and Schaffner, F., Eds., Grune and Stratton, New York, 1976, 5, 699.

48. **Esser, H. O., Mucke, W., and Alt, K. O.,** Der Abbau des Insektizides GS 13005 in der Ratte. Strukturaufklarung der wichtgsten Metabolite, *Helv. Chim. Acta,* 51, 513, 1968.

49. **Metivier, J.,** Chemical structure and biological activity relationship. Mode of action and selectivity of insecticides and acaricides, in *Pesticides Chemistry Proceedings. Second International IUPAC Congress,* Tahori, A. S., Ed., Gordon and Breach, London, 1972, 325.

50. **Cage, J. C.,** Metabolism of menazon (o,o-dimethyl S-(4,6-diamino-S-triazin-2-ylmethyl)-phosphorodithioate) in the rat, *Food Cosmet. Toxicol.,* 5, 349, 1967.

51. **Dupuis, G., Muecke, W., and Esser, H. O.,** Metabolic behaviour of the insecticidal phosphorus ester GS 13005, *J. Econ. Entomol.,* 64, 588, 1971.

52. **Mc Bain, J. B., Hoffman, L. J., and Menn, J. J.,** Dyfonate metabolism studies. II. Metabolic pathway of o-ethyl S-phenyl ethylphosphorodithioate in rats, *Pest Biochem. Physiol.,* 1, 356, 1971.

53. **Mc Bain, J. B. and Menn, J. J.,** S-methylation, oxidation, hydroxylation and conjugation of thiophenol in the rat, *Biochem. Pharmacol.,* 18, 2282, 1969.

54. **Williams, R. T.,** *Detoxification Mechanism,* 2nd ed., John Wiley and Sons, New York, 1959, 520.
55. **Debaun, J. R., Bova, D. L., Tseng, C. K., and Menn, J. J.,** Metabolism of (ring ^{14}C) ordram (Molinate) in the rat. 2. Urinary metabolite identification, *J. Agric. Food Chem.,* 26, 1098, 1978.
56. **Ando, M., Nakagawa, M., Nakamura, T., and Tomita, K.,** Metabolism of isoxathion o,o-diethyl o-(5-phenyl-3-isoxazolyl) phosphorothioate in the rats, *Agric. Biol. Chem.,* 30, 803, 1975.
57. **Hutson, D. H.,** Glutathione conjugates in, *Bound and Conjugated Pesticide* Symposium Series 29, American Chemical Society, Washington, D.C., 1976, 103.
58. **Usui, K., Shishido, T., and Fukami, J.,** Glutathione S-transferase of rat liver active on organophosphorus triesters, *Agric. Biol. Chem.,* 41, 2491, 1977.
59. **Yang, R. S. H., Hodgson, E., and Dauterman, W. C.,** Metabolism *in vitro* of diazinon and diazoxon in rat liver, *J. Agric. Food Chem.,* 19, 10, 1971.
60. **Crawford, M. J., Hutson, D. H., and King, P. A.,** Metabolic demethylation of the insecticide dimethylvinphos in rats, in dogs and *in vitro,* Xenobiotica, 6, 745, 1976.
61. **Roncucci, R., Verry, M., and Jeanniot, J. P.,** Interactions between nutrition, food, and drugs in man, *Wld. Rev. Nutr. Diet,* 43, 140, 1984.
62. **Durham, W. F.,** The interaction of pesticides with other factors, *Residue Rev.,* 18, 21, 1967.
63. **Quinn, G. P., Axelrod, J., and Brodie, B. B.,** Species, strain and sex differences in metabolism of hexobarbitone, amidopyrine and aniline, *Biochem. Pharmacol.,* 1, 152, 1958.
64. **Cram, R. L., Juchau, M. R., and Fouts, J. R.,** Differences in hepatic drug metabolism in various rabbit strains before and after pretreatment with phenobarbital, *Proc. Soc. Exp. Biol. Med.,* 118, 872, 1965.
65. **Chhabra, R. S. and Fouts, J. R.,** Stimulation of hepatic drug metabolizing enzymes by DDT, polycyclic hydrocarbons or phenobarbital in adrenalilectonized or castrated mice, *Toxicol. Appl. Pharmacol.,* 28, 465, 1974.
66. **Wassermann, M., Gon, M., Wassermann, D., and Zellermayer, L.,** DDT and DDE in body fat of people in Israel, *Arch. Environ. Health,* 11, 375, 1965.
67. **Hayes, W. J. Jr., Dale, W. E., and Burse, V. W.,** Chlorinated hydrocarbon pesticides in the fat on people in New Orleans, *Life Sci.,* 4, 1611, 1965.
68. **Brodeur, J. and Du Bois, K. P.,** Comparison of acute toxicity of anticholinesterase insecticides to weanling and adult male rats, *Proc. Soc. Expt. Biol. Med.,* 114, 509, 1963.
69. **Lu, F. C., Jessup, D. C., and Lavellee, A.,** Toxicity of pesticides in young rats versus adult rats, *Food Cosmet. Toxicol.,* 3, 591, 1965.
70. **Dutton, G. J. and Burchell, B.,** Newer aspects of glucuronidation, *Prog. Drug Metab.,* 2, 1, 1977.
71. **Dutton, G. J.,** Developmental aspects of drug conjugation, *Annu. Rev. Pharmcol. Toxicol.,* 18, 17, 1978.
72. **Conney, A. H. and Burns, J. J.,** Factors influencing drug metabolism, *Adv. Pharm.,* 1, 31, 1962.
73. **Murphy, S. D. and Du Bois, K. P.,** Enzymatic conversion of the dimethoxy ester of benzotriazine dithiophosphoric acid to an anticholinesterase agent, *J. Pharmacol. Expt. Ther.,* 119, 572, 1957.
74. **Truhaut, R. and Ferrando, R., Eds.,** *Toxicology and Nutrition,* World Review of Nutrition and Dietetics, S. Karger, Basel, 1978, 29.
75. **Debry, G.,** *Nutrition Food and Drug Interactions in Man,* World Review of Nutrition and Dietetics, S. Karger, Basel, 1984, 43.
76. **Boyd, E. M.,** *Protein Deficiency and Pesticide Toxicity,* Charles Thomas, Springfield, IL, 1972.
77. **Dixon, R. L., Shultice, R. W., and Fouts, J. R.,** Factors affecting drug metabolism by liver microsomes. IV. Starvation, *Proc. Soc. Expt. Biol. Med.,* 103, 333, 1960.
78. **Boyd, E. M. and Krijnen, C. J.,** Toxicity of dicophanae (DDT) in relation to dietary protein intake, *Ind. Med. Surg.,* 39, 229, 1970.
79. **Boyd, E. M., Du Bois, I., and Krijnen, J.,** Endosulfan toxicity and dietary protein, *Arch. Environ. Health,* 21, 15, 1970.
80. **Chadwick, R. W., Cranmer, M. F., and Peoples, A. J.,** Metabolic alterations in the squirrel monkey induced by DDT administration and ascorbic acid deficiency, *Toxicol. Appl. Pharmacol.,* 20, 308, 1971.
81. **Craig, F. N., Rales, P. D., and Frankel, H. M.,** Lethality of sarin in a warm environment, *J. Pharmacol. Exp. Ther.,* 127, 35, 1959.
82. **Frawley, J. P., Cook, J. W., Blake, J. R., and Fitzhugh, O. G.,** Insecticide stability effect of light on chemical and biological properties of parathion, *J. Agric. Food Chem.,* 6, 28, 1958.
83. **Gaines, T. B.,** The acute toxicity of pesticides to rats, *Toxicol. Appl. Pharmacol.,* 14, 515, 1969.
84. **Kimmerle, G. and Lorke, D.,** Toxicity of insecticidal organophosphate, Bayer-21, *Farbenfabricken,* Bayer AG, Leverkusen, 1968.
85. **Frawley, J. P., Fuyat, H. N., Hagan, E. C., Blake, J. R., and Fitzhugh, O. G.,** Marked potentiation in mammalian toxicity from simultaneous administration of two anticholinesterase compounds, *J. Pharmacol. Exp. Ther.,* 121, 96, 1957.
86. **Murphy, S. D., Anderson, R. L., and Du Bois, K. P.,** Potentiation of toxicity of malathion by triorthotolylphosphate, *Proc. Soc. Expt. Biol. Med.,* 100, 483, 1959.

87. **Ottoboni, A. and Ferguson, J. I.,** Evidence for conversion of DDT to TDE in rat liver, I. Liver/body fat ratios of TDE, *Bull. Environ. Contam. Toxicol.,* 3, 296, 1968.

88. **Ottoboni, A., Gee, R., Stanley, R. L., and Goetz, M. E.,** Evidence for conversion of p,p'-DDT to p,p'-DDT to p,p'-TDE in rat liver. II. Conversion of p,p'-DDT to p,p'-TDE in axenix rats, *Bull. Environ. Contam. Toxicol.,* 3, 302, 1968.

89. **Hassal, K. A.,** Species and sex differences in the reductive dechlorination of DDT by supplemented liver preparations, *Pestic. Biochem. Physiol.,* 5, 126, 1975.

90. **Datta, P. R. and Nelson, J. M.,** p,p'-DDT detoxication by isolated perfused rat liver and kidney, *Ind. Med. Surg.,* 39, 190, 1970.

91. **Datta, P. R., Lang, P., and Klein, A. K.,** Conversion of p,p'-DDT to p,p'-DDD in the liver of the rat, *Science,* 145, 1052, 1964.

92. **Peterson, J. E. and Robison, W. H.,** Metabolic products of p,p'-DDT in the rat, *Toxicol. Appl. Pharmacol.,* 6, 321, 1964.

93. **Woolley, D. E. and Talens, G. M.,** Distribution of DDT, DDD and DDE in tissues of neonatal rats and in milk and other tissues of mother rats chronically exposed to DDT, *Toxicol. Appl. Pharmacol.,* 18, 907, 1971.

94. **Fang, S. C., Fallin, E., and Freed, V. H.,** Maternal transfer of ^{14}C p,p'-DDT *via* placenta and milk and its metabolism in infant rats, *Arch. Environ. Contam. Toxicol.,* 5, 427, 1977.

95. **Krechniak, J. and Hawk, R. E.,** Fate of DDT in the organism. III. Distribution and elimination of DDT and its metabolites in rats treated with DDT in their diet, *Bromatol. Chem. Toksykol.,* 7, 481, 1974.

96. **Esaac, E. G. and Matsumura, F.,** Mechanism of reductive dechlorination of DDT by rat liver microsomes, *Pestic. Biochem. Physiol.,* 13, 81, 1980.

97. **Esaac, E. G. and Matsumura, F.,** Metabolism of insecticides by reductive systems in *Differential Toxicities of Insecticides and Halogenated Aromatics,* Matsumura, F., Ed., Pergammon Press, Oxford, *Encyc. Pharm. Ther.,* 113, 265, 1984.

98. **Baker, M. T. and van Dyke, R. A.,** Metabolism dependent binding of the chlorinated insecticide DDT and its metabolite DDD, to microsomal protein and lipids, *Biochem. Pharmacol.,* 33, 255, 1984.

99. **Burns, E. C., Dahm, P. A., and Lindquist, D. A.,** Secretion of DDT metabolites in the bile of rats, *J. Pharmacol. Exp. Ther.,* 121, 55, 1957.

100. **Jensen, J. A., Cueto, C., Dale, W. E., Rothe, C. F., Pearce, G. W., and Mattson, A. M.,** DDT metabolites in feces and bile of rats, *J. Agric. Food Chem.,* 5, 919, 1957.

101. **Pinto, J. D., Camien, M. N., and Dunn, M. S.,** Metabolic fate of p,p'-DDT in rats, *J. Biol. Chem.,* 240, 2148, 1965.

102. **Gingell, R.,** Enterohepatic circulation of bis(chlorophenyl) acetic acid in rat, *Drug Metab. Disp.,* 3, 42, 1975.

103. **Fail, V. J., Lamoureux, C. H., Styrvoky, E., Zaylskie, R. G., Thacker, E. J., and Holman, G. M.,** Metabolism of p,p'-DDT in rats, *J. Agric. Food Chem.,* 21, 1072, 1973.

104. **Reif, V. D. and Sinsheimer, J. E.,** Metabolism of o,p'-DDT in rats, *Drug Metab. Disp.,* 3, 15, 1975.

105. **Sundstrom, G.,** Metabolic hydroxylation of the aromatic rings of 1,1-dichloro-2,2-bis-(4-chlorophenyl)ethylene (p,p'-DDE) by the rat, *J. Agric. Food Chem.,* 25, 18, 1977.

106. **Kujawa, M., Macholz, R. M., Plass, R., Knoll, R., and Engst, R.,** The enzymatic degradation of DDT. 3. Metabolism of DDT, *Nahrung,* 29, 405, 1985.

107. **Kujawa, M., Macholz, R. M., and Lewerens, H. J.,** The enzymatic degradation of DDT. 4. Degradation of DDD, *Nahrung,* 29, 411, 1985.

108. **Gold, B. and Brunk, G.,** Metabolism of 1,1,1-trichloro-2,2-bis(p-chlorophenyl)ethane and 1,1-dichloro-2,2-bis (p-chlorophenyl)ethane in the mouse, *Chem. Biol. Interact.,* 41, 327, 1982.

109. **Wallcave, L., Bronczyk, S., and Gingell, R.,** Excreted metabolites of 1,1,1-trichloro-2,2-bis (p-chlorophenyl)ethane in the mouse and hamster, *J. Agric. Food Chem.,* 22, 904, 1974.

110. **Gingell, R.,** Metabolism of ^{14}C DDT in the mouse and hamster, *Xenobiotica,* 6, 15, 1976.

111. **Gold, G. and Brunk G.,** Metabolism of 1,1,1-trichloro-2,2-bis(p-chlorophenyl)ethane (DDT), 1,1-dichloro-2,2-bis(p-chlorophenyl)ethane and 1-chloro-2,2-bis-(p-chlorophenyl) ethane in the hamster, *Cancer Res.,* 43, 2644, 1983.

112. **Fawcett, S. C., Bunyan, P. J., Huson, L. W., King, L. J., Stanley, P. I.,** Excretion of radioactivity following the intraperitoneal administration of ^{14}C-DDT, ^{14}C-DDD, ^{14}C-DDE and ^{14}C-DDMU to the rat and Japanese quail, *Bull. Environ. Contam. Toxicol.,* 27, 386, 1981.

113. **Sundstrom, G., Hutzinger, O., Safe, S., and Platonow, N.,** The metabolism of p,p'-DDT and p,p'-DDE in the pigs, in *Fate of Pesticide in Large Animals,* Ivie, G. W. and Dorough, H. W., Eds., Academic Press, New York, 1977, 175.

114. **Ahdaya, S. and Guthrie, F. E.,** Stomach absorption of intubated insecticides in fasted mice, *Toxicology,* 22, 311, 1982.

115. **Skalsky, H. L. and Guthrie, F. E.,** Binding of insecticides to human serum proteins, *Toxicol. Appl. Pharmacol.,* 43, 229, 1978.

116. **Hayes, W. J., Quinby, G. E., Walker, K. C., Elliott, J. W., and Upholt, W. M.,** Storage of DDT and DDE in people with different degrees of exposure to DDT, *Arch. Environ. Health,* 18, 398, 1958.

117. **Ericksson, P.,** Age dependent of ¹⁴C-DDT in the brain of the postnatal mouse, *Toxicol. Lett.,* 22, 323, 1984.

118. **Deichmann, W. B., Keplinger, I., Dressler, I., and Sala, F.,** Retention of dieldrin and DDT in the tissue of dogs fed aldrin and DDT individually and as a mixture, *Toxicol. Appl. Pharmacol.,* 14, 205, 1969.

119. **Lillard, D. A. and Knoles, R. K.,** Effect of forced molting and induced hyperthyroidism on the depletion of DDT residues from the laying hen, *Poultry Sci.,* 52, 222, 1973.

120. **Daha, P. R. and Nelson, M. J.,** Enhanced metabolism of methylprylon, meprobamate and chloridazepoxide hydrochloride after chronic feeding of low dietary level DDT to male and female rats, *Toxicol. Appl. Pharmacol.,* 13, 346, 1968.

121. **Durham, W. F., Ortega, P., and Hayes, W. J.,** The effect of various dietary levels of DDT on liver function, cell morphology and DDT storage in the rhesus Monkey, *Arch. Int. Pharmacodyn.,* 141, 111, 1963.

122. **Davies, J. E., Edmunson, J. E., Maceo, A., Irvin, G. L., Cassady, J., and Barquet, A.,** Reduction par la diphenylhydantoine des residus de pesticides presents dans le tissu adipeux, *Food Cosmet. Toxicol.,* 9, 413, 1971.

123. **Kapor, J. R., Metcalf, R. L., Hirwe, A. S., Lu, P. Y., Coats, J. R., and Nystrom, R. F.,** Comparative metabolism of methoxychlor, Methiochlor and DDT in mouse, insect and in a model ecosystem, *J. Agric. Food Chem.,* 18, 1145, 1970.

124. **Reynolds, P. J., Lindahl, I. L., Cecil, H. C., and Betman, J.,** A comparison of DDT and methoxychlor accumulation and depletion in sheep, *Bull. Environ. Contam. Toxicol.,* 16, 240, 1976.

125. **Davidson, K. L., Feil, V. J., and Lamoureux, C. H.,** Methoxychlor metabolism in goats, *J. Agric. Food Chem.,* 30, 130, 1982.

126. **Bulger, W. H., Temple, J. E., and Kupfer, D.,** Covalent binding of ¹⁴C methoxychlor metabolites to rat liver micrisomal components, *Toxicol. Appl. Pharmacol.,* 68, 367, 1983.

127. **Orton, T. C., Sorman, A. E., Crisp, D. N., and Sturdie, A. P.,** Dynamics of xenobiotic metabolism by isolated rat hepatocytes using a multichannel perfusion system, *Xenobiotica,* 13, 743, 1983.

128. **Forsell, J. H., Jesse, B. W., and Shull, L. R.,** A technique for isolation of bovine hepatocytes, *J. Anim. Sci.,* 60, 1597, 1985.

129. **Tee. L. B., Seddon, T., Boobis, A. R., and Davies, D. S.,** Drug metabolising activity of freshly isolated human hepatocytes, *Br. J. Clin. Pharmacol.,* 19, 279, 1985.

130. **Ludwig, G., Weis, J., and Korte, F.,** Excretion and distribution of aldrin ¹⁴C and its metabolites after oral administration of a long period of time, *Life Sci.,* 3, 123, 1964.

131. **Oda, J. and Muller, W.,** Identification of a mammalian breakdown product of dieldrin, in *Environmental Quality and Safety,* Vol. 1, Coulston, F. and Korte, F., Eds., Academic Press, New York, 1972, 248.

132. **Hutson, D. H.,** Comparative metabolism of dieldrin in the rat (CFG) and in two strains of mouse (CF1 and CACG), *Food Cosmet. Toxicol.,* 14, 577, 2976.

133. **Korte, F. and Arent, H.,** Metabolism of insecticides. Isolation and identification of dieldrin metabolites from urine of rabbits after oral administration of ¹⁴C dieldrin, *Life Sci.,* 4, 2017, 1965.

134. **Robinson, J., Roberts, M., Baldwin, M., and Walder, A. I. T.,** The pharmacokinetics of HEOD (dieldrin) in rats, *Food Cosmet. Toxicol.,* 7, 317, 1969.

135. **Baldwin, M. K. and Robinson, J.,** Metabolism in the rat of the photoisomerization products of dieldrin, *Nature,* 224, 283, 1969.

136. **Nohynek, G. J., Muller, W. F., Coulston, F., and Korte, F.,** Metabolism excretion and tissue distribution of ¹⁴C photodieldrin in nonhuman primates following oral administration and intravenous injection, *Ecotoxicol. Environ. Safety,* 3, 1, 1979.

137. **Brooks, G. T. and Harrison, A.,** Metabolism and toxicity of the cyclodiene insecticides, *Biochem. J.,* 87, 5, 1963.

138. **Hutson, D. H., Baldwin, M. K., and Hoadley, E. C.,** Detoxication and bioactivation of endrin in the rats, *Xenobiotica,* 5, 697, 1975.

139. **Baldwin, M. K., Crayford, J. V., Hutson, D. H., and Street, D. L.,** The metabolism and residues of ¹⁴C endrin in lactating cows and laying hens, *Pestic. Sci.,* 7, 575, 1976.

140. **Bedford, C. T., Harrod, R. K., Hoadley, E. C., and Hutson, D. H.,** The metabolic fate of endrin in the rabbit, *Xenobiotica,* 5, 485, 1975.

141. **Ohsawa, T., Knox, J. R., Khalifa, S., and Casida, J. E.,** Metabolic dechlorination of toxaphene in rats, *J. Agric. Food Chem.,* 23, 98, 1975.

142. **Khalifa, S., Holmstead, R. L., and Casida, J. E.,** Toxaphene degradation by ion (II) protoporphyrins systems, *J. Agric. Food Chem.,* 24, 277, 1976.

143. **Chandurkar, P. S. and Matsumura, F.,** Metabolism of toxaphene components in rats, *Arch. Environ. Contam. Toxicol.,* 8, 1, 1979.

144. **Chandurkar, P. S. and Matsumura, F.,** Metabolism of toxicant bond toxicant C of toxaphene in rats, *Bull. Environ. Contam. Toxicol.,* 21, 539, 1979.

145. **Pollock, G. A. and Kilgore, W.,** Excretion and storage of ^{14}C toxaphene fractions, *J. Toxicol. Environ. Health,* 6, 127, 1980.

146. **Pollock, G. A. and Hiustrand, R.,** The elimination distribution and metabolism of ^{14}C toxaphene in the pregnant rat, *J. Environ. Sci. Health (B),* 17, 635, 1982.

147. **Mohammed, A., Anderson, O., Biessmann, A., and Slanina, P.,** Fate and specific tissue retention of toxaphene in mice, *Arch. Toxicol.,* 54, 311, 1983.

148. **Mohammed, A., Hallberg, E., Rydstrom, J., and Slanina, P.,** Toxaphene: accumulation in the adrenal cortex and effect on ACTH stimulated cortico steroid synthesis in the rat, *Toxicol. Lett.,* 24, 137, 1985.

149. **Keating, M. I.,** Excretion of toxaphene and dioxathion in the milk of dairy cows, *Bull. Anim. Health Prod. Afr.,* 27, 279, 1979.

150. **Steele, L. A., Nelson, H. A., Furr, A. A., Osheim, D. L., and Ross, P. F.,** Toxaphene residues in the bovine after oral exposure, *Vet. Hum. Toxicol.,* 22, 312, 1980.

151. **Mehendale, H. M., Fishbein, L., Fields, M., and Mathews, H. B.,** Fate of mirex ^{14}C in the rat and plants, *Bull. Environ. Contam. Toxicol.,* 8, 200, 1972.

152. **Charles, A. K., Rosembaum, D. P., Aohok, K., and Abraham, R.,** Uptake and disposition of mirex in hepatocytes and subcellular fractions in CD1 mouse, *J. Toxicol. Environ. Health,* 15, 395, 1985.

153. **Wiener, M., Pittman, K. A., and Stein, V. B.,** Mirex kinetics in the rhesus monkey. 1. Disposition and excretion, *Drug. Metab. Dispos.,* 4, 281, 1976.

154. **Pittman, K. A., Wiener, M., and Treble, D. H.,** Mirex kinetics in the rhesus monkey. 2. Pharmacokinetic model, *Drug Metab. Dispos.,* 4, 288, 1976.

155. **Chu, I., Villeneuve, D. C., and Vieau, A.,** Tissue distribution and elimination of photomirex in squirrel monkeys, *Bull. Environ. Contam. Toxicol.,* 29, 434, 1982.

156. **Morgan, D. P., Sandifer, S. H., Hetzler, H. L., Slach, E. F., Brady, C. D., and Colcolough, J.,** Test for *in vivo* conversion of mirex to kepone, *Bull. Environ. Contam. Toxicol.,* 22, 238, 1979.

157. **Egle, J. L., Fernandez, S. B., Guzelian, P. S., and Borzelleca, J. F.,** Distribution and excretion of chlordecone (kepone) in the rat, *Drug. Metab. Dispos.,* 6, 91, 1978.

158. **Schwartz, C. C., Soine, P. J., Blanke, R. V., and Guzelian, P. S.,** Preferential binding of chlordecone to the protein and high density lipoprotein fractions of plasma from humans and other species, *J. Toxicol. Environ. Health,* 9, 107, 1982.

159. **Soine, P. J. and Blanke, R. V.,** High density lipoproteins decrease in the biliary concentration of chlordecone in isolated perfused pig liver, *J. Toxicol. Environ. Health,* 14, 318, 1984.

160. **Soine, P. J., Blanke, R. V., and Schwartz, C. C.,** Chlordecone metabolism in the pig, *Toxicol. Lett.,* 17, 35, 1983.

161. **Dorough, H. W., Huhtanen, K., Marshall, T. C., and Bryant, H. E.,** Fate of endosulfan in rat and toxicological consideration of apolar metabolites, *Pestic. Biochem. Physiol.,* 8, 241, 1978.

162. **Dikshith, T. S. S., Raizada, R. B., Srivastava, M. K., and Kaphalia, B. S.,** Response of rats to repeated oral administration of endosulfan, *Ind. Health,* 22, 295, 1984.

163. **Ansari, R. A., Siddiqui, M. K. J., and Gutta, P. K.,** Toxicity of endosulfan distribution of alpha and beta isomers of racemic endosulfan following oral administration in rats, *Toxicol. Lett.,* 21, 29, 1984.

164. **Poonawalla, N. H. and Korte, F.,** Metabolism of insecticides. VIII. Excretion, distribution and metabolism of ^{14}C chlordane by rats, *Life Sci.,* 3, 1497, 1964.

165. **Street, J. C. and Blau, S. E.,** Oxychlordane: accumulation in rat adipose tissue in feeding chlordane isomers of technical chlordane, *J. Agric. Food Chem.,* 20, 395, 1972.

166. **Tashiro, S. and Matsumura, F.,** Metabolic route of cis and trans chlordane in rats, *J. Agric. Food Chem.,* 25, 872, 1977.

167. **Brimfield, A. A., Street, J. C., Futrell, J., and Chartfied, D. A.,** Identification of products arising from the metabolism of cis and trans chlordane in rat liver microsomes *in vitro*: outline of a possible metabolic pathway, *Pestic. Biochem. Physiol.,* 9, 84, 1978.

168. **Ewing, A. D., Kadry, A. M., and Dorough, W.,** Comparative disposition and elimination of chlordane in rats and mice, *Toxicol. Lett.,* 26, 233, 1985.

169. **Tashiro, S. and Matsumura, F.,** Metabolism of trans-nonachlor and related chlordane components in rats and man, *Arch. Environ. Contam. Toxicol.,* 7, 113, 1978.

170. **Rozman, K.,** Phase II enzyme induction reduces body burden of heptachlor in rats, *Toxicol. Lett.,* 20, 5, 1984.

171. **Scheufler, E. and Rozman, K.,** Enhanced total body clearance of heptachlor from rats by trans stilbene oxide, *Toxicology,* 32, 93, 1984.

172. **Fitzloff, J. F., Portig, J., and Stein, K.,** Lindane metabolism by human and rat liver microsomes, *Xenobiotica,* 12, 197, 1982.

173. **Yamamoto, T., Egashira, T., Yamanaka, Y., Yoshida, T., and Kuroiwa, Y.,** Initial metabolism of γ-hexachlorocyclohexane by rat liver microsomes, *J. Pharmacobiodyn.,* 6, 721, 1983.

174. **Tanaka, K., Kurihara, N., and Nakajima, M.,** Oxidative metabolism of lindane and its isomers with microsomes from rat liver and house fly abdomen, *Pestic. Biochem. Physiol.,* 10, 96, 1979.

175. **Tanaka, K., Kurihara, N., and Nakajima, M.,** Oxidative metabolism of tetrachlorocyclohexenes, pentachlorocyclohexenes and hexachlorocyclohexenes with microsomes from rat liver and house fly abdomen, *Pestic. Biochem. Physiol.,* 10, 79, 1979.

176. **Gopalaswamy, U. V. and Aiyar, A. S.,** Biotransformation of lindane in the rat, *Bull. Environ. Contam. Toxicol.,* 32, 148, 1984.

177. **Baker, M. T., Nelson, R. M., and Van Dyke, R. A.,** The formation of chlorobenzene and benzene by the reductive metabolism of lindane in rat liver microsomes, *Arch. Biochem. Biophys.,* 1, 236, 1985.

178. **Fukam, J. I.,** Metabolism of several insecticides by glutathione-S-transferase, in *Differential Toxicities of Insecticides and Halogenated Aromatics,* Matsumura, F., Ed., Pergamon Press, *Encyc. Pharm. Ther.,* 113, 223, 1984.

179. **Macholz, R. M., Knoll, R., Lewerenz, H. j., Petrizka, M., and Engst, R.,** Metabolism of alpha hexachlorocyclohexane. Free metabolites in urine and organs of rats, *Xenobiotica,* 12, 227, 1982.

180. **Portig, J., Kraus, P., Stein, K., Koransky, W., Noack, G., Gross, B., and Sodomann, S.,** Glutathione conjugate formation from hexachlorocyclohexane and pentachlorocyclohexane by rat liver, *in vitro, Xenobiotica,* 9, 353, 1979.

181. **Lay, J. P., Klein, W., Korte, F., and Richter, E.,** Metabolism of beta hexachlorocyclohexane ^{14}C in rats following low dosing in the daily diet, *J. Environ. Sci. Health B,* 16, 227, 1981.

182. **Eichler, D., Heupt, W., and Paul, W.,** Comparative study on the distribution of alpha and gamma HCH in the rat with particular reference to the problem of isomerization, *Xenobiotica,* 13, 639, 1983.

183. **Srinivasan, K. and Radhakrishanamurty, R.,** Studies on the distribution of beta and gamma isomers of HCH in rat tissues, *J. Environ. Sci. Health B,* 18, 401, 1983.

184. **Krishna, J. G. and Casida, J. E.,** Fate in rats of the radiocarbon from ten variously labeled methyl and dimethylcarbamate ^{14}C insecticide chemicals and their hydrolysis products, *J. Agric. Food Chem.,* 14, 98, 1966.

185. **Dorough, H. W. and Casida, J. E.,** Nature of certain carbamate metabolites of the insecticide sevin, *J. Agric. Food Chem.,* 12, 294, 1964.

186. **Knaak, J. B., Tallant, M. J., Bartley, W. J., and Sullivan, L. J.,** The metabolism of carbaryl in the rat, guinea pig and man, *J. Agric. Food Chem.,* 13, 537, 1965.

187. **Sullivan, L. J., Eldridge, J. M., Knaak, J. B., and Tallants, M. J.,** 5,6-Dihydro-5,6-dihydroxycarbaryl glucuronide as a significant metabolite of carbaryl in the rat, *J. Agric. Food Chem.,* 20, 980, 1972.

188. **Hassan, A., Zayed, S. M., and Abdul-Hamid, F. M.,** Metabolism of sevin in the rat, *Biochem. Pharmacol.,* 15, 2045, 1966.

189. **Knaak, J. B. and Sullivan, J.,** Metabolism of carbaryl in the dog, *J. Agric. Food Chem.,* 15, 1125, 1967.

190. **Dorough, H. W.,** Carbaryl ^{14}C metabolism in a lactating cow, *J. Agric. Food Chem.,* 15, 261, 1967.

191. **Fukuto, T. R.,** Metabolism of carbamate insecticides, *Drug. Metab. Rev.,* 1, 117, 1972.

192. **Bend, J. R., Holder, G. M., Protos, G. M., and Ryan, A. J.,** Water soluble metabolites of carbaryl in mouse liver preparation and in the rat, *Aust. J. Bil. Sci.,* 24, 535, 1971.

193. **Knaak, J. B., Tallant, M. J., Kozbelt, S. J., and Sullivan, L. J.,** Metabolism of carbaryl in man, monkey, pig and sheep, *J. Agric. Food Chem.,* 16, 465, 1968.

194. **Declume, C. and Derache, R.,** Passage placentaire d'un carbamate anticholinesterasique à activité insecticide: le carbaryl, *Chemosphere,* 2, 141, 1977.

195. **Declume, C. and Benard, P.,** Etude autoradiographique de la distribution d'un agent anticholinesterasique, le 1-naphthyl-N-methyl (^{14}C) carbamate chez la ratte gestante, *Toxicol. Appl. Pharmacol.,* 39, 451, 1977.

196. **Declume, C. and Benard, P.,** Foetal accumulation of ^{14}C carbaryl in rats and mice: autoradiographic study, *Toxicol.,* 8, 95, 1977.

197. **Benard, P., Cambon, C., and Declume, C.,** Passage of radioactivity into the milk of rats treated with ^{14}C carbaryl, *Toxicol. Lett.,* 4, 149, 1979.

198. **Strother, A. and Wheeler, L.,** Excretion and disposition of ^{14}C carbaryl in pregnant, non pregnant and foetal tissues of the rat after acute administration, *Xenobiotica,* 10, 113, 1980.

199. **Fernandez, Y., Falzon, M., Cambon-Gros, C., and Mitjavila, S.,** Carbaryl tricompartmental toxicokinetics and anticholinesterase activity, *Toxicol. Lett.,* 13, 253, 1982.

200. **Cambon, C., Fernandez, Y., Falzon, M., and Mitjavila, S.,** Variations of the digestive absorption kinetics of carbaryl with the nature of the vehicle, *Toxicology,* 22, 45, 1981.

201. **Falzon, M., Fernandez, Y., Cambon Gros, C., and Mitjavila, S.,** Influence of experimental hepatic impairment on the toxicokinetics and the anticholinesterase activity of carbaryl in the rat, *J. Appl. Toxicol.,* 3, 87, 1983.

202. **Ohkawa, H., Kohara, T., Yoshihara, R., and Miyamoto, J.,** Metabolism of N-methylcarbamate insecticides, *Noyaku Kagatu,* 1, 86, 1973.

203. **Ohkawa, H., Yoshihara, R., Kohara, T., and Miyamoto, J.,** Metabolism of tsumacide in rats, houseflies and bean plants, *Agric. Biol. Chem.,* 38, 1035, 1974.

204. **Miyamoto, J., Yamamoto, K., and Matsumoto, T.,** Metabolism of 3,4-dimethylphenyl N-methylcarbamate in white rats, *Agric. Biol. Chem.,* 33, 1060, 1969.

205. **Miyamoto, J.,** A feature of detoxification of carbamate insecticides in mammals, in *Biochemical Toxicology of Insecticides,* O'Brien, R. D. and Yamamoto, I., Eds., Academic Press, New York, 1970, 180.

206. **Miyamoto, J.,** Metabolism of organophosphorous compounds and carbamate insecticides, *Fate of Pesticides in Environment,* Tahari, A. S., Ed., Gordon and Breach, London, 1972, 319.

207. **Baron, R. L. and Doherty, J. D.,** Metabolism and excretion of an insecticide (6-chloro-3,4-dimethyl phenyl N-methylcarbamate) in the rat, *J. Agric. Food Chem.,* 15, 830, 1967.

208. **Krechmiak, J. and Foss, W.,** Distribution, biotransformation and elimination of propoxur following its intoxication in repeated doses, *Bromatol. Chem. Toksykol.,* 16, 205, 1983.

209. **Miskus, P. R., Andrews, T. L., and Look, M.,** Metabolic pathways affecting toxicity of N-acetyl Zectran, *J. Agric. Food Chem.,* 17, 842, 1969.

210. **Williams, E., Meikle, R. W., and Redemann, C. T.,** Identification of metabolites of Zectran insecticide in dog urine, *J. Agric. Food Chem.,* 12, 457, 1964.

211. **Strother, A.,** Comparative metabolism of selected N-methylcarbamates by human and rat liver fractions, *Biochem. Pharmacol.,* 19, 2525, 1970.

212. **Strother, A.,** *In vitro* metabolism of methylcarbamate insecticides in the human and rat liver, *Arch. Environ. Health,* 13, 257, 1966.

213. **Oonnithan, E. S. and Casida, J. E.,** Metabolites of methyl- and dimethylcarbamate insecticide chemical as formed by rat liver microsomes, *Bull. Environ. Contam. Toxicol.,* 1, 59, 1966.

214. **Dorough, H. W.,** Metabolism of Furadan in rats and houseflies, *J. Agric. Food Chem.,* 16, 319, 1968.

215. **Metcalf, R. L., Fukuto, T. R., Collins, C., Borack, K., El-Aziz, A., Munoz, R., and Cassil, C. C.,** Metabolism of 2,2-dimethyl-2,3-dichlorobenzofuranyl-7-N-methylcarbamate in plants, insects and mammals, *J. Agric. Food Chem.,* 16, 300, 1968.

216. **Gill, S. S.,** *In vitro* metabolism of carbofuran by liver microsomes of the padifiel fish, *Bull. Environ. Contam. Toxicol.,* 25, 697, 1980.

217. **Ferguson, P. W., Dey, M. S., Jewell, S. A., and Krieger, R. J.,** Carbofuran metabolism and toxicity in the rat, *Fundam. Appl. Toxicol.,* 4, 14, 1984.

218. **Ivie, G. W. and Dorough, H. W.,** Furadan ^{14}C metabolism in lactating cows, *J. Agric. Food Chem.,* 16, 849, 1968.

219. **Black, A. L., Chiu, Y. C., Fukuto, T. R., and Miller, T. A.,** Metabolism of 2,2-dimethyl-2,3-dihydroxybenzo-7-N-methyl-N-(2-toluensulfenyl) carbamate in the housefly and white mouse, *Pestic. Biochem. Physiol.,* 3, 435, 1973.

220. **Robbins, J. D., Bakke, J., and Feil, V. J.,** Metabolism of 4-benzothienyl N-methylcarbamate (Mobam) in rats: balance study and urinary metabolite separation, *J. Agric. Food Chem.,* 17, 236, 1969.

221. **Robbins, J. D., Bakke, J. E., and Feil, V. J.,** Metabolism of Mobam in dairy goats and a lactating cow, *J. Agric. Food Chem.,* 18, 130, 1970.

222. **Andrawes, N. R., Dorough, H. W., and Lindquist, D. A.,** Degradation and elimination of temik in rats, *J. Econ. Entomol.,* 60, 979, 1967.

223. **Dorough, H. W. and Ivie, G. W.,** Temik-S^{35} metabolism in a lactating cow, *J. Agric. Food Chem.,* 16, 460, 1968.

224. **Harvey, J., Jelinek, A. G., and Sherman, H.,** Metabolism of methomyl in the rat, *J. Agric. Food Chem.,* 21, 769, 1973.

225. **Huhtanen, K. and Dorough, H. W.,** Isomerization and Beckman rearrangement reactions in the metabolism of methomyl in rats, *Pestic. Biochem. Physiol.,* 6, 571, 1976.

226. **Hutson, D. H., Hoadley, E. C., and Pickering, B. A.,** Metabolism of S-2-cyanoethyl-N-(methylcarbamoyl)oxy) thio-acetimidate, an insecticidal carbamate in the rats, *Xenobiotica,* 1, 179, 1971.

227. **Challis, I. R. and Adcock, J. W.,** The metabolism of the carbamate insecticide Bendiocarb in the rat and in man, *Pestic. Sci.,* 12, 638, 1981.

228. **Page, A. C., Loeffler, J. E., Hendrickson, H. R., Huston, C. K., and Devries, D. M.,** Metabolic fate of dichlorvos in swine, *Arch. Toxicol.,* 30, 19, 1972.

229. **Huston, D. H. and Hoadley, E. C.,** The comparative metabolism of ^{14}C vinyldichlorvos in animals and man, *Arch. Toxicol.,* 30, 9, 1972.

230. **Huston, D. H. and Hoadley, E. C.,** The metabolism of ^{14}C-methyldichlorvos in the rat and mouse, *Xenobiotica,* 2, 107, 1972.

231. **Blair, D., Hoadley, E. C., and Hutson, D. H.,** The distribution of dichlorvos in tissues of mammals after its inhalation or intravenous administration, *Toxicol. Appl. Pharmacol.,* 31, 263, 1975.

232. **Potter, J. C., Boyer, A. C., Marxmiller, R. L., Young, R., and Loeffler, J. E.,** Radioisotope residues of dichlorvos and its metabolites dichlorvos ^{14}C and dichlorvos ^{36}Cl formed as PVC pellets, *J. Agric. Food Chem.,* 21, 734, 1973.

233. **Leoffler, J. E., Potter, J. C., Scordelis, S. L., Hendrickson, H. R., Hutson, C. K., and Page, A. C.,** Long term exposure of swine to a ^{14}C-dichlorvos atmosphere, *J. Agric. Food Chem.*, 24, 267, 1976.

234. **Elrich, M. and Cohen, S. D.,** Effect of DDVP in mouse liver glutathione levels and lack of potentiation by methyl iodide and TOTP, *Biochem. Pharmacol.*, 26, 997, 1977.

235. **Hutson, D. H., Holmes, D. S., and Crawford, J. M.,** The involvement of glutathione in the reductive dechlorination of a phenacyl halide, *Chemosphere*, 5, 79, 1976.

236. **Hutson, D. H., Akintonwa, D. A. A., and Hathway, D. E.,** The metabolism of 2-chloro-1(2',4'-dichlorophenyl)vinyl diethyl phosphate in the dog and rat, *Biochem. J.*, 102, 133, 1967.

237. **Akintonwa, D. A. A.,** The correlation between theorical and experimental biotransformation of 2-chloro-1-(2',4' dichlorophenyl) vinyl diethyl phosphate (chlorfenvinphos) in the dog and rat, *J. Theor. Biol.*, 114, 103, 1985.

238. **Crawford, M. J., Hutson, D. H., and King, P. A.,** Metabolic demethylation of the insecticide dimethylvinphos in rats, in dogs and *in vitro*, *Xenobiotica*, 6, 745, 1976.

239. **Akintonwa, D. A. A. and Hutson, D. H.,** Metabolism of 2-chloro-1-(2,4,5-trichlorophenyl) vinyldimethylphosphate in the dog and rat, *J. Agric. Food Chem.*, 15, 632, 1967.

240. **Donninger, C., Hutson, D. H., and Pickering, B. A.,** The oxidative dealkylation of phosphoric acid triesters by mammalian liver enzymes, *Biochem. J.*, 126, 701, 1972.

241. **Hutson, D. H., Pickering, B. A., and Donninger, C.,** Phosphoric acid triester: glutathione alkyl transferase. A mechanism for the detoxication of dimethyl phosphoric acid triesters, *Biochem. J.*, 127, 285, 1972.

242. **Donninger, C. D., Nobbs, B. T., and Wilson, K.,** An enzyme catalyzing the hydrolysis of phosphoric acid diesters in rat liver, *Biochem. J.*, 122, 51, 1971.

243. **Casida, J. E., Knaak, J. B., Lance, R. D., and Niedermeier, R. P.,** Bovine metabolism of organophosphate insecticides. Subacute feeding studies with o,o-dimethyl 1-carbomethoxy-1-propen-2-ylphosphate, *J. Agric. Food Chem.*, 6, 658, 1958.

244. **Morello, A., Vardanis, A., and Spencer, E. Y.,** Mechanism of detoxication of some organophosphorus compounds, the role of glutathione dependent demethylation, *Can. J. Biochem.*, 46, 885, 1968.

245. **Spencer, E. Y.,** Biochemistry and structure of organophosphorus pesticides in *Toxicology, Biodegradation and Efficacy of Livestock Pesticides,* Khan, M. and Haufe, W. O., Eds., Swets and Zeitlinger, Amsterdam, 1972, 23.

246. **Menzer, R. E. and Casida, J. E.,** Nature of toxic metabolites formed in mammals, insects and plants from 3-(dimethoxyphosphinyloxy)-N,N-dimethyl ciscrotonamide and its N-methyl analog, *J. Agric. Food Chem.*, 13, 102, 1965.

247. **Bull, D. L. and Lindquist, D. A.,** Metabolism of 3-hydroxy-N,N-dimethylcrotonamide dimethyl phosphate by cotton plants, insects and rats, *J. Agric. Food Chem.*, 12, 310, 1964.

248. **Menzer, R. E. and Dauterman, W. C.,** Metabolism of some organophosphorus insecticides, *J. Agric. Food Chem.*, 18, 103, 1970.

249. **Bull, D. L. and Lindquist, D. A.,** Metabolism of 3-hydroxy-N-methyl-cis-crotonamide dimethyl phosphate (Azodrin) by insects and rats, *J. Agric. Food Chem.*, 14, 105, 1966.

250. **Clemons, G. P. and Menzer, R. E.,** Oxidative metabolism of phosphamidon in rats and goats, *J. Agric. Food Chem.*, 16, 312, 1968.

251. **Lucier, G. W. and Menzer, R. E.,** Nature of neutral phosphorus ester metabolites of phosphamidon formed in rats and liver microsomes, *J. Agric. Food Chem.*, 19, 1249, 1971.

252. **Diggle, W. M. and Gage, J. C.,** Cholinesterase inhibition *in vitro* by o,o-diethyl, o,p-nitrophenyl thiophosphate (parathion), *Biochem. J.*, 49, 491, 1951.

253. **Kubistova, J.,** Parathion metabolism in female rats, *Arch. Intern. Pharmacodyn.*, 118, 308, 1959.

254. **Linchtenstein, E. P., Fuhremann, T. W., Hochberg, A. A., Zahlten, R. N., and Stratman, W.,** Metabolism of ^{14}C paraoxon with fractions and subfractions of rat liver cells, *J. Agric. Food Chem.*, 21, 416, 1973.

255. **Hollingworth, R. M., Alstott, R. L., and Litzenberg, R. D.,** Glutathione S-aryltransferase in the metabolism of parathion and its analogs, *Life Sci.*, 13, 191, 1973.

256. **Shishido, R., Usui, K., and Fukami, J.,** Oxidative metabolism of diazinon by microsomes from rat liver and cockroach, fat body, *Pestic. Biochem. Physiol.*, 2, 27, 1972.

257. **Appleton, H. T. and Nakatsugawa,** Paraoxon diethylation in the metabolism of parathion, *Pestic. Biochem. Physiol.*, 2, 286, 1972.

258. **Sultatos, L. G. and Minor, L. D.,** Biotransformation of paraoxon and p-nitrophenol by isolated perfused mouse liver, *Toxicology*, 36, 159, 1985.

259. **Shishido, T. and Fukami, J.,** Studies on the selective toxicities of organic phosphorus insecticides. II. The degradation of ethyl parathion, methyl parathion, methyl paraoxon and sumithion in mammals, insect and plant, *Botyu Kagaku*, 28, 69, 1963.

260. **Fukami, J. and Shishido, T.,** Studies on the selective toxicities of organic phosphorus insecticides. III. The characters of enzyme system in cleavage of methyl parathion to desmethyl parathion in the supernatant of several species of homogenate, *Botyu-Kagaku,* 28, 77, 1963.

261. **Hollingsworth, R. M.,** Dealkylation of organophosphorus esters by mouse liver enzymes *in vitro* and *in vivo, J. Agric. Food Chem.,* 17, 978, 1969.

262. **Fukami, J. and Shishido, T.,** Nature of soluble glutathione dependent enzyme system active in cleavage of methyl parathion to desmethyl parathion, *J. Econ. Entomol.,* 59, 1338, 1966.

263. **Miyamoto, J.,** Mechanism of low toxicity of sumithion towards animals, *Residue Rev.,* 25, 251, 1969.

264. **Negherbon, M. U.,** *Handbook of Toxicology Insecticides,* Vol. III, W. B. Saunders, Philadelphia, 1959.

265. **Hollingworth, R. M., Metcalf, R. L., and Fukuto, T.,** The selectivity of sumithion compounds with methyl parathion metabolism in the white mouse, *J. Agric. Food Chem.,* 15, 242, 1967.

266. **Hollingworth, R. M., Fukuto, T. R., and Metcalf, R. L.,** Selective toxicity of sumithion compared with methyl parathion, *J. Agric. Food Chem.,* 15, 235, 1967.

267. **Braeckman, R. A., Audenaert, F., Willems, J. L., Belpaire, F. M., and Bogaert, M. G.,** Toxicokinetics of methylparathion and parathion in the dog after intravenous and oral administration, *Arch. Toxicol.,* 54, 71, 1983.

268. **Miyamoto, J., Wakimura, A., and Kadota, T.,** Biodegradation of cyanophos in rats, in *Environmental Quality and Safety,* Vol. 1, Coulston, F, and Korte, F., Eds., Georg Thieme, Stuttgart, 1972, 235.

269. **Bradway, T. M., Shafik, T. M., and Lores, E. M.,** Comparison of cholinesterase activity residue levels and urinary metabolites excretion of rats exposed to organophosphorus pesticides, *J. Agric. Food Chem.,* 25, 1353, 1977.

270. **Metcalf, R. L., Fukuto, T. R., and Winton, M. Y.,** Metabolism of fenthion, *Bull. World Health Org.,* 29, 219, 1963.

271. **Plapp, F. W. and Casida, J. E.,** Bovine metabolism of organophosphorus insecticides. Metabolic fate of O,O-dimethyl-O-(2,4,5-trichlorophenyl) phosphorothioate in rats and cow, *J. Agric. Food Chem.,* 6, 662, 1958.

272. **Niessen, H., Tietz, H., and Frehse, F.,** On the occurrence of biologically active metabolites of the active ingredient S 1752 after application of lebycid, *Pflanzenschutz-Nachr.,* 15, 125, 1962.

273. **Francis, J. I. and Barnes, J. M.,** Studies on the mammalian toxicity of fenthion, *Bull. World Health Org.,* 29, 205, 1963.

274. **Emteres, R., Abdelghani, A., and Anderson, A. C.,** Determination of the half-life of fenthion in New Zealand white rabbits using three routes of administration, *J. Environ. Sci. Health,* 20, 577, 1985.

275. **Bakke, J. E., Feil, W. J., and Price, C. E.,** Rat urinary metabolites from o,o-diethyl-o-(3,5,6-trichloro-2-pyridyl) phosphorothionate, *J. Environ. Sci. Health,* 311, 225, 1976.

276. **Sultatos, L. G. and Murphy, S. D.,** Hepatic microorsmal detoxication of paraoxon and chlorpyrifos oxon in the mouse, *Drug. Metab. Disp.,* 11, 232, 1983.

277. **Sultatos, L. G. and Murphy, S. D.,** Kinetic analyses of the microsomal biotransformation of the phosphorothioate insecticides chlorpyrifos and parathion, *Fundam. Appl. Toxicol.,* 3, 16, 1983.

278. **Sultatos, L. G., Shao, M., and Murphy, S. D.,** The role of hepatic biotransformation in mediating the acute toxicity of chlorpyrifos, *Toxicol. Appl. Pharmacol.,* 73, 60, 1984.

279. **Shishido, T., Usui, L., Sato, M., and Fukami, J.,** Enzymatic conjugation of diazinon and diazinon in rat liver and cockroach fat body, *Pestic. Biochem. Physiol.,* 2, 51, 1972.

280. **Mount, M. E.,** Diagnostic value of urinary dialkyl phosphate measurement in goats exposed to diazinon, *Am. J. Vet. Res.,* 45, 817, 1984.

281. **Yang, R. S. H., Hogson, E., and Dauterman, W. C.,** *In vitro* metabolism of diazinon and diazoxon in susceptible and resistant houseflies, *J. Agric. Food Chem.,* 19, 14, 1971.

282. **Shishido, T. and Fukami, J.,** Enzymatic hydrolysis of diazinon by rat tissue homogenate, *Pestic. Biochem. Physiol.,* 2, 39, 1972.

283. **Machin, A. F., Auick, M. P., Rogers, H., and Anderson, P. H.,** Conversion of diazinon to hydroxy-diazinon in the guinea pig and sheep, *Bull. Environ. Contam. Toxicol.,* 6, 26, 1971.

284. **Miyazaki, H., Tojinbara, T., Watanabe, Y., Osaka, T., and Okui, S.,** Metabolism of diazinon in animals plants, *Proc. Symp. Drug. Metab. Action,* Pharmaceutical Society of Japan, 1969, 135.

285. **Janes, N. F., Machin, A. F., Quick, M. P., Rogers, H., Munoy, D. E., and Cross, J. A.,** Toxic metabolites of diazinon in sheep, *J. Agric. Food Chem.,* 21, 121, 1973.

286. **Tomokuni, K. and Hasegawa, T.,** Diazinon concentration and blood cholinesterase activities in rats exposed to diazinon, *Toxicol. Lett.,* 25, 7, 1985.

287. **Fukuto, T. R., Metcalf, R. L., March, R. B., and Maxon, M. G.,** Chemical behaviour of systox isomers in biological systems, *J. Econ. Entomol.,* 48, 347, 1955.

288. **Heath, D. F. and Vandekar, M.,** Some spontaneous reactions of O,O-dimethyl S-ethylthioethyl phosphorothiolate and related compounds in water and on storage, and their effects on the toxicological properties of the compounds, *Biochem. J.,* 67, 187, 1957.

289. **Knaak, J. B. and O'Brien, R. D.,** Insecticide potentiation: effects of EPN on *in vivo* metabolism of malathion by the rat and dog, *J. Agric. Food Chem.,* 8, 198, 1960.

290. **Seume, F. W. and O'Brien, R. D.,** Metabolism of malathion by rat tissue preparations and its modification by EPN, *J. Agric. Food Chem.,* 8, 36, 1960.

291. **Bradway, D. E. and Shafik, T. M.,** Malathion exposure studies determination of mono-dicarboxylic acids and alkyl phosphates in urine, *J. Agric. Food Chem.,* 25, 1342, 1977.

292. **Ryan, D. L. and Fukuto, T. R.,** The effect of isomalathion and O,S,S-trimethyl phosphonodithioate on the *in vivo* metabolism of malathion in rats, *Pestic. Biochem. Physiol.,* 21, 349, 1984.

293. **Gupta, R. C., Welsch, F., Thornburg, J. E., and Paul, B. S.,** Effect of chloramphenicol pretreatment on malathion induced acute toxicity in the rat, *J. Toxicol. Environ. Health,* 11, 897, 1983.

294. **Fukuto, T. R.,** Toxicological properties of trialkylphosphotothionate and dialkyl alkyl and arylphosphon-othioates esters, *J. Environ. Sci. Health,* 18, 89, 1983.

295. **Ryan, D. L. and Fukuto, T. R.,** The effects of impurities on the toxicokinetics of malathion in rats, *Pestic. Biochem. Physiol.,* 23, 413, 1985.

296. **Malik, J. K. and Summer, K. H.,** Toxicity and metabolism of malathion and its impurities in isolated rat hepatocytes. Role of glutathione, *Toxicol. Appl. Pharmacol.,* 66, 69, 1982.

297. **North, H. H. and Menzer, R. E.,** Biotransformation of dimethoate by cell culture systems, *Pestic. Biochem. Physiol.,* 2, 278, 1972.

298. **Uchida, T. and O'Brien, R. D.,** Dimethoate degradation by human liver and its significance for acute toxicity, *Toxicol. Appl. Pharmacol.,* 10, 89, 1967.

299. **Uchida, T., Dauterman, W. C., and O'Brien, R. D.,** The metabolism of dimethoate by vertebrate tissues, *J. Agric. Food Chem.,* 12, 48, 1964.

300. **Chen, P. R. S. and Dauterman, W. C.,** Studies on the toxicity of dimethoate analogs and their hydrolysis by sheep liver amidase, *Pestic. Biochem. Physiol.,* 1, 340, 1971.

301. **Kaplanis, J. N., Robbins, W. E., Darson, D. I., Hopkins, D. E., Monroe, R. E., and Treiber, G.,** The metabolism of dimethoate in cattle, *J. Econ. Entomol.,* 52, 1190, 1959.

302. **Dauterman, W. C., Casida, J. E., Knaak, J. B., and Kowalczyk, T.,** Bovine metabolism of organo-phosphorus insecticides. Metabolism and residues associated with oral administration of dimethoate rats and three lactating cows, *J. Agric. Food Chem.,* 1, 188, 1959.

303. **Chamberlain, F. W., Gatterdam, P. E., and Hopkins, D. E.,** The metabolism of ^{32}P-labeled dimethoate in sheep, *J. Econ. Entomol.,* 61, 733, 1961.

304. **Bowman, J. S. and Casida, J. E.,** Further studies on the metabolism of Thimet by plants, insects and mammals, *J. Econ. Entomol.,* 51, 838, 1958.

305. **Bull, D. L.,** Metabolism of disyston by insects isolated cotton leaves and rat, *J. Econ. Entomol.,* 58, 249, 1965.

306. **Takade, D. Y., Allsup, T., Khasawinah, A., Kao, T. S., and Fukuto, T. R.,** Metabolism of o,o-dimethyl S(alpha-(carboethoxy)benzyl) phosphorodithioate (Phenthoate) in the white mouse and house flies, *Pestic Biochem. Physiol.,* 6, 267, 1976.

307. **Debaun, J. R. and Menn, J. J.,** Sulfoxide reduction in relation to organophosphorus insecticide detoxi-cation, *Science,* 191, 187, 1976.

308. **Menn, J. J., Debaun, J. R., and McBain, J. B.,** Recent advances in the metabolism of organophosphorus insecticides, *Fed. Proc.,* 35, 2598, 1976.

309. **Harned, W. H. and Casida, J. E.,** Dioxathion metabolites, photoproducts and oxidative degradation products, *J. Agric. Food Chem.,* 24, 689, 1976.

310. **Ford, J. M., Menn, J. J., and Meyding, G. D.,** Metabolism of imidan-^{14}C: balance study in the rat, *J. Agric. Food Chem.,* 14, 83, 1966.

311. **McBain, J. B., Menn, J. J., and Casida, J. E.,** Metabolism of carbonyl-^{14}C-labelled imidan in rats and cockroaches, *J. Agric. Food Chem.,* 16, 813, 1968.

312. **Vononina, V. M., Popov, T. A., and Kagan, I.,** Effect of mixed function oxidase on phthalophos transformation in rat liver, *U.K.R. Biokhim. Zh.,* 53, 26, 1981.

313. **Chopade, H. M. and Dauterman, W. C.,** Studies on the *in vitro* metabolism of methidathion by rat and mouse liver, *Pestic. Biochem. Physiol.,* 15, 105, 1981.

314. **Everett, L. J., Anderson, C. A., and Mac Doughall, D.,** Nature and extent of guthion residues in milk and tissues resulting from treated forage, *J. Agric. Food Chem.,* 14, 47, 1966.

315. **Motoyama, N. and Dauterman, W. C.,** *In vitro* metabolism of azinphosmethyl by mouse liver, *Pestic Biochem. Physiol.,* 2, 170, 1972.

316. **Bauriedel, W. R. and Swank, M. G.,** Residue and metabolism of radioactive 4-tert-butyl-2-chlorophenyl methyl N-methylphosphoramidate administered as a single oral dose to sheep, *J. Agric. Food Chem.,* 10, 150, 1962.

317. **Bakke, J. E., Feil, V. J., Price, C. E., and Zaylskie, R. G.,** Metabolism of ^{14}C-crufomate (4-tert-butyl-2-chlorophenyl methyl methyl phosphoramidate) by sheep, *Biomed. Mass Spectrom.,* 3, 299, 1976.

318. **Metcalf, R. L., Fukuto, T. R., and March, R. B.,** Toxic action of dipterex and DDVP to the housefly, *J. Econ. Entomol.,* 52, 44, 1959.

319. **Miyamoto, J.,** Non-enzymatic conversion of dipterex into DDVP and their inhibitory action on enzymes, *Botyu-Kagaku,* 24, 130, 1959.

320. **Miyamoto, J.,** Studies on the mode of action of dipterex. II. New glucuronides obtained from the urine of rabbit following administration of dipterex, *Agric. Biol. Chem.,* 25, 266, 1961.

321. **Hassan, A., Abdel-Hamid, F. M., and Mohammed, S. I.,** Metabolism of ^{14}C-leptophos in the rat, *Arch. Environ. Contam. Toxicol.,* 6, 447, 1977.

322. **Holmsead, R. L., Fukuto, T. R., and March, R. B.,** The metabolism of leptophos in white mice and cotton plants, *Arch. Environ. Contam. Toxicol.,* 1, 133, 1974.

323. **Sugiyama, S., Igarashi, T., Ueno, K., Satoh, T., and Kitagawa, H.,** NAD coupled enzymatic oxidation of o-ethyl-o-p-nitrophenyl phenylphosphonothionate (EPN) to its oxygen analog with liver microsomes of rats, *Jpn. J. Pharmacol.,* 37, 245, 1985.

324. **Abou-Donia, M. B., Kinnes, C. G., Abdo, K. M., and Bjornssom, T. D.,** Physiological disposition and metabolism of o-ethyl-o-4-nitrophenyl phenylphosphonothionate in male rats following a single dermal administraiton, *Drug. Metab. Dispos.,* 11, 31, 1983.

325. **Abou-Donia, M. B., Reichert, B. L., and Ashry, M. A.,** The absorption, distribution, excretion and metabolism of a single oral dose of o-ethyl o-4-nitrophenyl phenylphosphonothionate in hens, *Toxicol. Appl. Pharmacol.,* 70, 18, 1983.

326. **Rhodes, C., Jones, B. K., Croucher, A., Hutson, D. H., Logan, C. J., Hopkins, R., Hall, B. E., and Vickers, J. A.,** The bioaccumulation and biotransformation of cis, trans cypermethrin in the rat, *Pest. Sci.,* 25, 471, 1984.

327. **Eadsforth, C. V., and Baldwin, M. K.,** Human dose-excretion studies with the pyrethroid insecticide, cypermethrin, *Xenobiotica,* 13, 67, 1983.

328. **Gray, A. J., and Rickard, J.,** The toxicokinetics of deltamethrin in rats after intravenous administration of a toxic dose, *Pestic Biochem. Physiol.,* 18, 205, 1982.

329. **Gray, A. J., Connors, T. A., Hoellinger, H., and Hoang-Nam, N.,** The relationship between the pharmacokinetics of intravenous cismethrin and bioresmethrin and their mammalian toxicity, *Pestic Biochem. Physiol.,* 13, 281, 1980.

330. **Ohkawa, H., Kameko, H., Tsuji, H., and Miyamoto, J.,** Metabolism of fenvalerate (sumicidin) in rats, *J. Pestic. Sci.,* 4, 143, 1979.

331. **Wszolek, P. C., Lafaunce, N. A., Wachs, T., and Lisk, D. J.,** Studies of possible bovine urinary excretion and rumen decomposition of fenvalerate insecticide and a metabolite, *Bull. Environ. Contam. Toxicol.,* 26, 262, 1981.

332. **Braun, W. H., Young, J. D., Blau, G. E., and Gehring, P. J.,** The pharmacokinetics and metabolism of pentachlorophenol in rats, *Toxicol. Appl. Pharmacol.,* 41, 395, 1977.

333. **Braun, W. H. and Sauerhoff, M. W.,** The pharmacokinetics profile of pentachlorophenol in monkeys, *Toxicol. Appl. Pharmacol.,* 38, 525, 1976.

334. **Gardiner, J. A., Kirland, J. J., Klopping, H. L., and Sherman, H.,** Fate of benomyl in animals, *J. Agric. Food Chem.,* 22, 419, 1974.

335. **Douch, P. G. C.,** Metabolism of benomyl fungicide in mammals, *Xenobiotica,* 3, 367, 1973.

336. **Franck, A.,** Metabolism of 2-(2-furyl)benzimidazole in certain mammals, *Acta Pharmacol. Toxicol.,* 29, 124, 1971.

337. **Tocco, D. J., Egerton, J. R., Bowers, W., Christensen, V. W., and Rosenblum, C.,** Absorption metabolism and elimination of thiabendazole in farm animals and a method for estimation in biological materials, *J. Pharmacol. Expt. Ther.,* 149, 263, 1965.

338. **Tocco, D. J., Rosemblum, C., Martin, M., and Robinson, H. J.,** Absorption metabolism, excretion of thiabendazole in man and laboratory animals, *Toxicol. Appl. Pharmacol.,* 9, 31, 1966.

339. **Noguchi, T., Ohkuma, K., and Kosaka, S.,** Chemistry and metabolism of thiophanate, *Proc. Int. Symp. Pesticide Terminal residues,* Tel Aviv, 1971, 235.

340. **Douch, P. G. C.,** Metabolism of thioureidobenzene fungicide in mice and sheep, *Xenobiotica,* 4, 457, 1974.

341. **Bratt, H., Daniel, J. W., and Monks, I. H.,** The metabolism of the systemic fungicide, dimethirimol by rats and dogs, *Food Cosmet. Toxicol.,* 10, 489, 1972.

342. **Waring, R. H.,** Metabolism of vitavax by rats and rabbits, *Xenobiotica,* 3, 65, 1973.

343. **Chin, W. T., Stone, G. M., Smith, A. E.,** *International Symposium on Pesticide Terminal Residues,* Tohori, A. S., Ed., Butterworths, London, 1971, 271.

344. **Ueyama, I., Kurogochi, S., Kobori, I., Hoshino, T., Ishii, Y., and Takase, I.,** Use of ion cluster analysis in a metabolic study of pencycuron, a phenylurea fungicide in rabbits, *J. Agric. Food Chem.,* 30, 1061, 1982.

345. **Piffaut, T. B. and Metche, M.,** Etude de la toxicité d' une dithioquinoxaline pour les plantules de concumbre et la microflore environnante, Contamination des Chaines Biologiques, *Recherche Environ.,* 14, 187, 1980.

346. **Carrera, G., Mitjavila, S., Lacombe, C., and Derache, R.,** Toxicocinetique d'un pesticide du groupe des thioquinoxalines: l'oxythioquinox, *Toxicology,* 6, 161, 1976.

347. **Carrera, G., Cambon-Gros, C., and Mitjavila, S.,** Oxythioquinone induced hepatomegaly, *Toxicol. Lett.,* 19, 159, 1983.

348. **Falzon, M., Carrera, G., and Mitjavila, S.,** Effets nutritionnels de l'oxythioquinox chez le rat, *Ann. Nutr. Metabl.,* 25, 109, 1981.

349. **Schlagbauer, B. G. L. and Schlagbauer, A. W. J.,** The metabolism of carbamate pesticides. A literature analysis, *Residue Rev.,* 42, 1, 1972.

350. **Fishbein, L.,** Environmental health aspects of fungicides 1-dithiocarbamates, *J. Toxicol. Environ. Health,* 1, 713, 1976.

351. **Vonk, J. W.,** Ethylenethiourea, a systemic decomposition product of nabam, *Med. Landbouwhogesch Genet.,* 36, 109, 1971.

352. **Mose, W., Munnecke, E., and Richardson, L. T.,** Cabonyl sulfide, volatile fungitoxicant from nabam in soil, *Nature,* 202, 831, 1964.

353. **Seidler, H., Hartig, M., Schnaak, W., and Engst, R.,** Metabolism of certain insecticides and fungicides in the rat. II. Distribution and degradation of carbon-14 labelled maneb, *Nahrung,* 14, 363, 1970.

354. **Truhaut, R., Fujita, M., Lich, N. P., and Chaigneau, M.,** Metabolism of zineb (zinc ethylene bis (dithiocarbamate) in rats, *C.R. Acad. Sci. Paris Ser.D,* 276, 229, 1973.

355. **Jordan, L. W. and Neal, R. A.,** Examination of the *in vivo* metabolism of maneb and zineb to ethylenethiourea (ETU) in mice, *Bull. Environ. Contam. Toxicol.,* 22, 271, 1979.

356. **Anon.,** Mancozebe, in *Evaluation de quelques Residues de Pesticides dans les Denrées Alimentaires,* Monogr., FAO/OMS, Geneva, 1970, 467.

357. **Ruddick, J. A., Williams, D. T., Hierlinhy, L., and Khera, K. S.,** (14C)-Ethylenethiourea; distribution, excretion and metabolism in pregnant rats, *Teratology,* 13, 35, 1976.

358. **Newsome, W. H.,** Excretion of ethylnethiourea by rat and guinea pig, *Bull. Environ. Contam. Toxicol.,* 11, 174, 1974.

359. **Ruddick, J. A., Newsome, W. H., and Iverson, F.,** Comparison of the distribution, metabolism and excretion of ethylenethiourea in the pregnant mouse and rat, *Teratology,* 16, 159, 1979.

360. **Savolainen, K. and Pyysalo, H.,** Identification of the main metabolite of ethylenethiourea in mice, *J. Agric. Food Chem.,* 27, 1177, 1979.

361. **Allen, J. R., Van Miller, J. P., and Seymour, J. L.,** Absorption tissue distribution and excretion of (14C) ethylenethiourea by the rhesus monkey and rat, *Res. Commun. Chem. Pathol. Pharmacol.,* 20, 109, 1978.

362. **Vekshtein, M. S. and Khitsenko, I. I.,** Ziram metabolism in warm blooded animals, *Giy. Sonit.,* 36, 23, 1973.

363. **Hodgson, J. R., Hoch, J. C., Castles, T. R., Helton, D. O., and Lee, C. C.,** Metabolism and disposition of Ferbam in the rat, *Toxicol. Appl. Pharmacol.,* 33, 505, 1975.

364. **Leng, M. L.,** Comparative metabolism of phenoxy herbicides, in *Fate of Pesticides in Large Animals,* Ivie, G. W. and Dorough, H. W., Eds., Academic Press, New York, 1977, 53.

365. **Clark, D. E., Young, J. E., Younger, R. L., Hunt, L. M., and McLaran, J. K.,** The fate of 2,4-dichlorophenoxyacetic acid in sheep, *J. Agric. Food Chem.,* 12, 43, 1964.

366. **Orberg, J.,** Observation on the 2,4-dichlorophenoxyacetic acid (2,4-D) excretion in the goat, *Acta Pharmacol. Toxicol. (Copenhagen),* 46, 78, 1980.

367. **Piper, W. N., Rose, J. Q., Leng, M. L., and Gehring, P. J.,** The fate of 2,4,5-trichlorophenoxyacetic acid (2,4,5-7) following oral administration to rats and dogs, *Toxicol. Appl. Pharmacol.,* 26, 33g, 1973.

368. **St. John, L. E., Wagner, D. G., and Lisk, D. J.,** Fate of atrazine, kuron, silvex and 2,4,5-T in the dairy cow, *J. Dairy Sci.,* 47, 1267, 1964.

369. **Hook. J. B., Bailie, M. D., and Johnson, J. T.,** *In vitro* analysis of transport of 2,4,5-trichlorophenoxyacetic acid by rat and dog kidney, *Food Cosmet. Toxicol.,* 12, 209, 1974.

370. **Eaton, D. L.,** Biliary excretion of 2,4,5-trichlorophenoxyacetic acid in the rat, *Toxicol. Lett.,* 14, 175, 1982.

371. **Courtney, K. D., Ebron, M. M. T., and Tucker, A. W.,** Distribution of 2,4,5-trichlorophenoxyacetic acid in the mouse fetus, *Toxicol. Lett.,* 1, 103, 1977.

372. **Koshakji, R. P., Bush, M. T., and Harbison, R. D.,** Metabolism and distribution of 2,4,5-trichlorophenoxyacetic acid in pregnant mice, *J. Environ. Sci. Health (C),* 13, 315, 1979.

373. **Colburn, W. A.,** A model for the dose-dependent pharmacokinetics of chlorophenoxy acid herbicides in the rat: the effect of enterohepatic recycling, *J. Pharmacoklin. Biopharm.,* 6, 417, 1978.

374. **Lemmerson, J. and Anderson, R. C.,** Metabolism of trifluralin in the rat and dog, *Toxicol. Appl. Pharmacol.,* 9, 84, 1966.

375. **Nelson, J. O., Kearney, P. C., Plimmer, J. R., and Menzer, R. E.,** Metabolism of trifluralin, profluralin and fluchloralin by rat liver microsomes, *Pestic. Biochem. Physiol.,* 7, 73, 1977.

376. **Crayford, J. V., Huston, D. H., and Stoydin, G.,** The metabolic fate of the herbicide nitralin in the rat, *Xenobiotica,* 14, 221, 1984.

377. **Heijboek, W. M., Muggleton, D. F., and Parke, D. V.,** Metabolism of the carbamate herbicide asulam in the rat, *Xenobiotica,* 14, 235, 1984.

378. **Paulson, G. D., Jacobsen, A. M., Zaylskie, R. G., and Feil, V. J.,** Isolation and identification of propham (isopropyl carbanilate) metabolites from the rat and the goat, *J. Agric. Food Chem.,* 21, 809, 1973.

379. **Fang, S. C., Fallin, E., Montgomery, M. L., and Freed, V. H.,** Metabolic studies of ^{14}C labelled propham and chlorpropham in the female rat, *Pestic Biochem. Physiol.,* 4, 1, 1973.

380. **Carrera, G., Dikshith, T. S. S., Periquet, A., and Mitjavila, S.,** Cytotoxocité du chlorpropham sur l'hepatocyte isolé de rat: influence d'une modulation de l'activite des sulfo et des glucuronconjugaisons, *Diab. Metab.,* 10, 341, 1984.

381. **Bobik, A., Holder, G. M., and Ryan, A. J.,** Excretory and metabolism studies of isopropyl N(3-chlorophenyl) carbamate in the rat, *Food Cosmet. Toxicol.,* 10, 163, 1972.

382. **Ishikawa, K., Okuda, J., and Kuwatsaka, S.,** Metabolism of benthiocarb. I. Metabolism of benthiocarb (4-chlorobenzyl N,N-diethylthiol carbonate) in mice, *Agric. Biol. Chem. (Japan),* 37, 165, 1973.

383. **Bakke, J. E., Larson, J. D., and Price, C. E.,** Metabolism of atrazine and 2-hydroxyatrazine by the rat, *J. Agric. Food Chem.,* 20, 602, 1972.

384. **Larsen, G. L., Bakke, J. E., and Feil, V. J.,** Metabolism of ^{14}C-terbutryn by rats and goats, *Biomed. Mass. Spectrom.,* 5, 382, 1978.

385. **Crayford, J. V. and Hutson, D. H.,** Metabolism of the herbicide, 2-chloro-4-(ethylamino)-6-(1-cyano-1-methylamino)-S-triazine in the rat, *Pestic Biochem. Physiol.,* 2, 295, 1972.

386. **Ernst, W. and Bohme, C.,** Uber den stoffwechsel von harnstoff-herbiciden in der ratte. 1. Mitteilung monuron und Aresin, *Food Cosmet. Toxicol.,* 3, 789, 1965.

387. **Bohme, C. and Ernst, W.,** Uber den stoffwechsel von harnstoff-herbiciden in der ratte. 2. Mitteilung Diuron and Afalon, *Food Cosmet. Toxicol.,* 3, 797, 1965.

388. **Hodge, H. C., Downs, W. L., Panner, B. S., Smith, B. W., Meynard, E. A., Clayton, G. W., and Rhodes, R. C.,** Oral toxicity and metabolism of Diuron in rats and dogs, *Food Cosmet. Toxicol.,* 5, 513, 1967.

389. **Ross, D., Farmer, P. B., Gescher, A., Hickman, J. A., and Threadgill, M. D.,** The formation and metabolism of N-hydroxymethyl compounds. 1. The oxidative N-demethylation of N-dimethyl derivatives of arylamines, aryltriazines, arylformamidines and arylurease including the herbicide Monuron, *Biochem. Pharmacol.,* 31, 3621, 1982.

390. **Hilbig, V., Lucas, K., and Sebek, V.,** Untersuchengen zur elimination und biotransformation von 3-(4-chlorophenyl) 1-methoxy-1-methylharnstoff (Monolinuron) beim schwein, *Zbl. Vet. Med. A.,* 24, 311, 1977.

391. **Westphal, D., Lucas, K., and Hilbig, V.,** Studies of the arylhydroxylation of monochlorophenylureas in the isolated perfused rat liver, *Food Cosmet. Toxicol.,* 19, 341, 1981.

392. **Sharp, C. W., Ottolenghi, A., and Posner, H. S.,** Correlation of paraquat toxicity with tissue concentrations and weight loss of the rat, *Toxicol. Appl. Pharmacol.,* 22, 241, 1972.

393. **Kurisaki, E. and Sato, H.,** Tissue distribution of paraquat, *Forensic Sci.,* 14, 165, 1979.

394. **Ingebrigtsen, K., Nafstat, I., and Andersen, R. A.,** Distribution and transplacental transfer of paraquat in rats and guinea pigs, *Gen. Pharmacol.,* 15, 201, 1984.

395. **Hawksworth, G. H., Bennett, P. N., and Davies, D. S.,** Kinetics of paraquat elimination in the dog, *Toxicol. Appl. Pharmacol.,* 57, 139, 1981.

396. **Waddell, W. J. and Marlowe, C.,** Tissue and cellular disposition of paraquat in mice, *Toxicol. Appl. Pharmacol.,* 56, 127, 1981.

397. **Gaudreault, P., Karl, P. I., and Friedman, P. A.,** Paraquat and putrescine uptake by lung slices of fetal and new-born rats, *Drug Metab. Dispos.,* 12, 550, 1985.

398. **Forman, H. J., Aldrich, T. K., Posmer, M. A., and Fisher, A. B.,** Differential paraquat uptake and redox kinetics of rat granular pneumocytes and alveolar macrophages, *J. Pharmacol. Exp. Ther.,* 221, 428, 1982.

399. **Richmond, R. and Halliwell, B.,** Formation of hydroxyl radicals from the paraquat radical cation demonstrated by a highly specific gas chromatographic technique: role of superoxide radical anion, hydrogen peroxide and glutathione reductase, *J. Inorg. Biochem.,* 17, 85, 1982.

400. **Hassan, H. M.,** Exacerbation of superoxide radical formation by paraquat, in *Oxygen Radicals in Biological Systems,* Packer L., Ed., Academic Press, Orlando, FL, 1984, 523.

401. **Aldrich, K. T., Fisher, A. B., Cadenas, E., and Chance, B.,** Evidence for lipid peroxidation by paraquat in the perfused rat lung, *J. Lab. Clin. Med.,* 101, 66, 1983.

Chapter 4

PESTICIDES AND LIPID PEROXIDATION

S. Mitjavila

TABLE OF CONTENTS

I. INTRODUCTION

Membrane lipid peroxidation is a degenerative process which takes place on the poly-unsaturated fatty acids from B position of phospholipids.[1-3] This oxidation is accompanied by the appearance of very different degradation products and of a profound modification of the membrane structure.[4,5] Damage to membrane proteins, DNA, and RNA induced by radicals and reactive species coming from the lipid peroxidation can explain the diversity of the generated toxicity form.[6-10] Oxygen, as a necessary element for life, can in this way, participate in extremely toxic reactions.[11,12] This toxicity is closely dependent on the aerobic life and on the oxidation processes which normaly take place in a controlled way in the organism.[13]

Mixed function oxidases localized in the endoplasmic reticulum certainly constitute the main oxidation path of xenobiotics. The pesticide containing an aromatic cycle is hydrox-ylated during phase I of the metabolism. Certain substrates can induce an uncoupling of this reaction and favor the appearance of an active form of oxygen.[14,15] Peroxidases can also catalyze the one electron oxidation of xenobiotics. In this way, the myeloperoxidase, lac-toperoxidase, catalase, and prostaglandin synthetase use substrates as lipid hydroperoxides and H_2O_2 for the cooxygenation of foreign compounds as aromatic amines, hydroxylamines, and hydrazines.[16] Various potential carcinogens such as benzo(a)pyrene can be cooxygenated during the metabolism of arachidonic acid,[17] and there is a good correlation between the promoter activity of a substance and the prostaglandin releasing potency.[18] Aromatic amines derived from the metabolism of a pesticide can undergo cooxygenation.

Several compounds such as the quinones, quinone-imines, nitroaromatics, azoaromatics, bipyridilium, and tetrazolium can suffer a one-electron reduction catalyzed by NADPH-cytochrome p-450 reductase, NADH-cytochrome b_5 reductase, xanthine dehydrogenase, cytochrome b_5, or cytochrome p-450 yielding a free radical and generating O_2.[16]

The electron transport chain of mitochondria and of endoplasmic reticulum normally generates small quantities of the active form of oxygen: superoxide anion (O_2^-) and hydrogen peroxide (H_2O_2). These reactive oxygen forms are controlled by defense enzymes, but an inactivation of these systems by foreign compounds or an increase of (O_2^-) flux due to their metabolism, can lead to an oxidative stress. Similarly, the repeated requirement of defense mechanism against the oxidative stress constitutes a pressure which can lead to progressive and irreversible loss of homeostasis.

Oxidative activation and lipid peroxidation are probably involved in many pathological processes like aging, diabetes provoked by alloxan, atherosclerosis, and heart diseases. The accumulation of high molecular weight proteins and chromolipids in nervous and mus-cular tissues is considered direct proof of the existence of peroxidation processes in the organism.[19]

Toxic processes due to lipid peroxidation started by foreign compounds, are subject to controversy.[20] In certain cases, it is difficult to define if the observed pathology is related to the initial state of the peroxidative aggression, or if it is a consequence of tissue injury or the depletion of endogenous compounds controlling the oxidative stress.[21] Moreover, the analytical methods used to prove the existence of a lipid peroxidation *in vivo* usually require fleeting and reactive intermediary metabolites not very representative of the processes. The measurement of alkanes in expired air reveals peroxidation reactions and constitutes a direct proof of their existence.[19] This allows us to follow, in a reliable manner the evolution of the peroxidation but, even in this case, it does not show, from a topographical point of view, the organelles or the membrane zones affected.

On the other hand, the existence of peroxidation processes initiated by xenobiotics on cellular or subcellular preparations, does not constitute proof of the existence of these processes *in vivo*. Unfortunately, the experimental conditions sometimes used only show evidence for the absence of coordinated regulatory mechanisms present in the whole organism.

In spite of this, it is clear that at whatever stage of aggression where the lipid peroxidation starts, the violence and the destructive force of this reaction on biological membranes can have consequences which contribute to the installation of a pathological process.

The importance of peroxidation processes in the toxicity of pesticides may be considered in two aspects:

- The repercussions of lipid peroxidation provoked by other substances on the toxicity of pesticides.
- The role of pesticides as protective agent or as agents acting directly or indirectly on the initiation of lipid peroxidation.

Concerning the first aspect, lipid peroxidation profoundly alters the structure of membranes and consequently modifies their enzymatic and transport activities. In this way, mitochondrial lipid peroxidation is characterized by extensive swelling and disintegration and is accompanied by a loss of their functional activity.[22-24] Spontaneous swelling of fetal mitochondria seems to be in relation to the low concentration of GSH and the low activity of catalase and glutathione peroxidase in fetal liver. Oxidative stress in lysosomes has been correlated with disintegration of lysosomal membranes.[25,26] Peroxide hemolysis of erythrocyte is observed during diverse pathological situations.[27,28]

The membrane of the endoplasmic reticulum, by its own activity, is quite exposed to peroxidation which leads to loss of microsomal enzymic and transport activities. Glucose-6-phosphatase, aminopyrine demethylase, cytochrome p-450, hydroxylases activity, and calcium uptake sharply decline during the preincubation of microsomes with agents initiating lipid peroxidation.[29-32]

Among the enzymes inhibited by the peroxidation, epoxide hydrolase presents a strong sensibility and deserves particular interest.[33] Its inhibition can provoke an accumulation of epoxides formed under the action of epoxidase. The latter enzyme participates in the detoxification of halogenated pesticides derived from cyclopentadiene (heptachlor, aldrin, isodrin) and compounds derived from halogenated ethylenes.[34] These epoxides can have covalent bonds with proteins or nucleic acids. This is used to explain the mutagenicity in bacterial tests and carcinogenicity in animal bioassays of halogenated ethylenes which are in relation to the structural characteristics of the halogenated pesticides and with the stability of the epoxide ring. This stability is considered to be the result of DNA binding and enzymatic detoxification.[35,36] An increase in the ratio of epoxidase activity to epoxide hydrolase activity favors the genotoxicity. By diminishing the functional activity of cellular organelles or of the enzymatic systems involved in the detoxification, the lipid peroxidation can affect the toxicity of foreign compounds either by limiting their metabolism or, by favoring the accumulation of toxic intermediates.

Concerning the participation of pesticides and related compounds to the processes of membrane peroxidation, several situations may be considered:

- Direct initiation by free radicals produced by the metabolism. In this way, CCl_3 derived from CCl_4 can take a hydrogen from other molecules (polyenoic fatty acids) and thus initiate a peroxidation chain.
- Indirect initiation by the production, during their metabolism of reactive forms of oxygen. For example, paraquat can activate O_2 by univalent reduction, to the superoxide anion (O_2^-).
- Inhibition of enzymatic systems of defense involved in the control of reactive oxidating entities. Thus, certain derived compounds of dithiocarbamates behave as inhibitors of superoxide dismutase (SOD).

● Destruction of natural antioxidants which control the reactions of peroxidation. For example, the reduction of the hepatocyte glutathione level induced by a fumigant (1,2-dibromoethane) is associated with the accumulation of malonicdialdehyde.

Besides the consequences of lipid peroxidation on the activity of membrane which we have already talked about, the eventual interaction of the intermediates with the DNA deserves particular attention. This interaction would be facilitated by the direct contact of the membrane of the endoplasmic reticulum with that of the nucleus and would allow a better understanding of the genotoxicity of foreign compounds by considering the migration of generated active forms of oxygen or of degradation products of lipoperoxides.

It has been postulated that promoters in particular may act through the generation of oxygen radical species. These radicals appear to be toxic because they act as initiators of lipid peroxidation.[10,37-39] During the peroxidation of lipids, substances such as hydroperoxides, endoperoxides, epoxides, or aldehydes appear. Some of them have been described as having a mutagenic and carcinogen potential.[40-42] Other foreign compounds provoke a proliferation of peroxisomes which is accompanied by an increase of hydrogen peroxide and other DNA damaging oxygen radicals.[10] Nevertheless, there are not many formal proofs of the carcinogenic activity of pesticides.

Environmental factors are considered as having an important incidence in the development of cancers. About 80% of human cancers would be in relation to these factors.[43-47] In spite of industrialization and changes in life styles, epidemiological studies do not reveal a clear implication of xenobiotics in cancer risk though some additive or contaminants of food products have exhibited carcinogenic properties.[44,48,49]

It is now important to understand the significance of the oxidative damage in the toxic processes concerning pesticides. It must be admitted that in spite of the interest on the subject this problem has not been tackled in a systemic way from an experimental point of view. Similarly, there are very few examples for the set of foreign compounds illustrating the importance of an oxidative activation and lipid peroxidation in toxic processes.

The chapter presents a brief overview on lipid peroxidation, explaining the observations made on different pesticides.

II. GENERALITIES ABOUT THE LIPID PEROXIDATION

A. THE REACTION OF LIPID PEROXIDATION

The peroxidation reaction of membrane phospholipids is of a radical nature. It is initiated by the abstraction of a methylenic hydrogen on the chain of a polyunsaturated fatty acid (RH). This homolytic cleavage gives rise to the formation of a fatty acid radical (R·). It follows rearrangement with the conjugation of double bonds, which can be confirmed by the appearance of an absorption peak at 233 nm. During the propagation stage, molecular oxygen quickly reacts with this radical constituting the lipid peroxy free radical (ROO·) which in turn acts, via a hydrogen abstraction on a methylene of a neighboring unsaturated fatty acid, yielding a lipid hydroperoxide (ROOH) and a new fatty acid free radical (R·).[4,50]

$$RH \longrightarrow R· + H·$$
$$R· + O_2 \longrightarrow ROO·$$
$$ROO· + RH \longrightarrow ROOH + R·$$

Chain branching is also possible

$$2 \ ROOH \rightarrow ROO^{\cdot} + RO^{\cdot} + H_2O$$

Yielding a new radical ($RO^{\cdot}$).

Vitamin E or α-tocopherol (α-TH) acts as a scavenger, which prevents the propagation of peroxidation reaction, by competing with a lipid peroxy free radical.[7,51,52]

$$ROO^{\cdot} + \alpha\text{-TH} \longrightarrow ROOH + \alpha\text{-T}^{\cdot}$$
$$2 \ \alpha\text{-T}^{\cdot} \longrightarrow \alpha\text{-T} - quinone$$

Diet poor in vitamin E favors the lipid peroxidation and potentiates, for example, the pulmonary toxicity of the paraquat.[53]

Glutathione peroxidase can reduce, at the expense of glutathione the lipid hydroperoxides to the corresponding hydroxide.[54]

$$ROOH + 2 \ GSH \longrightarrow R\text{-OH} + GS\text{-}SG + H_2O$$

Lipid hydroperoxides are unstable and can also be decomposed through reactions catalyzed by transition metal ions (M^{n+}) as ferrous or manganous or by heme pigments.[4,55]

$$ROOH + M^{n+} \rightarrow RO^{\cdot} + OH^- = M^{(n+1)+}$$
$$ROOH + M^{(n+1)+} \rightarrow ROO^{\cdot} + H^+ + M^{n+}$$

The superoxide anion can participate in the decomposition of fatty acid hydroperoxides according to the following reaction:[56]

$$ROOH + O_2^{\dot{-}} \rightarrow RO^{\cdot} + \dot{O}H + O_2$$

New free radicals ($RO^{\cdot}$, $ROO^{\cdot}$) appear which establish new peroxidation chains.

The β-cleavage of $RO^{\cdot}$ originated from ω-6 hydroperoxides and ω-3 hydroperoxides and gives rise to the formation of pentane and ethane respectively.[57,58]

$$RO^{\cdot} \xrightarrow{\ \beta\text{-cleavage}\ } R - CHO + CH_3 - CH_2^{\cdot}$$
$$CH_3 - CH_2^{\cdot} + RH \longrightarrow R^{\cdot} + CH_3 - CH_3$$

Through these reactions, these fatty acids and hydroperoxides are reduced to hydroxy fatty acids or broken down to more simple compounds such as alkanes, alkenals, malonicdialdehyde.[59]

During the termination phase several rections lead to the annihilation or $R^{\cdot}$, $ROO^{\cdot}$, $RO^{\cdot}$ radicals giving condensation products. Other reactions give rise to cross-linking of fatty acids and proteins.

B. EVIDENCE OF LIPID PEROXIDATION PROCESSES

Several methods, based on the above-described reactions, confirm the existence of a lipid peroxidation process and follow its evolution on subcellular, cellular, tissue, or whole animal preparations.

The most widely used method for measurement of lipid peroxidation is the reaction of thiobarbituric acid with one of the oxidative degradation products of lipids, the malonicdialdehyde.[60] This method yields excellent results *in vitro* nevertheless, this aldehyde is rapidly metabolized and reacts with proteins and nucleic acids. The absence of a positive reaction *in vivo* is not a proof of the absence of lipid peroxidation.

Diene conjugation is an important step during the lipid peroxidation process. After *in vivo* treatment with toxicants initiating peroxidation, lipid extract of liver shows a characterisitic ultraviolet difference spectra with intense absorption at 233 nm.[4,61,62] This method has been improved by utilizing tetracyanoethylene ^{14}C in a Diels-Adler condensation reaction with conjugated dienes which gives a more sensitive and specific measurement.[63]

The peroxidation of unsaturated fatty acids gives rise to the formation of ethane and pentane.[64] These two alkanes can be easily determined by gas chromatography in the head space of cellular or subcellular preparations incubated in aerobiose. Besides, it is also possible to evaluate *in vivo* the induced peroxidation by the xenobiotics determining the ethane and pentane of the expired gases, without needing to sacrifice the animal.[19]

C. BASES FOR THE PARTICIPATION OF XENOBIOTICS TO THE INITIATION OF LIPID PEROXIDATION

Peroxidation of membrane phospholipids can be directly initiated by certain pollutants such as nitrogen dioxide and ozone,[65] or by radicals arising from the microsomal metabolism. Thus, the CCl_4 used along with fumigants to reduce fire hazard, is reductively dehalogenated by cytochrome p-450 and gives the CCl_3 radicals.[66,67] This radical or the $CCl_3OO^{\cdot}$ radical formed in the presence of oxygen induced the abstraction of hydrogen on methylene carbons of polyenoic fatty acids which is the first stage leading to peroxidation.[7,68-70]

Other xenobiotics indirectly initiate the peroxidation through the reactive forms of singlet oxygen ($^1O_2$), superoxide anion ($O_2^{\cdot}$), hydroxy radical ($OH^{\cdot}$), and hydrogen peroxide (H_2O_2) which originate during their oxidation in the organism. Mixed-function oxidase is a system consisting of cytochrome p-450 (the terminal oxygen transferase), cytochrome p-450 reductase (containing FAD and FMN), phosphatidyl choline, and it is linked to a source of electrons (NADPH). This system catalyzes the activation of oxygen needed for the hydroxylation of natural substrates and a variety of environmental chemicals as pesticides. Coupled to superoxide dismutase and catalase, this system can also have a role in the detoxification of oxygen.[12,71] Prior to activation of the oxygen, the prosthetic group of cytochrome p-450 undergoes a conformational change from a low spin state, with six ligands, to a high spin state, with five ligands. Some toxic drugs give a stable ligand complex with the hemoprotein and, in these conditions, instead of the normal hydroxylation function, it catalyzes autooxidative processes.[72,73]

Different forms of oxygen can appear in the tissues during diverse biological reactions catalyzed by hemoproteins, flavoproteins, cytochrome p-450, and even iron. The metabolism of several pesticides leads to the formation of phenols. These compounds can react with oxyhemoglobin yielding a phenoxy free radical and the methemoglobin -H_2O_2 system which possesses a high peroxidative acitvity.[16]

Finally, the xenobiotics which interefere with the activity of the enzymes involved in oxygen detoxification favor the initiation of the peroxidation by these active forms of oxygen. The implication of active oxygen sources in both nonenzymatic as well as enzymatic oxidation in biological systems has been the main theme of the review on the active forms of oxygen as initiators of lipid peroxidation.[74]

The relative importance of $^1O_2$, $O_2^{\cdot}$, $OH^{\cdot}$, and H_2O_2 in the processes of peroxidation is widely discussed. In the ground state, molecular oxygen possesses two unpaired electrons. It can react with free radicals through reactions using one electron only, but it cannot take part in ionic reactions. In order to participate in oxidation reactions, a high activation energy must be supplied. Coupled to certain transition metals, oxygen behaves like an ion species. It is in this way that it participates in the metabolic reactions in the respiratory cycle. Most cellular oxidations use the cytochrome c reductase which simultaneously transports the four necessary electrons for the reduction of the oxygen molecule.

$$\cdot O - O \cdot + 4H^+ + 4e^- \longrightarrow 2\,H_2O$$

In aerobic cells 95% of oxygen is directly reduced in this way through the respiratory chain localized in the mitochondria. Among 25 molecules an electron from the ubiquinone escapes to the respiratory chain giving rise to a superoxide ion radical. An electron transport chain not accompanied by energy conversion is localized in the endoplasmic reticulum. It can use the oxidation of NADHP and NADH by the flavoproteins as electron source to reduce molecular oxygen by transporting electrons one by one. Lipid peroxidation of microsomes will not occur if proper substrate for terminal hydroxylation by cytochrome p-450 is present. In these conditions, the global reaction is

$$RH + O_2 + 2H^+ + 2e^- \longrightarrow ROH + H_2O$$

The uncoupling of such a reaction can take place in the presence of certain substrates which shift the redox potential making the reduction of cytochrome p-450 easier. In this case the reaction catalyzes the formation of hydrogen peroxide.

$$RH + O_2 + 2H^+ + 2e^- \longrightarrow RH + H_2O_2$$

The *in vivo* production of hydrogen hydroperoxide in the smooth endoplasmic reticulum is small. However, isolated microsomes use very well the oxidation of NADPH as an electron source to reduce molecular oxygen producing hydrogen peroxide.[15,75] If an electron acceptor such as cytochrome c or ferricyanide is added to the medium, it reduces the cytochrome p-450 and lipid peroxidation is abolished.[76]

It is probable that the reduction of active forms of oxygen, produced by uncouplings, also produces water. In fact, the step by step reduction of oxygen would be

oxygen	superoxide radical	hydroxygen peroxide	hydroxyl radical
E' volt - 0.33	0.87	0.38	2.33

The first step of reduction shows a redox couple of -0.33 V confirming that oxygen is a poor one-electron oxidant.

The implication of the superoxide radical anion in the intiation of peroxidation processes has been discussed.[77-79] In fact, the superoxide radical is a toxic byproduct of aerobic organisms, and SOD acts as a defense mechanism against this toxicity by catalyzing its dismutation:[80]

$$2O_2^{\overline{\cdot}} + 2H^+ \xrightarrow{\text{SOD}} O_2 + H_2O_2$$

This protection is efficient and makes it difficult to show the direct role of $O_2^{\overline{\cdot}}$ in the

126   *Toxicology of Pesticides in Animals*

peroxidation. Furthermore, the detection methods are not very specific and may only be used in highly purified systems.[81]

In fact, the O_2^- is believed not to be very reactive in aqueous medium and it would be unable on its own to start the peroxidation of membranes.[82,83] However the O_2^- can be activated by other stable free radicals which link covalently with superoxide. The decomposition of this adduct could generate a strong oxidant, the singlet oxygen.[84]

To sum up, the reaction characteristics of superoxide anion do not correspond to the observed effects. Other oxygenated intermediates have been considered in order to explain the initiation of peroxidation. The one electron reduction of hydrogen hydroperoxide by a superoxide radical is favorable from the thermodynamic point of view (0.71 V). This reaction is known as the Haber-Weiss reaction.

$$O_2^- + H_2O_2 \longrightarrow OH^\cdot + OH^- + O_2$$

It gives rise to the hydroxyl radical (OH$^\cdot$), considered to be one of the most powerful oxidants in aqueous medium.[85] It has been proposed to be a potential initiator of lipid peroxidation.[86] Several scavengers of the hydroxy radical are known (ethanol, benzoate, manitol). The inhibition of paraquat-stimulated lipid peroxidation by another scavenger (dimethylurea) is favored in the intervention of this radical.[87]

From the point of view of kinetics the Haber-Weiss reaction is extremely slow and it cannot explain the observed phenomena. It has been proved that the presence of iron considerably increases the speed of the reaction:[88,89]

$$O_2^- + Fe^{3+} \longrightarrow O_2 + Fe^{2+}$$
$$H_2O_2 + Fe^{2+} \longrightarrow OH^\cdot + OH^- + Fe^{3+}$$

The Fe^{2+} catalyzes the decomposition of hydrogen peroxide (Fenton reaction) which is very stable at ambient temperature. However, physiological reductants such as ascorbate have been proved to be more effective than superoxide to maintain iron in its reduced state.[90] This form of iron could be reoxidized in the presence of O_2^-

$$Fe^{2+} + O_2^- + 2H^+ \longrightarrow Fe^{3+} + H_2O_2$$

inhibiting the production of OH$\cdot$. Moreover, in the presence of an O_2^- generating system (xanthine oxidase) the Fe^{3+}-DETAPAC is not reduced, which shows the complexity of this catalysis.[91] The participation of iron in the peroxidation process is further complicated by the fact it catalyzes the homolytic cleavage of the hydroperoxides

$$ROOH + Fe^{2+} \longrightarrow RO^\cdot + OH^- + Fe^{3+}$$
$$ROOH + Fe^{3+} \longrightarrow ROO^\cdot + H^+ + Fe^{2+}$$

giving rise to new free radicals which will start other peroxidation chains.

It is unlikely that the protein-bound iron such as ferritin and transferrin participates in the production of OH$^\cdot$. However, a catalyzed Haber-Weiss reaction as described for Fe^{3+}-EDTA[89-92] could explain certain observed peroxidation *in vitro* because buffers and reagents can supply sufficient iron (1 μM) to induce the destruction of hydrogen peroxide. Nevertheless, two arguments oppose the intervention of the hydroxyl radical in the initiation of the peroxidative process: on the one hand from a theoretical point of view and because of its strong reactivity, this radical should be quickly scavenged by other biological molecules. On the other hand the formation of OH$^\cdot$ has been shown with erythrocytes incubated in the presence of xanthine oxidase, but the absence of lyse shows the incapacity of this radical to induce the peroxidation of membranes. It is also likely that the OH· is consumed by $O_2^{\cdot-}$.[93]

$$O_2^{\cdot-} + H_2O_2 \longrightarrow O_2 + OH^- + OH^·$$
$$OH^· + O_2^{\cdot-} \longrightarrow OH^- + O_2$$

The role of metal chelating agents remains ambiguous. In this way, even though Fe^{3+}-EDTA actively participates in the Haber-Weiss reactions, the addition of small concentrations of EDTA to the microsomal preparations, complexes metals and completely prevents the endogenous peroxidation reaction.[94]

The participation of forms of cellular iron other than those noted has been considered, in particular ADP-Fe^{3+}. In the presence of ADP-Fe^{3+} a rapid erythrocyte lyse is observed with production of malonaldehyde. The mentioned reaction uses the production of OH·:

$$ADP\text{-}Fe^{3+} + O_2^{\cdot-} \longrightarrow ADP\text{-}Fe^{2+} + O_2$$
$$ADP\text{-}Fe^{2+} + H_2O_2 \longrightarrow ADP\text{-}Fe^{3+} + OH^· + OH^-$$

but the following mechanism seems more attractive[95,96]

$$ADP\text{-}Fe^{3+} + O_2^{\cdot-} \longrightarrow ADP\text{-}Fe^{3+}\text{-}O_2^{\cdot-}$$

in this case, the lipid peroxidation would be directly initiated by the attack of the perferryl radical on the polyenoic fatty acids.[97,98]

The presence in singlet oxygen of spin-paired electrons gives it a strong reactivity as an oxidant. In this way, it can quickly act on the polyenoic fatty acids by a Diels-Adler reaction giving rise to hydroperoxy fatty acids.[99,100] Studies carried out on the lyse of incubated erythrocytes in the presence of an $O_2^{\cdot-}$ generating system (xanthine oxidase) and of several scavengers confirm that $^1O_2$ would be a responsible agent for the intiation of lipid peroxidation.[101,102] Singlet oxygen may come either from the nonenzymatic decrease of a superoxide radical[103]

$$2O_2^{\cdot-} + 2H^+ \longrightarrow H_2O_2 + {}^1O_2$$

or of a Haber-Weiss type reaction.

$$O_2^{\cdot-} + H_2O_2 \longrightarrow OH^· + OH^- + {}^1O_2$$

Carotenoids and vitamin E are capable of quenching $^1O_2$[104] and the administration of β-carotene protects the mouse, against $^1O_2$-mediated toxicity.[105]

D. ENZYMATIC SYSTEMS OF DEFENSE AGAINST LIPID PEROXIDATION

Several enzymatic systems control and direct the evolution of active oxygen produced in the organism. These are in particular the superoxide dismutase, the catalase, and the complex glutathione peroxidase, glutathione reductase, and G-6-P dehydrogenase. Glutathione peroxidase can reduce at the expense of reduced glutathione, the hydroperoxides and hydrogen hydroperoxide formed during the oxidative process by the reaction:

$$2GSH + R\text{-}OOH \longrightarrow GS\text{-}SG + H_2O + R\text{-}OH$$
$$2\ GSH + HOOH \longrightarrow GS\text{-}SG + 2H_2O$$

Glutathione peroxidase is present in animals in two different forms, a selenium dependent enzyme active on organic hydroperoxides and H_2O_2[106] and a selenium independent enzyme which uses as substrates the organic hydroperoxides only. The later is, in fact, a glutathione-S-transferase.[107] The selenium dependent glutathione peroxidase represents and carries out the most important global activity. It is cytosolic and from this fact its main function is the destruction of hydrogen hydroperoxide.[108] However, it could play a role *in vivo* (by the digestive mucosa) in the reduction of lipid hydroperoxides present in food,[109] and as inhibitor of the initiation of peroxidation.[110] In rat liver homogenate it inhibits the formation of malon aldehyde during aerobic oxidation.[111]

Glutathione peroxidase, glutathione reductase, and G-6-P-dehydrogenase constitute a coupled system whose activity increases in oxidative stress[11] and works in the following pattern:

$$\left(\begin{array}{l} \text{NADPH} \\ \text{G-6-P} \\ \text{dehydrogenase} \\ \text{NADP}^+ \end{array}\right) \left(\begin{array}{l} \text{CSSG} \\ \text{GSH} \\ \text{reductase} \\ \text{2GSH} \end{array}\right) \cdot \left(\begin{array}{l} \text{2H}_2\text{O} \\ \text{GSH} \\ \text{peroxidase} \\ \text{H}_2\text{O}_2 \end{array}\right)$$

Glutathione plays a central role in chemical detoxification through conjugation reactions with electrophilic compounds, for example, as reductor agent protector of peroxidative processes. The glutathione concentration in rat liver is about 8 mM, but only half of this quantity is available for detoxification. A depletion of over 10% of reserves seriously compromises the control of the lipid peroxidation rate and any diminution favors peroxidation.[113-115] It is obvious that the alteration of the GSH level induced by the metabolism of xenobiotics would be of considerable toxicological interest. Certain pesticides such as malathion and parathion reduce the level of glutathione when incubated with a hepatic supernatant fraction (78,000 × g) whereas malaoxon and paraoxon do not.[116] On the other hand, induced genotoxicity by several pesticides can be removed by the addition of thiol-derived compounds with antioxidant activity.[117] Similarly, after administration of paraquat, the hepatic glutathione rate decreases and after depletion of glutathione by the diethyl maleate this pesticide attacks more specifically the liver.[118]

The simultaneous presence of superoxide radical and hydrogen hydroperoxide gives rise to the hydroxyl radical. The physiological role of superoxide dismutase coupled with the catalase is to avoid the formation of this radical. The peroxisomes play a central role in the production of hydrogen peroxide and substrates of peroxisomal flavoproteins (glycolate, urate, and D-amino acids) and increase the production of H_2O_2 which behaves as an inhibitor of the SOD.[119,120]

The catalase enzyme present in high concentration in liver catalyzes the detoxification reaction of the hydrogen hydroperoxide.[121]

$$2H_2O_2 \longrightarrow O_2 + 2H_2O$$

The inhibition of the catalase can provoke a dangerous increase in the concentration of H_2O_2. Aminotriozole is recognized as a powerful inhibitor of this enzyme.[122] Similarly, the microsomal oxidative demethylation of xenobiotics leads to the formation of formate which is another inhibitor.[123] It is also interesting to note that certain compounds related to carbamate pesticides, for example, sodium diethyl dithio carbamate and disulfiram are powerful inhibitors of SOD and have been found to potentiate the toxicity of compounds supposed to induce the production of the superoxide radical as oxygen and paraquat.[124,125] Conversely the SOD inhibits the inflammatory processes generated by the production of O_2^- during the phagocytic activation.[88]

III. PESTICIDES AND RELATED COMPOUNDS INDUCING LIPID PEROXIDATION

In this section, the pesticides are individually studied, as well as their metabolites and related compounds for which *in vivo* or *in vitro* experimental data exist concerning their participation in lipid peroxidation processes.

A. ORGANOPHOSPHORUS PESTICIDES

Pesticides belonging to the organophosphates or dithionates series have been extensively used due to their high insecticidal activities. Evidently, the effect of these pesticides on cholinesterase activity is considered to be the most important from a toxicological point of view. Several organophosphorus insecticides are well-known as alkylating agents and hepatic drug metabolism has been found to be decreased by alteration of the mixed function oxidase system.[126] There is a paucity of information concerning the effect of these insecticides on microsomal activation and very few data are available concerning their effect on lipid peroxidation.

1. Nitroaromatic Compounds

Various organophosphosphorus insecticides include in their molecules a nitroaromatic function (parathion, methylparathion, chlorthion, dicapthion, paraoxon). The hydrolysis of the arylphosphoester bond by an esterase is the first step of their metabolism, and yields a nitroaromatic compound which can be reduced by microsomal nitroreductases:

$$R - NO_2 \xrightarrow{e^-} R - NO_2^{\dot{-}} \xrightarrow[4H^+]{3\,e^-} R - NHOH \xrightarrow[2H^+]{2\,e^-} R - NH_2$$

The first stage is a one-electron reduction and leads to the formation of a nitro anion radical. Nitroreductases are inhibited by oxygen which under aerobic conditions acts as electron acceptors according to the following reaction:

$$R - NO_2^{\dot{-}} + O_2 \longrightarrow R - NO_2 + O_2^{\dot{-}}$$

The nitro anion radical is rapidly oxidized and catalyses the production of the superoxide anion radical.[127] This reaction is catalyzed by the NADPH-cytochrome p-450 reductase and the futile redox cycle of these nitroaromatic compounds leads to the uncontrolled oxidation of NADPH.[128]

This mechanism presents an analogy with that suggested for paraquat which induces lipid peroxidation.[125] This analogy is confirmed by the fact that during nitrofurantoin therapy, several cases of pulmonary edema and fibrosis have been observed which resemble the effects of paraquat poisoning.[129] Similarly, several nitrophenyl compounds and nitrofurazone stimulate the consumption of oxygen by cellular preparations according to the dismutation of $O_2^{\dot{-}}$. This stimulation is partially decreased when superoxide dismutase and catalase are added to the medium.[16]

When reaction conditions are present the superoxide anion produced in these reactions should be able to initiate a lipid peroxidation. Unfortunately, there are no clear examples of peroxidations induced by organophosphorus compounds having a nitroaromatic ring.

A nitroreduction has also been suggested to explain the mechanism of action of compounds derived from 5-nitrothiazol, having an interesting antiparasitic activity.[128] It seems likely that under aerobic conditions, a futile redox cycle leads to the $O_2^{\dot{-}}$ production.[19]

2. Vinyl Derivatives

Pesticides derived from vinylphosphate such as mevinphos, phosphamidon, dicrotophos, tetrachlorvinphos, and temivenphos constitute another series which, due to their metabolism, could induce favorable situations for the peroxidation of phospholipids. These compounds are metabolized conjugated with glutathione. A metabolite which is common to several compounds, the 2,4-dichlorophenylacyl chloride, in fact, spontaneously reacts with glutathione.[130] The glutathione conjugate is subject to nucleophilic attack by another molecule of glutathione. The result is the formation of GS-SG and hence a depletion of glutathione which leads to a loss of the defense capacity against lipid peroxidation.

3. Tick-20

The first results concerning the susceptibility to lipid peroxidation after the administration of organophosphorus compounds relate to Tick-20 (O,O-dimethylmalathion) a common household insecticide. This organophosphorus compound was injected intraperitoneally in rats (150 mg/kg body weight) for two successive days employing corn oil as a carrier. The animals were sacrificed 24 h after the last injection and NADPH-linked lipid peroxidation was assayed in the liver microsomal fraction. Lipid peroxidation was increased by 23% due to the injection of Tick-20.[131] However, it was decreased in animals with pretreated phenobarbital though this compound is known to increase the degree of liver microsomal lipid peroxidation. Later studies by the same group gave variable results depending on the administered dose of insecticide. Nevertheless, these studies confirm the induction of both enzymatic and nonenzymatic lipid peroxidation on microsomal liver preparations of female and male rat exposed to Tick-20.[132,133]

4. Parathion and Malathion

Parathion, malathion, and their oxygenated derivatives, paraoxon and malaoxon, were comparatively studied for their ability to bind covalently to cytochrome p-450 and to induce enzymatic or nonenzymatic peroxidation in microsomes.[116] These organophosphorus insecticides which behave as noncompetitive inhibitors of the metabolism of type I compounds, have a great affinity for the cytochrome p-450, but the latter is not converted in an irreversible way into cytochrome p-420. Paraoxon increases endogenous lipid peroxidation observed in the absence of NADPH, whereas malathion decreases it. The four insecticides are completely ineffective on the NADPH-dependent lipid peroxidation and the results strongly suggest that heme destruction is not associated with lipid peroxidation.[116]

5. Thiodemeton

The alteration in drug metabolizing enzymes and lipid peroxidation has been studied in mice which had received intraperitoneally thiodemeton (O,O-diethyl S-2(ethyl-thio) ethyl phosphorodithionate) at the dose of 1 mg/kg body weight for 3 days.[134] Lipid peroxidation linked to NADPH or promoted by ascorbate was tried in liver microsomal fractions. Thiodemeton stimulated both, and NADPH and ascorbate promoted lipid peroxidation. Treatment of animals with phenobarbital prior to thiodemeton intoxication increases lipid peroxidation.[134] The activities of aminopyrine N-demethylase and acetanilide hydroxylase and the levels of cytochromes were significantly lowered due to thiodemeton.

6. Trichlorfon and Sumithion

A comparative study of induced lipid peroxidation of two organophorus compounds, the trichlorfon (O,O-dimethyl, 1-hydroxy-2,2,2-trichloroethyl phosphonate) and sumithion (fenitrothion: O,O'-dimethyl-4-nitrophenyl triphosphoric acid ester) has been carried out on controlled rats and on vitamin A or vitamin E-deficient rats.[135,136] The toxicants were administered intraperitoneally at the dose of 150 and 800 mg/kg for trichlorfon and sumithion respectively. Cholinesterase activity, lipid peroxidation and the activity of mainly antioxidant enzymes (superoxide dismutase and catalase) were measured in liver homogenates prepared 150 min after trichlorfon administration or 240 min after sumithion administration. Trichlorfon which is the weaker cholinesterase blocker increases lipid peroxidation and the activity of the antioxidant enzymes more strongly than sumithion. Pretreatment of deficient animals with vitamin E before the experiment leads to higher lipid peroxide and superoxide dismutase values in the liver, but catalase values were decreased. Vitamin E pretreatment did not prove effective in preventing the trichlorfon induced increases in the antioxidant enzyme activities and lipid peroxidation but it compensated the activity changes caused by sumithion.

B. ORGANOHALOGENATED PESTICIDES AND RELATED COMPOUNDS

Some organohalogenated pesticides have been described for their ability to cause oxidative deterioration in membranes or because of their eventual participation, as oxygen acceptors in microsomal oxidations giving birth to active oxygenated derivatives. Among these compounds we can name, halogenated alkanes used in agriculture as fumigants (1,2-dibromoethane, 1,2-dichloroethane, 1,3-dichloropropane, 1,2-dichloropropane, 1,2-dibromo-3-chloropropane) or as stabilizing agents (1-chloro-2,3-epoxiethane) or even as derived products known to reduce the fire hazard (CCl_4) are linked to the use of fumigants. Others belong to the group of aromatic halogenated hydrocarbon pesticides such as DDT aldrin, mirex, and hexachlorobenzene. Finally, some others are organohalogenated-derivated products present in marketed preparations of pesticides as impurities of synthesis (dibenzodioxins, dibenzofurans) or formed during the metabolism of different pesticides (chloroanilines).

1. Halogenated Alkanes

Halogenated ethylene has been widely used in agriculture as fumigants (against pests of stored products), soil nematicides, and fungicides. Sometimes they are mixed with other haloalkanes as epichlohydrin (1-chloro-2,3) epoxyethane) or carbon tetrachloride. Rats treated with these compounds showed a significant decrease in cytochrome p-450 in microsomes of different organs and more significantly in the liver.[137] Some of these pesticides are finally very toxic. Carbon tetrachloride and ethylene dibromide cause a characteristic centrilobular necrosis of the liver[138] and are considered as mutagens and carcinogens.[139] In the pathogenesis of the cell necrosis, the involvement of lipid peroxidation seems probable but other mechanisms may certainly interfere.

Lipids extracted from the liver of rats intoxicated with dibromoethane show an increase in conjugated dienes.[140] In isolated hepatocytes treated with dibromoethane, lipid peroxidation measured by malonicdialdehyde accumulation is stimulated.[141] Peroxidation is associated with an increase in the leakage of lactate dehydrogenase causing a serious cellular damage. Antioxidants, such as tocopherol, N,N'-phenyl-phenylenediamine and promethazine, added to the incubation medium, reduced malonicdialdehyde formation without interfering with the covalent binding of dibromoethane. In the same way, the diethyldithiocarbamate and other free radical scavengers effective in preventing lipid peroxidation, did not inhibit ethylene dibromide-induced liver damages.[142] An analogous compound related to thiocarbamate pesticides, disulfiram potentiates the carcinogenicity of 1,2-dibromoethane probably by the inhibition of this microsomal oxidation.[143] The metabolic oxidation of 1,2-dibromoethane induces the formation of a hydroxyethyl-glutathione conjugate. Under the action of the disulfiram an active compound appears: the S-2-bromoethylglutathione which could account for the enhanced carcinogenic effect.[144] In any case glutathione plays an important role in the detoxication of dibromoethane[145] and during intoxication, glutathione contents in the target organs are rapidly depleted.[146,147] A significant decrease in glutathione content is also observed *in vitro* on hepatocytes incubated with this fumigant.[148] This depletion in glutathione may favor the lipid peroxidation. Thus, related compounds such as 1,1-dibromoethane and 1,2-dichloroethane did not cause either lipid peroxidation or GSH depletion.[149]

Carbon tetrachloride, used as coadjuvant to the fumigants, is a hepatotoxic agent which has been extensively studied and discussed in several reviews.[150-153] The liver necrosis caused by the CCl_4 is related to its bioactivation by the cytochrome p-450 of the endoplasmic reticulum. The initial event is the homolytic cleavage of the chlorine-carbon bond which produces trichloromethyl radical.[66,150,154]

$$CCl_4 \xrightarrow{+e^-} CCl_3^{\cdot} + Cl^-$$

The trichloromethyl radical can covalently bind to lipids and macromolecules. This binding is considered as one of the mechanisms responsible for CCl_4-induced hepatic damage.[155-157] This free radical can also initiate the attack on the hydrogen of a methylene carbon of a polyenoic fatty acid (RH).[158,159]

$$RH + CCl_3^{\cdot} \longrightarrow R^{\cdot} + CHCl_3$$

The new fatty acid free radical $R^{\cdot}$ will react with molecular oxygen giving birth to peroxy-fatty acid free radical ($ROO^{\cdot}$) thus initiating the lipid peroxidation which is a key event in CCl_4 hepatotoxicity.[159]

Through this mechanism the $CCl_3^{\cdot}$ enhances the microsomal lipid peroxidation observed both *in vitro* and *in vivo*.[160-162] Chloroform formed in the previous reaction may undergo further metabolism to phosgene ($COCl_2$).[163] But this compound does not appear to play a major role in CCl_4 toxicity.[164] Trichloromethyl radical reacts with oxygen to form a trichloromethyl peroxy free radical.[165] The trichloromethyl radical may also undergo one-electron reduction to yield the trichloromethyl carbanion, and then, after dechlorination, the dichlorocarbene anion:

$$CCl_3^{\cdot} \xrightarrow{+e^-} CCl_3^- \xrightarrow{-Cl^-} CCl_2^-$$

Dichlorocarbene is an electrophilic compound which easily reacts with the Fe^{2+} of the cytochrome p-450, giving a stable carbenic complex which explains the destruction of the hemoprotein. It is now known that covalent binding and lipid peroxidation both takes place in the smooth endoplasmic reticulum of CCl_4-poisoned adult rats. In fetal liver microsomes only covalent binding is observed.[166]

Several findings are in favor of the participation of the lipid peroxidation in the toxic processes induced by the CCl_4. The administration of lipid antioxidants, selenium, and free radical scavengers protects against CCl_4 hepatotoxicity[68,167] and decreases the CCl_4-induced ethane production.[58] A protection aginst lipid peroxidation is observed with competitive inhibitors of microsomal mixed-function oxidases.[68,168] On the contrary, compounds which induce this activity increase the susceptibility to CCl_4 and increase the degree of lipid peroxidation.[169,170] Exposure to DDT and chlordecone also potentiates the hepatotoxicity of CCl_4.[170,171] Therefore, chlordecone treatment apparently failed to significantly enhance microsomal lipid peroxidation.[170]

In vitro stimulation of lipid peroxidation by CCl_4 requires the presence of NADPH and is followed by an increase of the malonicdialdehyde. It was also proved that the decrease of cytochrome p-450 of rabbit liver microsomes can be initiated by endogenous peroxidation and is accelerated further by CCl_4. A good correlation was found between the rate of lipid peroxidation and the decrease of cytochrome p-450.[172] It is also quite obvious from the *in vivo* study that in destructing the cytochrome p-450 the pretreatment with a low dose of CCl$_4$ makes the animal resistant to a next dose of CCl$_4$.[76] Under *in vitro* anaerobic conditions, there is a strong covalent binding and a loss of cytochrome p-450[173,174] but lipid peroxidation is much more effective in the destruction of the cytochrome.[175]

Apart from the cytochrome p-450, other microsomal activities such as the calcium sequestration capacity or membrane enzymes seem quite sensitive to lipid peroxidation.[94,152,160,161,176,177] Some of these activities, such as aminopyrine demethylase and glucose 6-phosphatase were unaffected during anaerobic metabolism of CCl$_4$ by rat liver microsomes, excluding a direct attack of these enzymes by a trichlormethyl radical.[175] Thus these results are in favor of the improtant role of the lipid peroxidation in the toxic effects induced by CCl$_4$.

2. Tetrachlorodibenzodioxin

2,3,7,8-Tetrachlorodibenzodioxin (TCDD) is a compound formed during the synthesis of the herbicide 2,4,5-trichloropehnoxy acetic acid. As with other carcinogenic polycyclic hydrocarbons, TCDD is an inducer of cytochrome p-448-related enzyme activities.[178]

The administration of TCDD to animals provokes the peroxidation of hepatic lipids.[179,180] Selenium and iron are two elements which are quite implied in the peroxidative damage due to TCDD. Iron is a necessary factor in the peroxidative processes induced by TCDD. This polyhalogenated aromatic compound is nontoxic in iron-deficient mice.[181,182] Optimum dietary selenium provides partial protection from the toxic effect of TCDD.[183] TCDD is a very effective inducer of some hepatic enzymes,[178,184] but inhibits the enzyme responsible for the destruction of the active forms of oxygen, more particularly, the glutathione peroxidase. In animal species, this enzyme is selenium-dependent and its activity increases with the level of selenium in the diet.[185]

3. Pentachlorophenol

Pentachlorophenol used to protect wood is considered as having a low toxicity. Therefore, the administration of technical product to rats for 14 weeks shows an increase in the activity of the superoxide dismutase in the glial cells, whereas the glutathione contents decreases.[186] Through these characteristics, the transient oxidative stress observed has been related to the presence in commercial product, of dibenzodioxin and dibenzofuran contaminants.[186]

4. Hexachlorobenzene

Hexachlorobenzene (HCB) is a fungicide known as a potent inducer of porphyria.[187] Free radicals are involved in the metabolism of HCB, but rats receiving intraperitoneally 1.33 g/kg body weight of HCB do not present any increase of malonicdialdehyde in liver.[187] The administration of iron with HCB goes with an important increase of hepatic malonicdialdehyde, an inhibition of the glucose-6-phosphatase and a cross-linking of membrane protein,[188] typical phenomena of a lipid peroxidation that go with an increase of the toxicity of the HCB. It is a new proof of the role of iron in the catalysis of the process of lipid peroxidation. It allows us also to foresee the participation of products of the degradation of polyenoic fatty acids in the pathogenesis of induced porphyria. Besides, in patients with porphyria cutanea tarda remissions have been observed after administration of vitamin E.

5. Other Aromatic Halogenated Pesticides

Among the aromatic halogenated pesticides, some examples exist, obviously, showing their intervention in the processess of lipid peroxidation. For instance, animals given a diet containing DDT, an increase of the malonicdialdehyde content in liver is clearly demonstrated.[189] A similar result has been observed with diets containing a contaminant (polychlorinated biphenyls) and in this case, the increase of malonicdialdehyde goes with a decrease in the activity of the glutathione peroxidase of rats or chickens.[189,190]

On the contrary, after administration of DDT intratracheally to rats (5 mg/100 g body weight for 3 consecutive days) an inhibition of the lipid peroxidation in lungs is seen.[191] However, under similar conditions, endosulfan does not appear to have any lipid peroxidative effect.[191] In some other studies made with mice brain microsomal fractions, DDT is also revealed as being a relatively effective inhibitor of lipid peroxidation at concentration levels about 3×10^{-2} mM.[192] It is suggested that similar damage caused in the hepatic endoplasmic reticulum *in vivo* by DDT leads to membrane changes hampering lipid peroxidation.[192,193]

Dieldrin, another chlorinated insecticide, administered orally to rats (30 mg/kg body weight) also caused a decrease in the endogenous lipid peroxidation of microsomal liver fraction when compared to the controls.[194] In fact, compounds which undergo NADPH-linked hydroxylations in endoplasmic reticulum, inhibit endogenous lipid peroxidation when they are present in the incubation medium of the microsome. Thus, we can expect that all the substrates of the mixed function oxidases behave *in vitro* as inhibitors of the endogenous lipid peroxidation.

6. Chloroanilines

Several pesticides of the phenylcarbamate series (chlorpropham, chlorbupham), the phenyl-urea series (linuron, monuron, neburon, monolinuron, metoxuron, diuron), or the acylanilide series (propanil, monalide) give rise, during their degradation in the ground, or in their metabolism by superior organisms, to derived compounds of chloroaniline.[195-198] The acute toxicity of these hydrolysis products is higher than that of the parent compound.[199] Some metabolic paths of chloroanilines tend towards detoxification. Others, conversely, tend towards an overtoxification, sometimes using peroxidative processes. In this manner, the N-oxidation of these anilines leads to the formation of azoic compounds,[200] whose carcinogenic activity is well known.[201] The azoic compounds can give rise to an azoanion radical under the action of microsomal azoreductase. This activation is accompanied by an oxidation of NADPH or an increase in the consumption of oxygen and the appearance of superoxide anion which can be at the origin of an oxidative stress.[16]

The N-oxidation of mono, di-, and tri-chloroanilines can be catalyzed by aniline oxidase or by a peroxidase, but the first enzyme does not transform monosubstituted anilines in ortho or meta positions.[202] The prostaglandin endoperoxide synthetase, an enzyme present in large quantities in kidney medulla catalyzes the peroxidation of arachidonic acid.[203] This peroxide can act as a mediator in the N-oxidation of arylamines. The induction of bladder cancers by these compounds is explained in this way.[204] Cooxygenation is a research field which has been rarely investigated in relation to the toxicity of pesticides. Similarly, lipo-peroxidation generated by the skin due to exposure to UV radiation can be the origin of the N-oxidation of arylamines, lipophiles known for inducing skin cancers.[201]

C. HERBICIDES
1. Aminotriazole

3-Amino-1,2,4-triazole is a nonselective herbicide inhibiting chlorophyl formation. Its activity is shown by the bleaching of pigments in light-grown plants. Aminotriazole is a good inhibitor of catalase.[205] This property has found an application in the cytochemical localization of catalase in microbodies or other organelles by the diaminobenzidine staining method.

Aminotriazole, when administered to animals inhibits endogenous catalase activity and can be used to demonstrate the effect of a xenobiotic on the proliferation of peroxisomes or the damage produced by oxygen radicals.[206] Administered intraperitoneally to mice at a dose of 60 mmol/kg, the aminotriazole leads to a complete inhibition of plasma catalase activity and a considerable increase in lipid peroxidation of the liver, kidney, and lung.[207] In relation to lipid peroxidation, it is interesting to note that the aminotriazole inhibits the formation of hydroxylated metabolites (HHT and PHD) of the prostaglandin cyclic endoperoxides PGG2 and PGH2 in the platelet microsomal fraction.[208] Aminotriazole is also known to be a powerful cataractogenic agent. After intravenous administration of this compound (1 g/kg body weight) an inhibition of catalase activity in eye tissues was observed, associated with a two- to threefold increase in hydrogen peroxide concentration of aqueous humor and vitreous humor. Glutathione peroxidase activity was unaltered. Catalase of eye tissues regulates the endogenous hydrogen peroxide in humors.[122]

2. Paraquat

Paraquat (1,1′-dimethyl-4,4′-bipyridilium dichloride), also known by the names of methyl viologen and gramoxone, is a widely used contact herbicide. Besides, its effect on plants, paraquat has been shown to be extremely toxic to animals too. The poisonous symptoms of paraquat are characterized by an anoxia due to serious pulmonary lesions that it induces, which lead to death. Various cases of human mortality have been registered following the intentional or accidental ingestion of this herbicide. In all cases a progressive and inexorable aggression of the respiratory system is noticed. Paraquat produces an acute damaging phase in the lung followed by a characteristic intra-alveolar fibrosis responsible for the anoxia.[209] Renal and hepatic lesions have also been reported, but the pulmonary attack seems to be the most specific.[210] It has been related to the selective accumulation of paraquat in the lungs due to the diamino transport process located in the alveolar epithelial cells. The higher partial pressure of oxygen in this organ also seems to play a role. In fact, it should be noticed that the toxicity of this herbicide is potentiated by oxygen.[211,212] Biochemical mechanisms of paraquat toxicity have been discussed in detail.[2,213,214]

The mode of action of paraquat in animals seems to be close to that described for plants. In the latter, paraquat is reduced to a radical anion in the chloroplasts due to an electron flow from the normal reduction of NADP+. During photosynthesis, this free radical is reoxidized by molecular oxygen, which by gaining an electron gives rise to the superoxide radical. The superoxide radical is at the origin of an oxidation chain which ends in the degradation of the polyunsaturated fatty acids, as shown by the malonicdialdehyde which is accumulated in the leaves of the plants.[215] In animals, a similar biochemical mechanism has been proposed to be the basis of the toxicity of paraquat by the induction of the phospholipid peroxidation.[125] It sets in action a futile oxido-reduction cycle localized in the smooth endoplasmic reticulum of lung cells, which leads to the production of superoxide ions. The reducing equivalents by one electron reduction of paraquat comes form the NADPH-NADPH cytochrome p-450 oxidoreducatase system. The formed cation radical bispyridinium reacts almost instantly with molecular oxygen giving the superoxide anion O_2^-, thus maintaining the redox cycle of paraquat.[16,216,217] The oxygenated compounds initiating the peroxidation of lipids are generated from this superoxide radical under the action of superoxide dismutase and through a metal catalyzed Haber-Weiss reaction. However, the *in vivo* increase of the lipid peroxidation by paraquat has not been shown with certainty.[218,219]

The different reactive species of oxygen, which are to take place in the cascade leading to peroxidation observed *in vitro* have been studied, but the relative importance of each of these species in the observed final effect is not well defined. The formation of O_2^- and of H_2O_2 has been shown in microsomal preparations of lungs incubated in the presence of paraquat and NADPH.[217,220,221] The superoxide radical seems to play a pivotal role since the addition of superoxide dismutase to a microsomal preparation inhibits paraquat-mediated lipid peroxidation.[125,222] However, the administration to animals of superoxide dismutase seems to have little effect to prevent the toxicity of paraquat.[223] Similarly, an inhibitor of superoxide dismutase, diethyl dithiocarbamate, sensitizes the lung tissue from paraquat.[224] The addition to the liver perfusion medium of copper complexes (Cu(tyr)$_2$ and Cu-penicillamine) having a superoxide dismutase activity reduces the lipid peroxidation induced by the presence of paraquat.[225] The hydroxyl radical formed during the Haber-Weiss reactions catalyzed by iron seems to be the direct initiator of the lipid peroxidation induced by paraquat. In fact, the dimethylurea, a hydroxyl radical scavenger, inhibits the peroxidation.[222]

The chlorofibrate is recognized as increasing the rate of catalase of hepatic peroxysomes. However, the administration of this compound to paraquat-intoxicated animals does not modify the lung antioxidant enzyme activities. Nevertheless, the chlorofibrate has been proved to be a good protector for rats which receive a lethal dose of paraquat.[226] On the other hand, the joint administration to mice of aminotriazole, a fairly specific inhibitor of catalase and the LD_{50} of paraquat leads to a more rapid death of the animals.[207] Even though the catalasic activity of hemolyzed blood is strongly inhibited by the aminotriazole, that of the lungs is not modified. However, an inhibition of the superoxide dismutase and a clear increase of lipid peroxidation is noticed in this organ.[207]

The facts in favor of a toxic mechanism involving lipid peroxidation are based on the observations concerning the lipid peroxidation of membrane preparations and on the increase of the pulmonary aggression in animals subjected to an oxygen atmosphere or diets poor in natural antioxidant vitamin E or in selenium.[53] These compounds decrease the glutathione peroxidase activity and facilitate the lipid peroxidation. However, rats having received a lethal dose of paraquat, placed in an oxygen atmosphere show an increase in the rate of expired ethane which indicates a lipid peroxidation, clearly insufficient to explain the toxicity of this herbicide.[219] It should be added that paraquat reduced the GSH content in mouse liver,[118] but the glutathione depletion favors the lipid peroxidation.[113]

In spite of the indications in favor of the hypothesis explaining the toxicity of paraquat through lipid peroxidation, the contradictory observations on the *in vitro* paraquat-mediated rat lung microsomal lipid peroxidation raises the question of the validity of this hypothesis. Besides, under similar incubation conditions rat lung microsomes are more resistant to lipid peroxidation than mouse lung microsomes. A higher rate of vitamin E in the rat microsomes could explain this difference, because the reactivity of superoxide ion is subject to the control by this radical scavenger.[227] Moreover, the activity of NADPH cytochrome p-450 reductase is more than two times higher in the microsomes of mice than in those of rats.[228,229] Finally, the ability of paraquat to stimulate lipid peroxidation was also dependent on the presence of adequate reducing equivalents (NADPH).[222] In fact, when the intoxication by paraquat takes place a strong decrease in the rate of NADPH in the lung is observed which cannot be balanced by the normal metabolic processes.[230] This NADPH depletion makes the alveolar cells more sensitive to the radical attack and to peroxidation.[231]

IV. CONCLUSIONS

At the present level of our knowledge, it would not be prudent to draw conclusions on the importance of the lipid peroxidation induced, directly or indirectly, by pesticides and the toxic process they generate. The experimental conditions are often quite different and the results for a given compound can be contradictory. The radical activation of numerous pesticides is now quite well-defined and some forms of toxicity are related to the reactivity of these radicals and to the formation of covalent linkages with macromolecules.

Nevertheless, what is called the oxidative stress where active forms of oxygen are generated during the metabolism of the pesticides, is a field of research rarely explored. These active forms of oxygen are detrimental to membrane functions, mainly when the cellular defense mechanisms are overwhelmed or when transition metals act as catalysts.

REFERENCES

1. **Tappel, A. L.,** Lipid peroxidation damage to cell components, *Fed. Proc.,* 32, 1870, 1973.
2. **Bus, J. S. and Gibson, J. E.,** Lipid peroxidation and its role in toxicology, in *Reviews in Biochemical Toxicology,* Vol. 1, Hodgson, E., Bend, J. R., and Philpot, R. M. Eds., Elsevier, Amsterdam, 1979, 125.
3. **Mead, J. F.,** Free radical mechanisms of lipid damage and consequences for cellular membrane, in *Free Radicals in Biology,* Vol. 1, Prvor, W. A. Ed., Academic Press, New York, 1976, 51.
4. **Holman, R. T.,** Autoxidation of fats and related substances, in *Progress in the Chemistry of Fats and Other Lipids,* Vol. 2, Holman, R. T., Lundberg, W. O., and Malkin, T., Eds., Academic Press, New York, 1954, 51.
5. **Dilliard, C. J. and Tappel, A. L.,** Volatile hydrocarbon and carbonyl products of lipid peroxidation: a comparison of pentane, ethane, hexane and acetone as *in vivo* indices, *Lipids,* 14, 989, 1979.
6. **Hicks, M. and Gebicki, J. M.,** A quantitative relationship between permeability and the degree of peroxidation in microsome membrane, *Biochem. Biophys. Res. Commun.,* 80, 704, 1978.
7. **Tappel, A. L.,** Vitamin E and selenium as inhibitors in *in vivo* lipid oxidation, in *Lipids and Their Oxidation,* Schultz, H. W., Ed., AVI Publ., Westport, CT, 1962, 367.
8. **Recknagel, R. O. and Glende, E. A. Jr.,** Lipid peroxidation: a specific form of cellular injury, in *Handbook of Physiology, Reactions to Environmental Agents,* Lee, D. H. K., Falk, H. L., Murphy, S. D., and Geiger, S. R., Eds., Williams and Wilkins, Baltimore, 1977, 591.
9. **Plaa, G. L. and Witschi, H.,** Chemicals, drugs and lipid peroxidation, *Annu. Rev. Pharmacol. Toxicol.,* 16, 125, 1976.
10. **Ames, B. N.,** Dietary carcinogens and anticarcinogens. Oxygen radicals and degenerative diseases, *Science,* 221, 1256, 1983.
11. **McCord, J. M. and Fridovich, I.,** The biology and pathology of oxygen radicals, *Ann. Int. Med.,* 88, 122, 1978.
12. **Franck, L. and Massaro, D.,** Oxygen toxicity, *Am. J. Med.,* 69, 117, 1980.
13. **Wickramsinghe, R. H. and Villee, R. A.,** Early role during chemical evolution for cytochrome p-450 in oxygen detoxication, *Nature,* 256, 509,1975.
14. **Debey, P. and Balny, C.,** Production of superoxide ions in rat liver microsomes, *Biochimie,* 55, 329, 1973.
15. **Hildebrandt, A. G., Tjoe, M., and Roots, I.,** Mono oxygenase linked hydrogen peroxide production and degradation in liver microsomal fractions, *Biochem. Soc. Trans.,* 3, 807, 1975.
16. **Mason, R. P. and Chignell, C. F.,** Free radicals in pharmacology and toxicology: selected topics, *Pharmacol. Rev.,* 33, 189, 1982.
17. **Marnett, L., Wlodawer, P., and Samuelsson, B.,** Cooxygenation of organic substrates by the prostaglandin synthetase of sheep vesicular gland, *J. Biol. Chem.,* 250, 8510, 1975.
18. **Brune, K., Kalin, H., Schmidt, R., Hecker, E.,** Inflammation tumor initiating and promoting activities of polycyclic aromatic hydrocarbons and diterpene esters in mouse skin as comapred with their prostaglandin releasing potency *in vitro, Cancer Lett.,* 4, 333, 1978.
19. **Tappel, A. L.,** Measurement of and protection from *in vivo* lipid peroxidation, in *Free Radicals in Biology,* Vol. IV, Pryor, W. A., Ed., Academic Press, New York, 1980, 1.
20. **Smith, M. R., Thor, H., and Orrenius, S.,** The role of lipid peroxidation in the toxicity of foreign compounds to liver cells, *Biochem. Pharmacol.,* 32, 763, 1983.
21. **Mitchell, J. R., Corcoran, G. B., Smith, C. V., Huques, H., Lauterburg, B. H., and Nelson, E. B.,** in *Drug Reactions and the Liver,* Davis, M., Tredquer, J. M., and Williams, R., Eds., Pitman Press, Bath, England, 1981, 130.
22. **Hoffsten, P. E. Hunter, F. E., Jr., Geqieki, J. M., and Weinstein, J.,** Formation of lipid peroxide under conditions which lead to swelling and lysis of rat liver mitochondria, *Biochem. Biophys. Res. Commun.,* 7, 276, 1962.
23. **Hunter, F. E., Scott, A., Weinstein, J., and Schneider, A.,** Effect of phosphate, arsenate and other substances on swelling and lipid peroxide formation when mitochondria are treated with oxidized and reduced glutathione, *J. Biol. Chem.,* 239, 622, 1964.
24. **Tappel, A. L. and Zalkin, H.,** Lipid peroxidation in isolated mitochondria, *Arch. Biochem. Biophys.,* 80, 326, 1959.
25. **Desai, I. D., Sawant, P. L., and Tappel, A. L.,** Peroxidative and radiation damage to isolated lysosomes, *Biochem. Biophys. Acta,* 86, 277, 1964.
26. **Wills, E. D. and Wilkinson, A. E.,** Release of enzymes from lysosomes by irradiation and the relation of lipid peroxide formation to enzyme release, *Biochem. J.,* 99, 657, 1966.
27. **Bunyan, J., Green, J., Edwin, E. E., and Diplock, A. T.,** Studies on vitamin E. 5. Lipid peroxidation in dialuric acid-induced hemolysis of Vitamin E-deficient erythrocytes, *Biochem. J.,* 76, 47, 1960.
28. **Lubin, B. and Chin, D.,** Properties of vitamin E-deficient erythrocytes following peroxidant injury, *Pediatr. Res.,* 16, 928, 1982.

29. **Wills, E. D.,** Lipid peroxide formation in microsomes. The role of nonheme iron, *Biochem. J.,* 113, 1969.
30. **Glende, E. A., Jr.,** On the mechanism of carbon tetrachloride toxicity — coincidence of loss of drug metabolising activity with peroxidation of microsomal lipid, *Biochem. Pharmacol.,* 21, 2131, 1972.
31. **Reiner, O., Athanossopoulos, S., Hellmer, K. H., Murray, R. E., and Uehleke, H.,** Bildung von chloroform aus tetrachlorkolenstoff in Lebermikrosomen, Lipid peroxidation und Zerstorung von cytochrome p-450, *Arch. Toxicol.,* 29, 219, 1972.
32. **Kamataki, T. and Kitagawa, H.,** Effects of lipid peroxidation on activities of drug-metabolizing enzymes in liver microsomes of rats, *Biochem. Pharmacol.,* 22, 3199, 1973.
33. **Watabe, T. and Akamatsu, K.,** Microsomal epoxidation of cis-stilbene decrease in epoxidase activity related to lipid peroxidation, *Biochem. Pharmacol.,* 23, 1079, 1974.
34. **Wong, D. T. and Terriere, L. C.,** Epoxidation of aldrin, isodrin and heptachlor by rat liver microsomes, *Biochem. Pharmacol.,* 14, 375, 1965.
35. **Bolt, H. M., Laib, R. J., and Filser, J. G.,** Reactive metabolites and carcinogenicity of halogenated ethylenes, *Biochem. Pharmacol.,* 31, 1, 1982.
36. **Jones, R. B. and Mackrodt, W. C.,** Structure-genotoxicity relationship for aliphatic epoxides, *Biochem. Pharmacol.,* 32, 2359, 1983.
37. **Demopoulos, H. B., Pietronigro, D. D., Flamm, E. S. and Seligman, M. L.,** The possible role of free radical reactions in carcinogenesis, *J. Environ. Pathol. Toxicol.,* 3, 273, 1980.
38. **Ames, B. N., Hollstein, M. C., and Cathcart, R.,** in *Lipid Peroxide in Biology and Medecine,* Yagi, K., Ed. Academic Press, New York, 1982, 339.
39. **Marx, J. L.,** Do promotors affect DNA after all?, *Science,* 219, 158, 1983.
40. **Rosen, G. M., Finkelstein, E., Rauckman, E. J., and Kitchell, B. B.,** Biological generation of free radicals and carcinogenesis, in *Safe Handling of Chemical Carcinogens, Mutagens, Teratogens, and Highly Toxic Substance,* Vol. II, Walters, D. B., Ed., Ann Arbor Science Publ., Ann Arbor, Mich., 1980, 469.
41. **Cutler, M. G. and Schneider, R.,** Sensitivity of function tests in detecting liver damage in the rat, *Food Cosmet. Toxicol.,* 12, 451, 1974.
42. **Waters, M. D., Simon, V. F., Mitchell, A. D., Jorgenson, T. A., and Valencia, R.,** A phased approach to the evaluation of environmental chemicals for mutagenesis and presumptive carcinogenesis, in *In Vitro Toxicity Testing for Environmental Agents,* Part 3, Kolber, A. R., Wong, T. K., Grant, L. D., Dewoskin, R. S., and Huges, T. J., Eds., Plenum Press, New York, 1983, 417.
43. **Wynder, E. L. and Gori, G. B.,** Contribution of the environment to cancer incidence: and epidemiologic exercise, *J. Natl. Cancer Inst.,* 58, 825, 1977.
44. **Hiatt, H. H., Watson, J. D., and Wistein, J. A., Eds.,** *Origins of Human Cancer,* Cold Spring Harbor Laboratory, Cold Spring Harbor, NY, 1977.
45. **Silverberg, E.,** Cancer statistics, 1981, Ca-A: *Cancer J. Clin.,* 31, 20, 1981.
46. **Demopoulos, M. D. and Mehlman, M. A., Eds.,** Cancer and the environment, *J. Environ. Pathol. Toxicol.,* 3, 1, 1980.
47. **Weisburger, J. H., Reddy, B. S., Hill, P., Cohen, L. A., and Springarn, J. E.,** Nutrition and cancer — on the mechanisms bearing on causes of cancer of the colon, breast, prostate, and stomach, *Bull. N.Y. Acad. Med.,* 56, 673, 1980.
48. **Searle, C. E., Ed.,** *Chemical Carcinogenesis,* American Chemical Society, Washington, D.C., 1976.
49. International Agency for Research on Cancer, *Chemicals and Industrial Processes Associated with Cancer in Humans,* IARC Mongr. Vols. 1—2, Suppl. 1, Lyon, 1979.
50. **Pryor, W. A.,** The role of free radical reactions in biological systems, in *Free Radicals in Biology,* Pryor, W. A., Ed., Vol. 1, Academic Press, New York, 1976, 1.
51. **Tappel, A. L.,** Vitamin E and free radical peroxidaiton of lipids, in *Vitamin E and its Role in Cellular Metabolism,* Nair, P. P. and Kayden, H. J., Eds., *Ann. N.Y. Acad. Sci.,* 203, 12, 1972.
52. **Witting, L. A.,** Vitamin E and lipid antioxidants in free radical initiated reaction in *Free Radical in Biology,* Vol. IV, Pryor, W. A., Ed., Academic Press, New York, 1980, 295.
53. **Bus, J. S., Aust, S. D., and Gibson, J. E.,** Lipid peroxidation: a possible mechanism for paraquat toxicity, *Res. Commun. Chem. Pharmacol.,* 11, 31, 1975.
54. **Little, C. and O'Brien, P. J.,** An intracellular GSH peroxidase with lipid peroxide substrate, *Biochem. Biophys. Res. Commun.,* 31, 145, 1968.
55. **Walling, C.,** Fenton's reaction revised *acc., Chem. Res.,* 8, 125, 1975.
56. **Peters, J. W. and Foote, C. S.,** Chemistry of superoxide ion. II. Reaction with hydroperoxides, *J. Am. Chem. Soc.,* 98, 873, 1976.
57. **Dillard, C. J., Dumelin, E. E., and Tappel, A. L.,** Effect of dietary vitamin E on expiration of pentane and ethane by the rat, *Lipids,* 12, 109, 1977.
58. **Hafeman, D. G. and Hoekstra, W. G.,** Protection against carbon tetrachloride induced lipid peroxidation in the rat by dietary vitamin E, selenium, and methionine as measured by ethane evolution, *J. Nutr.,* 107, 656, 1977.

59. **Esterabauer, H.,** Aldehylic products of lipid peroxidation, in *Free Radicals, Lipid Peroxidation and Cancer,* McBrien, D. C. H. and Slater, T. C., Eds., Academic Press, New York, 1982, 102.

60. **Yu, T. C. and Sinnhuber, R. O.,** Further observations on the 2-thiobartituric acid method for measurement of oxidative randicity, *J. Am. Oil. Chem. Soc.,* 41, 540, 1964.

61. **Recknagel, R. O. and Ghoshal, A. K.,** Lipid peroxidation as a factor in carbon tetrachloride hepatotoxicity, *Lab. Invest.,* 15, 132, 1966.

62. **Judah, J. D. and Rees, K. R.,** Mechanism of action of carbon tetrachloride, *Fed. Proc.,* 18, 1013, 1959.

63. **Waller, R. L. and Recknagel, R. O.,** Determination of lipid conjugated dienes with tetracyanoethylene-14C: significance for the pathology of lipid peroxidation, *Lipids,* 12, 914, 1977.

64. **Riely, C. A., Cohen, G., and Lieberman, M.,** Ethane evolution: a new index of lipid peroxidation, *Science,* 183, 914, 1974.

65. **Menzel, D. B.,** The role of free radicals in the toxicity of air pollutants (nitrogen dioxide and ozone), in *Free Radical Biology,* Vol. 2, Pryor, W. A., Eds., Academic Press, New York, 1976, 181.

66. **Butler, T. C.,** Reduction carbon tetrachloride *in vivo* and reduction of carbon tetrachloride and cholorform *in vitro* by tissues and tissue constituents, *J. Pharmacol. Exp. Ther.,* 134, 311, 1961.

67. **Recknagel, R. O.,** Carbon tetrachloride hepatotoxicity, *Pharmacol. Rev.,* 19, 145, 1967.

68. **Recknagel, R. O. and Glende, E. A., Jr.,** Carbontetrachloride hepatotoxicity: an example of lethal cleavage, *Crit. Rev. Toxicol.,* 2, 263, 1973.

69. **Packer, J. E., Slater, T. F., and Willson, R. L.,** Reactions of the carbon tetrachloride-related peroxy free radical (CCl_3O_2) with amino-acids: pulse radiolysis evidence, *Life Sci.,* 23, 2617, 1978.

70. **Slater, T. F.,** Free radical mechanisms in tissue injury, *Biochem. J.,* 222, 1, 1984.

71. **White, R. E. and Coon, M. J.,** Oxygen activation by cytochrome p-450, *Annu. Rev. Biochem.,* 49, 315, 1980.

72. **Parke, D. V.,** The endoplasmic reticulum. Its role in physiological functions and pathological situations, in *Concepts in Drug Metabolism,* Part B, Jenner, P. and Tests, B., Eds. Marcel Dekker, New York, 1981, 1.

73. **McCay, P. B. and Poyer, J. L.,** Enzyme-generated free radicals as initiators of lipid peroxidation in biological membranes, in *The Enzymes of Biological Membranes,* Vol. 4, Plenum Press, New York, 1976, 239.

74. **Paine, A. J.,** Excited states of oxygen in biology: their possible involvement in cytochrome p-450 linked oxidations as well as in the induction of the p-450 system by many diverse compounds, *Biochem. Pharmacol.,* 27, 1805, 1978.

75. **Hildebrant, A. G. and Roots, I.,** NADPH dependent formation and breakdown of hydrogen peroxide during mixed function oxidation reactions in liver microsomes, *Arch. Biochem. Biophys.,* 171, 385, 1975.

76. **Glende, E. A., Jr.,** Carbon tetrachloride-induced protection against carbon tetrachloride toxicity: role of the liver microsomal drug-metabolizing system, *Biochem. Pharmacol.,* 21, 1697, 1972.

77. **Fong, K., McCay, P. B., Poyer, J. L., Keele, B. B., and Misra, H.,** Evidence that peroxidation of lysosomal membranes is initiated by hydroxyl free radicals produced during flavin enzyme activity, *J. Biol. Chem.,* 248, 7792, 1973.

78. **McCord, J. M., Keele, B. B., and Fridovich, I.,** An enzyme based theory of obligate anaerobiosis: the physiological function of superoxide dismutase, *Proc. Natl. Acad. Sci.,* 68, 1024, 1971.

79. **McCay, P. B., Fong, K., King, M., Lai, E., Weedle, C., Poyer, L., and Hornbrook, K. R.,** Enzyme-generated free radicals and singlet oxygen as promoters of lipid peroxidation in cell membrane, *Lipids,* 1, 157, 1976.

80. **McCord, J. M. and Fridovich, I.,** Superoxide dismutase: an enzymic function for erythrocuprein (hemocuprein), *J. Biol. Chem.,* 244, 6049, 1969.

81. **Finkelstein, E., Rosen, G. M., and Rauckman, E. J.,** Spin trapping of superoxide and hydroxyl radical: practical aspects, *Arch. Biochem. Biophys.,* 200, 1, 1980.

82. **Fee, J. A., and Valentine, J. S.,** Chemical and physical properties of superoxide in *Superoxide and Superoxide Dismutases,* Michelson, A. M., McCord, J. M., and Fridovich, I., Eds., Academic Press, New York, 1977, 19.

83. **Bielski, B. H. J. and Richter, H. W.,** A study of the superoxide radical chemistry by stopped flow radiolysis and radiation induced oxygen consumption, *J. Am. Chem. Soc.,* 99, 3019, 1977.

84. **Ando, W., Kabe, Y., Kobayashi, S., Takyu, C., Yamagishi, A., and Inaba, H.,** Formation of sulfinyl oxide and singlet oxygen in the reaction of thianthrene cation radical and superoxide ion, *J. Am. Chem. Soc.,* 102, 4526, 1980.

85. **Beauchamp, C. and Fridovich, I.,** A mechanism for the production of ethylene from methional. The generation of the hydroxyl radical by xanthine oxidase, *J. Biol. Chem.,* 245, 4641, 1970.

86. **Lai, C. and Piette, L. H.,** Hydroxyl radical production involved in lipid peroxidation of rat liver microsomes, *Biochem. Biophys. Res. Commun.,* 78, 51, 1977.

87. **Heikkila, R. E. and Cabbat, F. S.,** Protection against alloxan-induced diabetes in mice by the hydroxyl radical scavenger dimethylurea, *Eur. J. Pharmacol.,* 52, 57, 1978.

88. **McCord, J. M. and Wong, K.,** Phagocyte produced free radicals: roles in cytotoxicity and in inflammation, in *Oxygen Free Radicals and Tissue Damage,* Ciba Foundation Symposium, 65, Excerpta Medica, Amsterdam, 1979, 343.

89. **McCord, J. M. and Day, E. D.,** Superoxide-dependent production of hydroxyl radical catalyzed by iron-EDTA complex, *FEBS Lett.,* 86, 139, 1978.

90. **Winterbourn, C. C.,** Comparison of superoxide with other reducing agents in the biological production of hydroxyl radical, *Biochem. J.,* 182, 625, 1979.

91. **Buettner, G. R., Oberley, L. W., and Leuthauser, S. W. H. C.,** The effect of iron on the distribution of superoxide and hydroxyl radicals as seen by spin trapping, *Photochem. Photobiol.,* 28, 693, 1978.

92. **Halliwell, B.,** Superoxide dependent formation of hydroxyl radicals in the presence of iron chelates, *FEBS Lett.,* 92, 321, 1978.

93. **Tyler, D. D.,** Role of superoxide radicals in the lipid peroxidation of intracellular membranes, *FEBS Lett.,* 51, 180, 175.

94. **Masuda, Y. and Murano, T.,** Carbon tetrachloride induced lipid peroxidation of rat liver microsomes *in vitro, Biochem. Pharmacol.,* 26, 2275, 1977.

95. **Aust, S. D., Roeriq, D. L., and Pederson, T. C.,** Evidence for superoxide generation by NADPH-cytochrome c reductase of rat liver microsomes, *Biochem. Biophys. Res. Commun.,* 47, 1133, 1972.

96. **Pederson, T. C. and Aust, S. D.,** NADPH-dependent lipid peroxidation catalysed by purified NADPH cytochrome c reductase from rat liver microsomes, *Biochem. Biophys. Res. Commun.,* 48, 789, 1972.

97. **Gutteridge, J. M. C., Halliwell, B., Treffry, A., Harrisson, P. M., and Blake, D.,** Effect of ferritin-containing fractions with different iron loading on lipid peroxidation, *Biochem. J.,* 209, 557, 1983.

98. **Halliwell, B. and Gutteridge, J. M. C.,** Oxygen toxicity, oxygen radicals transition metals, and disease, *Biochem. J.,* 219, 1, 1984.

99. **Rawls, H. C. and Van Santen, P. J.,** Singlet oxygen: a possible source of the original hydroperoxides in fatty acids, *Ann. N.Y. Acad. Sci.,* 171, 135, 1970.

100. **Anderson, S. M., Krinsky, N. I., Stone, M. J., and Clagett, D. C.,** Effect of singlet oxygen quenchers on oxidative damage to liposomes initiated by photosensitization or by radiofrequency discharge, *Photochem. Photobiol.,* 20, 65, 1974.

101. **Kellog, E. W. and Fridovich, I.,** Superoxide, hydrogen peroxide, and singlet oxygen in lipid peroxidation by a xanthine oxidase system, *J. Biol. Chem.,* 250, 8812, 1975.

102. **Kellog, E. W. and Fridovich, I.,** Liposome oxidation and erythrocyte lysis by enzymically generated superoxide and hydrogen peroxide, *J. Biol. Chem.,* 252, 6721, 1977.

103. **Khan, A. U.,** Singlet molecular oxygen from superoxide anion and sensitized fluorescence of organic molecules, *Science,* 168, 476, 1970.

104. **Foote, C. S.,** Quenching of singlet oxygen, *Ann. N.Y. Acad. Sci.,* 171, 139, 1970.

105. **Mattews, M.,** Protective effects of beta-carotene lethal photosensitization by haematoporphyrin, *Nature,* 203, 1092, 1964.

106. **Cohen, G. and Hochstein, P.,** Glutathione peroxidase: the primary agent for the elimination of hydrogen peroxide in erythrocytes, *Biochem. J.,* 2, 1420, 1963.

107. **Prohaska, J. R. and Ganther, H. E.,** Glutathione peroxidase activity of glutathion S-transferase purified from rat liver, *Biochem. Biophys. Res. Commun.,* 76, 437, 1977.

108. **McCay, P. B., Gibson, D. D., Fong, K., and Hornbrook, K. R.,** Effect of glutathione peroxidase activity on lipid peroxidation in biological membranes, *Biochim. Biophys. Acta,* 431, 459, 1976.

109. **Boigegrain, R. A., Derache, P. H., and Mitjavila, S.,** Deperoxydation de l'-acide hydroxylinoleique par la muqueuse intestinale, *Food Chem. Toxicol.,* 21, 181, 1983.

110. **Reed, D. J. and Beatty, P. W.,** Biosynthesis and regulation of glutathione: toxicological implications, in *Reviews in Biochemical Toxicology,* Vol. 2, Hodgson, E., Bend, J. R., and Philpot, R. M., Eds., Elsevier/North-Holland, New York, 1980, 213.

111. **Christophersen, B. O.,** Oxidation of reduced glutathione by subcellular fraction of rat liver, *Biochem. J.,* 100, 95, 1966.

112. **Chow, C. K. and Tappel, A. L.,** An enzymatic protective mechanism against lipid peroxidation damage to lung on ozone-exposed rats, *Lipid,* 7, 518, 1972.

113. **Younes, M. and Siegers, C. P.,** Mechanistic aspects of enhanced lipid peroxidation following glutathione depletion, *Chem. Biol. Interact.,* 34, 257, 1981.

114. **Hoqberg, J., Orrenius, S., and Larson, R. E.,** Lipid peroxidation in isolated hepatocytes, *Eur. J. Biochim.,* 50, 595, 1975.

115. **Stacey, N. and Priestly, B. G.,** Lipid peroxidation in isolated hepatocytes: relationship to toxicity of CCl4, ADP/Fe+++ and diethyl maleate, *Toxicol. Appl. Pharmacol.,* 45, 41, 1978.

116. **Stevens, J. T.,** The role of binding in inhibition of hepatic microsomal metabolism by parathion and malathion, *Life Sci.,* 14, 2215, 1974.

117. **Moriya, M., Kato, K., and Shirasu, Y.,** Effect of cysteine and a liver metabolic activation system on the activities of mutagenic pesticides, *Mutat. Res.,* 57, 259, 1978.

118. **Bus, J. S., Cagen, S. Z., Olgaard, M., and Gibson, J. E.,** A mechanism of paraquat toxicity in mice and rats, *Toxicol. Appl. Pharmacol.,* 35, 501, 1976.

119. **Oshino, N. and Chance, B.,** Properties of glutathion release observed during the reduction of organic hydroperoxide, demethylation of aminopyrine and oxidation of some substances in perfused rat liver and their implications for physiological function of catalase, *Biochem. J.,* 162, 509, 1977.

120. **Bray, R. C., Cockle, S. A., Fielden, E. M, Roberts, P. B., Rotilio, G., and Calabrese, L.,** Reduction and inactivation of superoxide dismutase by hydrogen peroxide, *Biochem. J.,* 139, 43, 1974.

121. **Summer, J. B. and Dounce, A. L.,** Crystalline catalase, *J. Biol. Chem.,* 121, 417, 1937.

122. **Bhuyan, K. C. and Bhuyan, D. K.,** Regulation of hydrogen peroxide in eye humors. Effect of 3-amino-1H-1,2,4-triazole on catalase and glutathion peroxidase of rabbit eye, *Biochim. Biophys. Acta,* 497, 641, 1977.

123. **Jones, D. P., Thor, H., Anderson, B., and Orrenius, S.,** Detoxification reactions in isolated hepatocytes, *J. Biol. Chem.,* 253, 6031, 1978.

124. **Frank, L., Wood, D. L., and Roberts, R. J.,** Effect of diethyldithiocarbamate on oxygen toxicity and lung enzyme activity in immature and adult rats, *Biochem. Pharmacol.,* 27, 251, 1978.

125. **Bus, J. S., Aust, S. D., and Gibson, J. E.,** Superoxide and singlet oxygen catalysed lipid peroxidation as a possible mechanism for paraquat (methyl viologen), *Biochem. Biophys. Res. Commun.,* 58, 749, 1974.

126. **Stevens, J. T., Stitzel, R. A. and McPhillips, J. J.,** Effect of anticholinesterase insecticides on hepatic microsomal metabolism, *J. Pharmacol. Exp. Ther.,* 181, 576, 1972.

127. **Wardman, P. and Clarke, E. D.,** Oxygen inhibition of nitroreductase: electron transfer from nitro radical-anions to oxygen, *Biochem. Biophys. Res. Commun.,* 69, 942, 1976.

128. **Mason, R. P. and Holtzman, J. L.,** The role of catalytic superoxide formation in the O_2 inhibition of nitroreductase, *Biochem. Biophys. Res. Commun.,* 67, 1267, 1975.

129. **Kutter, E., Machleidt, H., Reuter, W., Sauter, R., and Wildfeuer, A.,** Comparative *in vitro* and *in vivo* structure activity studies of antiparasitic 2-methylene-amino-5-nitrotiazoles, in *Biological Correlations, The Hansch Approach,* Gould, R. F., Ed., Am. Chem. Soc., Washington, D.C., 1972, 98.

130. **Hutson, D. H., Holmes, D. S., and Crawford, M. J.,** The involvement of glutathione in the reductive dechlorination of a phenacylhalide, *Chemosphere,* 5, 79, 1976.

131. **Makhija, S. J. and Pawar, S. S.,** Effect of insecticide Tick-20 (O,O-dimethyl malathion) on hepatic drug metabolism and lipid peroxidation in young growing rats, *Indian J. Biochem. Biophys.,* 11, 266, 1974.

132. **Pawar, S. S. and Makhija, S. J.,** Hepatic aminopyrine N-demethylase, acetanilide hydroxylase and lipid peroxidation in young growing rats during the treatment of insecticides, *Bull. Environ. Contam. Toxicol.,* 14, 714, 1975.

133. **Makhija, S. J. and Pawar, S. S.,** Hepatic drug metabolizing enzymes and lipid peroxidation in young growing male rats during treatment with an organophosphorus insecticide Tick-20 (O,O-dimethyl malathion), *Indian J. Med. Res.,* 63, 1402, 1975.

134. **Fawade, M. M. and Pawar, S. S.,** Effect of phenobarbital pretreatment on mixed function oxidases and lipid peroxidation during thiodemeton toxicity, *Indian J. Exp. Biol.,* 18, 646, 1980.

135. **Matkowice, B., Szabo, L., Mindszenty, L., and Ivan, J.,** The effects of organophosphate pesticides on some liver enzyme and lipid peroxidation, *Gen. Pharmacol.,* 11, 353, 1980.

136. **Matkowics, B., Szabo, L., Ivan, L., and Gaal, I.,** Some further data on the effects of two organophosphate pesticides on the oxidative metabolism in the liver, *Gen. Pharmacol.,* 14, 689, 1983.

137. **Moody, D. E., Clawson, G. A., Woo, C. H., and Smuckler, E. A.,** Cellular distribution of cytochrome p-450 loss in rats of different ages treated with alkyl halides, *Toxicol. Appl. Pharmacol.,* 66, 278, 1982.

138. **Broda, C., Nachtomi, E., and Alumot, E.,** Differences in liver morphology between rats and chicks treated with ethylene dibromide, *Gen. Pharmacol.,* 7, 344, 1976.

139. **Fishbein, L.,** Industrial mutagens and potential mutagens. I. Halogenated aliphatic derivatives, *Mutat. Res.,* 32, 267, 1976.

140. **Nachtomi, E. and Alumot, E.,** Comparison of ethylene dibromide and carbon tetrachloride toxicity in rats and chicks: blood and liver levels: lipid peroxidation, *Exp. Mol. Pathol.,* 16, 71, 1972.

141. **Albano, E., Poli, G., Tomasi, A., Bini, A., Vannini, V., and Dianzani, M. U.,** Toxicity of 1,2-dibromoethane in isolated hepatocytes: role of lipid peroxidation, *Chem. Biol. Interact.,* 50, 255, 1984.

142. **Nachtomi, E. and Sarma, D. S. R.,** Repair of rat liver DNA *in vivo* damaged by ethylenedibromide, *Biochem. Pharmacol.,* 26, 1941, 1977.

143. **Plotnick, H. B., Weigel, W. W., Richards, D. E., and Cheever, K. L.,** The effect of dietary disulfiram upon the tissue distribution and excretion of ^{14}C-1,2-dibromoethane in the rat, *Res. Commun. Chem. Pathol. Pharmacol.,* 26, 535, 1979.

144. **VanBladeren, P. J., Hoogeterp, J. J., Breimer, D. D., and Van der Gen, A. S.,** The influence of disulfiram and other inhibitors of oxidative metabolism on the formation of 2-hydroxyethyl-mercapturic acid from 1,2-dibromoethane by the rat, *Biochem. Pharmacol.,* 30, 2983, 1981.

145. **Nachtomi, E.,** The metabolism of ethylene dibromide in the rat: the enzymic reaction with glutathione *in vitro* and *in vivo, Biochem. Pharmacol.,* 19, 2853, 1970.

146. **Nachtomi, E., Alumot, E., and Bondi, A.,** Metabolism of ethylene dibromide in the rat. Identification of detoxification products in the urines, *Israel J. Chem.,* 4, 239, 1966.
147. **Kluwe, W. M., McNish, R., Smithson, K., and Hook, J. B.,** Depletion by 1,2-dibromoethane 1,2-dibromo-3-chloropropane, tris (2,3-dibromopropyl) phosphate and hexachloro-1,3-butadiene of reduced non-protein sulphydryl groups in target and non-target organs, *Biochem. Pharmacol.,* 30, 2265, 1981.
148. **Sundheimer, D. W., White, D. E., Brendel, K., and Sipes, I. G.,** The bioactivation of 1,2-dibromoethane in rat hepatocytes: covalent binding to nucleic acids, *Carcinogenesis,* 3, 1129, 1982.
149. **Van Bladeren, P. J., Breimer, D. D., Rotteveel-Smijjls, G. M. T., de Knijff, P., Mohn, G. R., Van Meeteren-Walchili, W. B., and Van der Gen, A.,** The relation between the structure of vicinal dihalogen compounds and their mutagenic activation via the conjugation with glutathione, *Carcinogenesis,* 2, 499, 1981.
150. **Recknagel, R. O.,** Carbon tetrachloride hepatotoxicity, *Pharmacol. Rev.,* 19, 145, 1967.
151. **Recknagel, R. O., Glende, E. A., Jr., and Hruszkewycz, A. M.,** Chemical mechanism in carbon tetrachloride toxicity, in *Free Radicals in Biology,* Vol. III, Pryor, W. A. Ed., Academic Press, New York, 1977, 97.
152. **Recknagel, R. O. Minireview:** a new direction in the study of carbon tetrachloride hepatotoxicity, *Life Sci.,* 33, 401, 1983.
153. **Slater, T. F.,** Activation of carbon tetrachloride: chemical principles and biological significance, in *Free Radicals, Lipid Peroxidation and Cancer,* McBrien, D. C. H. and Slater, T. F., Eds., Academic Press, New York, 243, 1982.
154. **Noquchi, T., Fong, K. L., Lai, E. K., Alexander, S. S., King, M. M., Olson, L., Poyer, J. L., and McCay, P. B.,** Specificity of phenobarbital-induced cytochrome p-450 for metabolism of carbon tetrachloride to the trichloromethyl radical, *Biochem. Pharmacol.,* 31, 615, 1982.
155. **Castro, J. A., Cignoli, E. V., de Castro, C. R., and de Fenos, O. M.,** Prevention by cystamine of liver necrosis and early biochemical alterations induced by carbontetrachloride, *Biochem. Pharmacol.,* 21, 49, 1972.
156. **Cignoli, E. V. and Castro, J. A.,** Lipid peroxidation, necrosis, and the *in vivo* depression of liver glucose-6-phosphatase by carbon tetrachloride, *Exp. Mol. Pathol.,* 14, 43, 1971.
157. **Diaz-Gomez, M. I., Castro, J. A., de Ferreyra, E. C., D'Acosta, N., and de Castro, C. R.,** Irreversible binding of ^{14}C from $^{14}CCl_4$ to liver microsomal lipids and proteins from rats pretreated with compounds altering microsomal mixed function oxygenase activity, *Toxicol. Appl. Pharmacol.,* 25, 534, 1973.
158. **Rao, K. S. and Recknagel, R. O.,** Early onset of lipoperoxidation in rat liver after carbon tetrachloride administration, *Exp. Mol. Pathol.,* 9, 271, 1968.
159. **Rao, K. S. and Recknagel, R. O.,** Early incorporation of carbon-labeled carbon tetrachloride into rat liver particulate lipids and proteins, *Exp. Mol. Pathol.,* 10, 219, 1969.
160. **Recknagel, R. O. and Lombardi, B.,** Studies of biochemical changes in subcellular particles of rat liver and their relationship to a new hypothesis regarding the pathogenesis of carbon tetrachloride fat accumulation, *J. Biol. Chem.,* 236, 564, 1961.
161. **Klaassen, C. D. and Plaa, G. L.,** Comparison of the biochemical alterations elicited in livers from rats treated with carbon tetrachloride, chloroform, 1,1-2-trichloroethane, and 1,1,1,-trichlorethane, *Biochem. Pharmacol.,* 18, 2019, 1969.
162. **Slater, T. F. and Sawyer, B. C.,** The stimulatory effect of carbon tetrachloride on peroxidative reactions in rat liver fractions *in vitro.* Interaction sites in the endoplasmic reticulum, *Biochem. J.,* 123, 815, 1971.
163. **Kubic, V. L. and Anders, M. W.,** Metabolism of carbon tetrachloride to phosgene, *Life Sci.,* 6, 2151, 1980.
164. **Waller, R. L. and Recknagel, R. O.,** On a possible role for phosgene in CCL_4 and $BrCl_3$ toxicity, *Fed. Proc.,* 39, 612, 1980.
165. **Ingall, A., Lott, K. A. K., Slater, T. F., Finch, S., and Stier, A.,** Metabolic activation of carbon tetrachloride to a free radical product: studies using a spin trap, *Biochem. Soc. Trans.,* 6, 962, 1978.
166. **Cambon-Gros, C., Deltour, P., Boigegrain, R. A., Fernandez, Y., and Mitjavila, S.,** Radical activation of carbon tetrachloride in foetal and maternal rat liver microsomes, *Biochem. Pharmacol.,* 35, 2041, 1986.
167. **Di Luzio, N. R. and Costales, F.,** Inhibition of the ethanol and carbon tetrachloride induced fatty liver by antioxidants, *Exp. Mol. Pathol.,* 4, 141, 1965.
168. **Rao, K. S., Glende, E. A., Jr., and Recknagel, R. O.,** Effects of drug pretreatment on CCl_4 induced lipid peroxidation, *Exp. Mol. Pathol.,* 12, 324, 1970.
169. **Stenger, R. J. and Johnson, E. A.,** Further observations upon the effects of phenobarbital pretreatment on the hepatotoxicity of carbon tetrachloride, *Exp. Mol. Pathol.,* 14, 220, 1971.
170. **Klingensmith, J. S. and Mehendale, H. M.,** Hepatic microsomal metabolism of CCl_4 after pretreatment with chlordecone, mirex, or phenobarbital in male rats, *Drug Metab. Disp.,* 11, 329, 1983.
171. **McLean, A. E. M. and McLean, E. K.,** Effect of diet and 1,1,1-trichloro2,2)bis(p-chlorophenyl)ethane (DDT) on microsomal hydroxylation enzymes and on sensitivity of rats to carbon tetrachloride poisoning, *Biochem. J.,* 100, 564, 1966.

172. **Reiner, O., Athanassopoulos, S., Hellmer, K. H., Murray, R. E., and Uehleke, H.,** Bildung von chloroform aus tetrachlorkolenstoff in lebermikrosomen, lipid peroxidation und zerstorung von cytochrom p-450, *Arch. Toxikol.,* 29, 219, 1972.

173. **Masuda, Y.,** Carbon tetrachloride-induced loss of microsomal glucose-6-phosphatase and cytochrome p-450 *in vitro, Jpn. J. Pharmacol.,* 31, 107, 1981.

174. **De Groot, H. and Haas, W.,** Self-catalysed, molecular oxygen-independent inactivation of NADPH- or dithionite-reduced microsomal cytochrome p-450 by carbon tetrachloride, *Biochem. Pharmacol.,* 30, 2343, 1981.

175. **Glende, E. A. Jr., Hruszkewycz, A. M., and Recknagel, R. O.,** Critical role of lipid peroxidation in carbon tetrachloride-induced loss of aminopyrin demethylase, cytochrome p-450 and glucose 6-phosphatase, *Biochem. Pharmacol.,* 25, 2163, 1976.

176. **Moore, L., Davenport, G. R., and Landon, E. J.,** Calcium uptake of rat liver microsomal subcellular fraction in response to *in vivo* administration of carbon tetrachloride, *J. Biol. Chem.,* 251, 1197, 1976.

177. **Cambon-Gros, C., Carrera, G., and Mitjavila, S.,** Inhibition of Ca^{++} sequestration in foetal liver microsomes by carbon tetrachloride and dibromotrichloromethane, *Biochem. Pharmacol.,* 33, 2605, 1984.

178. **Poland, A. and Glover, E.,** Comparison of 2,3,7,8-tetrachlorodibenzo-p-dioxine a potent inducer of arylhydrocarbon hydroxylase with 3-methylchlolanthrene, *Mol. Pharmacol.,* 10, 349, 1974.

179. **Stohs, S. J., Hassan, M. O., and Murray, W. J.,** Lipid peroxidation as a possible cause of TCDD toxicity, *Biochem. Biophys. Res. Commun.,* 111, 854, 1983.

180. **Hassan, M. O., Stohs, S. J., and Murray, W. J.,** Comparative ability of TCDD to induce lipid peroxidation in rats, guinea pigs, and Syrian golden hamsters, *Bull. Environ. Contam. Toxicol.,* 31, 649, 1983.

181. **Sweeney, G. D., Jones, K. G., Cole, F. M., Basford, D., and Krestynski, H.,** Iron deficiency prevents liver toxicity of 2,3,7,8-tetrachlorodibenzo-p-dioxin, *Science,* 204, 332, 1979.

182. **Jones, K. G., Cole, F. M., and Sweeney, G. D.,** The role of iron in the toxicity of 2,3,7,8-tetrachloro-p-dibenzodioxin (TCDC), *Toxicol. Appl. Pharmacol.,* 61, 74, 1981.

183. **Hassan, M. O., Stohs, S. J., Murray, M. J., and Birt, D. F.,** Dietary selenium glutathione, peroxidase activity an toxicity of 2,3,7,8-tetrachlorodibenzodioxin, *J. Toxicol. Environ. Health,* 15, 405, 1985.

184. **Greig, J. B. and De Matteis, H.,** Effect of 2,3,7,8-tetrachlorodibenzo-p-dioxin on drug metabolism and hepatic microsome of rats and mice, *Environ. Health Perspect.,* 5, 211, 1973.

185. **Sunde, R. A. and Hoekstra, W. G.,** Structure, synthesis and function of glutathione peroxidase, *Nutr. Rev.,* 38, 265, 1980.

186. **Savolainen, H. and Pekari, K.,** Neurochemical effects of peroral administration of technical pentachlorophenol, *Res. Commun. Chem. Pathol. Pharmacol.,* 23, 97, 1979.

187. **Courtney, K. D. and Andrew, J. E.,** Mobilization of hexachlorobenzene (HCB) during gestation, *Toxicol. Lett.,* 3, 357, 1979.

188. **Alleman, M. A., Koster, J. F., Wilson, J. H. P., Edixhoven-Bosdijk, A., Slee, R. G., Kroos, M. J., and Ejik, H. G.,** The involvement of iron and lipid peroxidation in the pathogenesis of HCB induced porphyria, *Biochem. Pharmacol.,* 34, 161, 1985.

189. **Kamohara, K., Yqi, N., and Itokawa, Y.,** Mechanism of lipid peroxide formation in polychlorinated biphenyls (PCB) and dichloro diphenyltrichloroethane (DDT) poisoned rats, *Environ. Res.,* 34, 18,1984.

190. **Scott, M. L.,** Effects of PCBS, DDT and mercury compound in chickens and Japanese quail, *Fed. Proc.,* 36, 1888, 1977.

191. **Satyanarayan, S., Bajpai, A., Chauhan, S. S., and Misra, U. K.,** Lipid peroxidation in lung and liver of rats given DDT and endosulfan intratracheally, *Bull. Environ. Contam. Toxicol.,* 34, 63, 1985.

192. **Konat, G.,** Endogenous microsomal phospholipid peroxidation in mouse brain, *J. Neurochem.,* 20, 1247, 1973.

193. **Konat, G. and Clausen, J.,** Activity of cytochrome p-450 complex in multiple intoxications of the mouse, *Environ. Physiol.,* 1, 72, 1971.

194. **Kohli, K. K., Maggon, K. K., and Venkitasubramanian, T. A.,** Induction of mixed function oxidases on oral administration of dieldrin, *Chem. Biol. Interact.,* 17, 249, 1977.

195. **Kearney, P. C. and Kaufman, D. D.,** Enzyme from soil bacterium hydrolyzes phenylcarbamate herbicides, *Science,* 147, 740, 1965.

196. **Herrett, R. A.,** Methyl and phenylcarbamates, in *Degradation of Herbicides,* Kearney, P. C. and Kaufman, D. D., Eds., Marcel Dekker, New York, 1969, 113.

197. **Geissbhiiler, H.,** The substituted ureas, in *Degradation of Herbicides,* Kearney, P. C. and Kaufman, D. D., Eds., Marcel Dekker, New York, 1969, 79.

198. **Lanzilotta, R. P. and Pramer, D.,** Herbicide transformation. II. Studies with an acylamidase of *Fusarium solani, Appl. Microbiol.,* 19, 307, 1970.

199. **Christensen, H. E.,** Registry of Toxic Effects of Chemical Substances, U.S. Department of Health, Education and Welfare, National Institute for Occupational Safety and Health, Rockville, MD, 1976, 1245.

200. **Bartha, R. and Pramer, D.,** Metabolism of acylanilide herbicides, *Adv. Appl. Microbiol.,* 13, 317, 1970.

201. **Lenk, W. and Sterzl, H.,** Difference in the ferrihemoglobin forming capabilities and carcinogenicities between monocyclic and policyclic N-acrylamines and their derivatives, *Rev. Drug Metab. Drug. Interact.,* 4, 171, 1982.

202. **Bordeleau, L. M. and Bartha, R.,** Biochemical transformations of herbicide derived anilines: requirements of molecular configuration, *Can. J. Microbiol.,* 18, 1873, 1972.

203. **Zenser, T. V., Mattammal, M. B., and Davis, B. B.,** Cooxidation of benzidine by renal medullary prostaglandin cyclooxygenase, *J. Pharmacol. Exp. Ther.,* 211, 460, 1979.

204. **Boyd, J. A., Harven, D. J., and Eling, T. E.,** The oxidation of 2-aminofluroene by prostaglandin endoperoxide sunthetase. Comparison with other peroxidases, *J. Biol. Chem.,* 258, 8246, 1983.

205. **Flinstein, R. N., Berliner, S., and Green, F. O.,** Mechanism of inhibition of catalase by 3-amino-1,2,4-triazole, *Arch. Biochem. Biophys.,* 76, 32, 1958.

206. **Kornburst, D. J., Barfnecht, T. R., Ingram, P., and Shelburne, J. D.,** Effects of di(2)ethylhexyl)phthalate on DNA repair and lipid peroxidation in rat hepatocytes and on metabolic cooperation in Chinese hamster V-79 cells, *J. Toxicol. Environ. Health,* 13, 99, 1984.

207. **Barabas, K., Berencsi, G., Szabo, L., Varqa, Sz, I., and Matkovics, B.,** Enhancing effect of amino-triazole on paraquat toxicity *in vivo, Gen. Pharmacol.,* 11, 569, 1980.

208. **Gerrard, J. M. White, J. G., Rao, G. H., and Townsend, D.,** Localization of platelet prostaglandin production in the platelet dense tubular system, *Am. J. Pathol.,* 83, 283, 1976.

209. **Copland, G. M., Kolin, A., and Shulman, H. S.,** Fatal pulmonary intra-alveolar fibrosis after paraquat ingestion, *N. Engl. J. Med.,* 291, 190, 1974.

210. **Thurlbeck, W. M. and Thurlbeck, S. M.,** Pulmonary effects of paraquat poisoning, *Chest,* 69(Suppl.), 267, 1976.

211. **Fisher, H. K., Clements, J., and Wright, R. R.,** Enhancement of oxygen toxicity by the herbicide paraquat, *Am. Rev. Respir. Dis.,* 107, 246, 1973.

212. **Kehrer, J. P., Haschek, W. M., and Witschi, H.,** The influence of hyperoxia on the acute toxicity of paraquat and diquat, *Drug. Chem. Toxicol.,* 2, 397, 1979.

213. **Smith, L. L., Rose, M. S., and Wyatt, I.,** The pathology and biochemistry of paraquat, in *Oxygen Free Radicals and Tissue Damage,* CIBA Foundation Symposium N 65, Exerpta Medica, Amsterdam, 1979, 321.

214. **Autor, A. P.,** *Biochemical Mechanisms of Paraquat Toxicity,* Academic Press, New York, 1977.

215. **Dodge, A. D.,** Oxygen radicals and herbicide action, *Biochem. Soc. Transact.,* 10, 73, 1982.

216. **Smith, P. and Heath, D.,** Paraquat, *Crit Rev. Toxicol.,* 4, 411, 1976.

217. **Montgomery, M. R.,** Interaction of paraquat with the microsomal fatty acid desaturase system, *Toxicol. Appl. Pharmacol.,* 36, 543, 1976.

218. **Steffen, C. and Netter, K. J.,** On the mechanism of paraquat action on microsomal oxygen reduction and its relation to lipid peroxidation, *Toxicol. Appl. Pharmacol.,* 47, 593, 1979.

219. **Steffen, C., Muliawan, H., and Kappus, H.,** Lack of *in vivo* lipid peroxidation in experimental paraquat poisoning, *Naunr. Schmiedebergs Arch. Pharmacol.,* 310, 241, 1980.

220. **Ilett, K. P., Stripp, G., Menard, R. H., Reid, W. D., and Gillette, J. R.,** Studies on the mechanism of the lung toxicity of paraquat: comparison of tissue distribution and some biochemical parameters in rats and rabbits, *Toxicol. Appl. Pharmacol.,* 28, 216, 1974.

221. **Talcott, R. E., Shu, H., and Wei, E. T.,** Dissociation of microsomal oxygen reduction and lipid peroxidation with the electron acceptors, paraquat and menadione, *Biochem. Pharmacol.,* 28, 665, 1979.

222. **Trush, M. A., Mimnaugh, E. G., Ginsburg, E., and Gram, T. E.,** *In vitro* stimulation by paraquat of reactive oxygen-mediated lipid peroxidation in rat lung microsomes, *Toxicol. Appl. Pharmacol.,* 60, 279, 1981.

223. **Patterson, C. E. and Rhodes, M. L.,** The effect of superoxide dismutase on paraquat mortality in mice and rats, *Toxicol. Appl. Pharmacol.,* 62, 65, 1982.

224. **Goldstein, B. D., Rozen, M. C., Quintavalla, J. C., and Amoruso, M. A.,** Decrease in mouse lung and liver glutathion peroxidase activity and potentiation of the lethal effects of ozone and paraquat by the superoxide dismutase inhibitor diethyldithiocarbamate, *Biochem. Pharmacol.,* 28, 27, 1979.

225. **Brigelius, R., Hashem, A., and Lengfelder, E.,** Paraquat-induced alterations of phospholipids and GSSG-release in the isolated perfused rat liver, and the effect of SOD-active copper complexes, *Biochem. Pharmacol.,* 30, 349, 1981.

226. **Frank, L., Neriishi, K., Sio, R., and Pascual, D.,** Protection from paraquat induced lung damage and lethality in adult rat pretreated with chlorofibrate, *Toxicol. Appl. Pharmacol.,* 66, 269, 1982.

227. **Kornbrust, D. J. and Mavis, R. D.,** The effect of paraquat on microsomal lipid peroxidation *in vitro* and *in vivo, Toxicol. Appl. Pharmacol.,* 53, 323, 1980.

228. **Litterst, C. L., Mimnaugh, E. G., Reagan, R. L., and Gram, T. E.,** Comparison of *in vitro* drug metabolism by lung, liver and kidney of several common laboratory species, *Drug. Metab. Dispos.,* 3, 259, 1975.

229. **Dutcher, J. S. and Boyd, M. R.,** Species and strain differences in target organ alkylation and toxicity by 4-ipomeanol. Predictive values of covalent binding in studies of target organ toxicities by reactive metabolites, *Biochem. Pharmacol.*, 28, 3367, 1979.
230. **Witschi, J., Kacew, S., Hirai, K. J., and Cote, M. G.,** *In vivo* oxidation of reduced nicotin-amido-adenine dinucleotide phosphate by paraquat and diquat in rat lung, *Chem. Biol. Interact.*, 19, 143, 1977.
231. **Rose, M. S., and Smith, L. L., and Wyatt, I.,** Evidence for energy dependent accumulation of paraquat into rat lung, *Nature*, 252, 314, 1974.

Chapter 5

HEPATOTOXIC EFFECTS OF PESTICIDES

T. S. S Dikshith

TABLE OF CONTENTS

I. INTRODUCTION

The liver is a singularly unique organ in its structure and function. It plays a major role in the ability of an animal to deal effectively with toxic chemicals. For example, the combination of apparent simplicity of liver cell with actual complexity of its function is a challenge to unravel the disorders and injury to liver caused by a host of xenobiotics. Once again, liver is unique in that over 80% of the blood it receives is venous in character which obviously makes the liver cells peculiarly liable to injury from anoxia and from toxic chemicals.

A variety of chemicals including pesticides produce pathological changes in the liver, which include necrosis, hepatoma, and other injuries. The necrosis may be (1) *diffuse* where all the cells in groups of lobules are affected, (2) *zonal* in which only the cells of a particular area in each lobule are injured, or (3) *focal* where small areas, unevenly, are affected. The zonal necrosis may be restricted to central, midzonal, and peripheral regions of the liver.

There is a growing evidence that several pesticides produce liver injury in animals and humans. For example, chlordecone, DDT, dieldrin, heptachlor, hexachlorocyclohexane, lindane, and mirex have produced pathomorphological and enzymatic changes in liver of experimental animals.[1-11] In fact, the ability of animals and humans to survive chronic low levels of pesticides through direct or indirect exposure(s) may depend in large measure on the adaptive mechanism of the liver.

II. METHODS OF STUDY

Liver is the major site of the metabolism of pesticides. In general, liver reacts to pesticide or to chemical stress by patterned responses, for instance, in increase of enzyme, in structural changes, in cellular organelles as well as in the alteration in the size of the cell and organ. There are different ways by which this organ can be studied. Each of the methods has its own relevance in the understanding of liver metabolism in intact animal. Thus, a variety of experimental models and toxicity tests has been utilized to characterize hepatotoxicity of chemicals *vis à vis* potential hepatotoxins.[12]

A. THE INTACT LIVER *IN SITU*

When a pesticide is administered into the hepatic portal vein most metabolites are excreted in a concentrated solution in the bile. They can be analyzed by direct application of bile by HPLC. These metabolites can be detected in several ways. For instance, by their radioactivity, absorption of light, and fluorescence. This has the unique advantage that the liver remains undisturbed and functions normally. And the metabolites so formed are sufficient for chemical characterization by microchemical methods, MS, and higher resolution NMR.

B. THE ISOLATED PERFUSED LIVER

The use of isolated perfused liver is more artificial than *in situ* preparation. This technique, however, has the special advantage that the pesticides bathing the sinusoids can be regulated. The metabolites of pesticides which are excreted through the sinusoids in a significant measure can also be estimated in these animals.

Isolated perfused liver preparation offer us several advantages over experimentation with whole animals. For example, one can retain the structural and functional integrity of the liver during experimentation. Details of isolated perfused liver techniques however, may be seen elsewhere.[13]

C. ISOLATED HEPATOCYTES

This method is essentially of less physiological condition than the use of the intact liver tissue. This is because of the breakage and repair of tight junctions between liver cells during their isolation. In fact, the liver cells so isolated exist in a different environment than the normal tissue architecture. The isolated liver cells, however, have experimental advantage as only small amounts of material are required and this can be obtained from a single animal.

D. DIVIDING HEPATOCYTES IN CULTURE

Although this is one of the experimental methods used in the screening of potential hepatotoxins this method is not recommended for general studies. This is because of the fact that dividing liver cells in culture are usually incompletely or abnormally differentiated.

III. MORPHOLOGICAL CHANGES

A. LIGHT MICROSCOPY

Morphologically, liver injury produced by a chemical can manifest itself in several ways.[14] The changes in hepatocyte morphology resulting from chronic organochlorine insecticide (OC) treatment appear to follow a general pattern, which often consists of the following: cellular hypertrophy, fatty degeneration, cellular margination, increased basophilia, increased fat granules, cytoplasmic vacuolization, necrosis, increase in smooth endoplasmic reticulum, presence of atypical mitochondria and golgi apparatus, scattered swollen degenerated hepatocytes, enlargement and pyknosis of nuclei, and hypertrophy of nucleoli and related changes.

Liver injury, observed in experimental animals exposed to pesticides, is a product of several factors. Essentially the injury depends on the nature of pesticide, its concentration, and whether or not the poisoning is acute or chronic. In the case of acute pesticide poisoning, the liver injury is characterized by the accumulation of lipid in the liver cells followed by cellular necrosis and hepatobiliary dysfunction. For instance, acute exposure to mirex produced liver cell enlargement and bile stasis in rats.[15] A single oral dose of mirex (365 mg/kg) to rates produced fatty metamorphosis in periportal hepatic zones and glycogen depletion.[16,17]

Earlier reports on the morphological changes produced by DDT in the liver of experimental animals were often equivocal.[18,19] However, studies of Ortega et al.[20] clearly demonstrated that DDT does produce histological changes in the liver of rats. These changes in the parenchymal cells of the liver consisted of an increased deposition of fat, margination of cytoplasmic granules, and hypertrophy of the cells. The most characteristic change was the formation of complex, lipoid cytoplasmic inclusion bodies termed, *lipospheres*.

Pesticides have caused liver injury leading to accumulation of lipid granules (steatosis). In several cases these degenerative processes have ended up in the death of the liver cell (necrosis). For example, chlordecone and CCl_4 produced necrotic changes in several liver cells.[21] The process of necrosis, if continued because of repeated long-term exposure to pesticides, may affect small groups of isolated parenchymal cells and result in focal necrosis. For example, feeding dieldrin to rats for 2 years produced focal necrosis and intrahepatic nodules in animals.[22] In fact, pesticides in high concentrations have virtually damaged all of the cells within hepatic lobule causing massive necrosis. Similarly, the accumulation of lipid in the liver cell can be more diffuse or zonal. Liver of mirex-fed rats for example, showed a definite pattern of periportal liposis and periportal necrosis[9] as compared to normal liver (Figure 1).

The major characteristic liver lesions observed after DDT administration to animals includes hepatocellular enlargement, central cytoplasmic hyalinization, peripheral migration of ergastoplasm, vacuolation, and necrosis of liver cells.[23,26] Interestingly, dietary DDT (100 to 2500 ppm) caused basic pathomorphological changes such as cellular hypertrophy and margination in liver cells of rats, yet produced no cellular necrosis.[24] In a general way, the intensity of DDT-related liver injury in experimental rats was directly proportional to the duration of exposure.

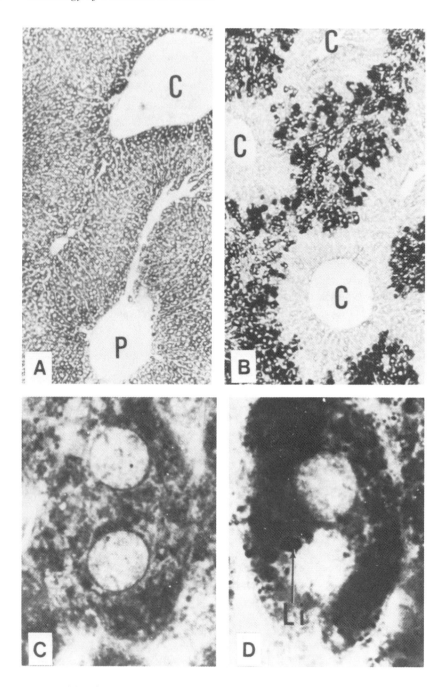

FIGURE 1.   (A) Light micrograph of a cryostat section of liver from a control rat receiving corn oil. Note hepatocytes surrounding the central vein (C) of a central zone and portal vein (P) of a periportal zone containing very low amounts of stainable lipid. (Sudan Black stain; magnification × 125.) (B) Light micrograph of a cryostat section of liver from a mirex-treated rat. Hepatocytes near central zones appear unaffected whereas periportal hepatocytes contain large amounts of lipid (C — central vein). This condition is termed periportal liposis. (Sudan Black Stain; magnification × 125.) (C) Light micrograph enlargement of hepatocyte from A. Only small amounts of lipid may be present. (Sudan Black stain; magnification × 3000.) (D) Light micrograph enlargement from hepatocyte periportal zone of large amount of lipid (Li) is stained black and indicates vast lipid accumulation. (Sudan Black stain; magnification × 3000.) (From Kendall, M. W., *Arch. Environ. Contam. Toxicol.*, 8, 25, 1979. With permission.)

In comparison to rats and rodents, dietary feeding of DDT (5 to 5000 ppm) to adult rhesus monkey for a prolonged period (8 to 40 months) produced no liver injury. The liver function test by bromosulfalein retention indicated no change in DDT-treated monkeys.

The unique pathomorphological alterations in the liver cells from rats given chlordecone alone and along with CCl_4 are of particular significance as potentiation of haloalkane hepatotoxicity occurred after chlordecone pretreatment. For instance, the increase in liver weight after CCl_4 exposure to chlordecone-treated rats could be explained by ingress of water. This in fact, is typically demonstrated by the dilation and vesiculation of the endoplasmic reticulum and the swelling of the mitochondria. The chlordecone and CCl_4 in combination also accentuated the hepatic storage of lipids.[21]

Different OCs, for example, chlordecone, dieldrin, lindane, and toxaphene in dietary doses for prolonged periods up to 9 months, produced liver injury in rats. The injury was distinctive as seen with centrolobular cell hypertrophy, peripheral migration of basophilic cytoplasmic granulations, and the presence of lipospheres.[22]

Pesticides in high doses consistently cause more liver injury in male rodents than in females.[23] The responses observed in liver of rats exposed to different doses of HCH, lindane, malathion, melthyl demeton, phosphamidon, and quinalphos follow a pattern that parallels the classic pathophysiological alterations. For instance, a generalized enlargment of the liver with an increase in the size of the liver parenchymal cells and accumulation of lipid droplets[10,11,27,28] were seen in these cases. Similarly, oral administration of phosphamidon (2.16 mg/kg/day) for 15 days, for instance, produced significant pathomorphological changes in the liver of female rabbits. The liver, for example, showed dilation and congestion of sinusoids, ballooning of hepatocytes with acentric pycnotic nuclei, and associated cytoplasmic changes[28] (Figure 2).

Oral administration of CCl_4 (0.5 ml/kg/day) for 7 days followed by quinalphos (3 and 6 mg/kg/day) for 2 days, however, produced appreciably severe liver injury and greater susceptibility of animals to the organophosphorus insecticide (OP). The pathomorphological changes in CCl_4-quinalphos treated liver include degenerative changes in the cytoplasm, presence of large coarse fat vacuoles, and proliferation of fibroblasts which obliterated some of the portal triads around the lobule[27] (Figures 3 and 4).

Daily feeding of chlordecone (10 ppm) for 15 days followed by a single i.p. challenge of CCl_4 (0.1 ml/kg) to rats produced significant liver injury. The entire lobule contained vacuolated hepatocytes and necrotic foci. There was an increase in the number of well-defined nodules consisting of necrosed liver cells and inflammatory cells scattered throughout the liver lobule[29] (Figures 5 and 6).

Feeding of low levels of chlordecone (10 ppm) in diet for 15 days produced no discernible gross changes in liver histology under light microscope. However, animals pretreated with chlordecone followed by a single i.p. challenge of CCl_4 elicited severe necrosis of the liver involving all zones of the lobular structure. The diffuse necrosis was associated with characteristic hepatocellular swelling and accumulation of lipid droplets in all the liver cells.[30] This, in fact, has shown the propensity of chlordecone to potentiate the hepatotoxicity of CCl_4. The pattern and sequel of liver injury is characterized by liver dysfunction, liver cell necrosis, and hepatic failure eventually leading to potentiated lethality. The assay of biliary excretion of phenolphthalein glucuronide and the rate of bile flow revealed that chlordecone did potentiate the dysfunction of liver in animals. Further, it has been observed that higher doses of CCl_4 in combination with chlordecone caused severe cholestatic response and totally disturbed the hepatobiliary function in animals.[29]

Oral doses of carbaryl (200 mg/kg 3 times/wk) for 90 days to male rats produced no significant liver injury.[31] However, combined treatment of carbaryl and CCl_4 for 90 days produced liver cell necrosis for example, hydropic changes and cytoplasmic swelling. Further, in the enlarged cells nuclear changes were very prominent suggesting necrosis. The

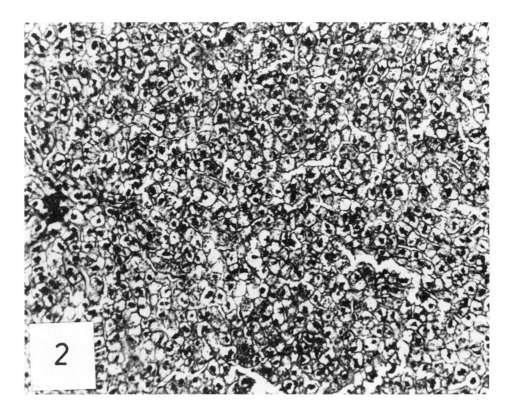

FIGURE 2. Liver from a phosphamidon-treated female rabbit (2.16 mg/kg/day for 15 days). Note vacuolated hepatocytes scattered throughout the lobule with necrotic foci. (Magnification × 320.)

liver cells showed for instance nuclear shrinkage, absence or loss of normal structural organization into nuclei, and granular chromatin. The majority of cells in the lobule showed extreme clumping of nuclear components.[32]

B. MORPHOMETRY

Volume density determinations of liver cells with glycogen, lipid, dilated RER, pycnotic nuclei, and mitoses revealed no significant differences between control group and chlordecone fed (10 ppm in diet for 15 days) animals. However, the cytoplasmic volume of swollen liver cells after CCl_4 treatment or chlordecone plus CCl_4 treatment showed a 2- to 4-fold increase. This increased cell volume decreased the total number of liver cells which occupied 1 ml of liver.

Numerical densities indicated no apparent difference between the number of liver cells per milliliter liver tissue in animals given normal diet and those fed with the chlordecone diet.

A combination of chlordecone and CCl_4 produced liver injury which became more severe with time. A progressive and increased loss of glycogen associated with lipid accumulation and a large number of swollen liver cells was very evident. In fact, the *in vivo* and *in vitro* investigations have indicated that bioactivation of CCl_4 is enhanced in liver of animals exposed to chlordecone.[33,34] Interestingly, pretreatment of chlordecone followed by CCl_4 administration showed progressive increase in the level of cytosolic Ca^{2+}, while no such change was seen after treatment of CCl_4 alone. However, more studies are needed to validate whether or not these hepatocellular alterations have any close relationship with the Ca^{2+} homeostasis mechanism.[29]

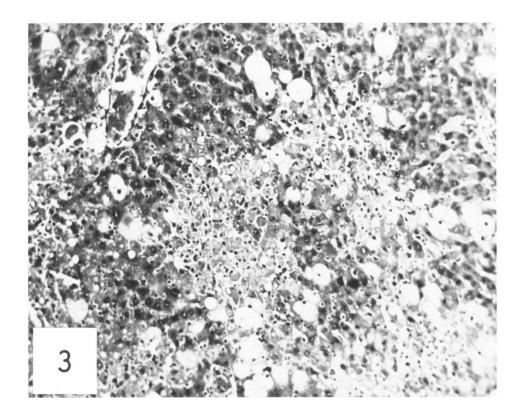

FIGURE 3. Liver from rat pretreated with CCl₄ (0.5 mg/kg) for 7 days followed by quinalphos (3 mg/kg/day) for 2 days. Note necrotic hepatocytes with a few vacuolated hepatocytes scattered all around the inflammatory cells. (Magnification × 425.)

Morphometric data revealed no significant difference between animals fed a normal diet and those exposed to a chlordecone diet. For example, the numerical density and volume density of liver cells, along with the levels of glycogen, lipid, dilated rough endoplasmic reticulum, pycnosis, or mitosis all remained almost the same and comparable.[29]

C. ULTRASTRUCTURE

The ultrastructure of normal cells shows the presence of numerous rosettes of glycogen and very few lipid vacuoles (Figure 7). In contrast, the liver cells in centrolobular zones from mirex-treated rats contain numerous ultrastructural changes, for example, the presence of discontinuous rough endoplasmic reticulum (RER) with dilated cisternae free ribosomes and increased proliferation of smooth endoplasmic reticulum (SER). The latter appeared dilated and distributed throughout the cytoplasm (Figures 8 to 10). Reports of Baker et al.[35] and Davison et al.[36] with mirex showed a dose response proliferation of SER in animals.

The liver cells from the periportal zone of mirex-exposed rats also contain myelin figures, which play a major role in the formation of liposomes (Figures 1 to 13), and large number of lipid droplets or giant liposomes, apparently in different phases of formation[9] (Figure 14).

In comparison to control (Figure 7), the mitochondria assumed apparently a normal profile in the mirex-treated rats (Figure 14). The microbodies (Figures 8 and 11) were surrounded by a single membrane with a peculiar, more electron-dense area which was acentric in location. These microbodies were far fewer in the control group of animals.

The intracellular, myelin-like figures that occur in the liver cells of a mirex-exposed rat

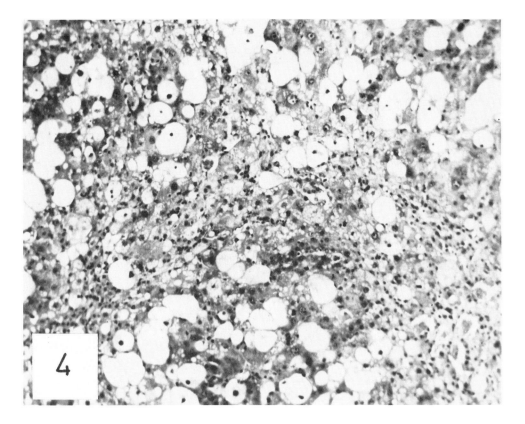

FIGURE 4.   Liver from rat pretreated with CCl$_4$ (0.5 mg/kg) for 7 days followed by quinalphos (6 mg/kg/day) for 2 days. Note vacuolated hepatocytes and necrotic foci scattered throughout the lobule. (Magnification × 425.)

is of special significance. This is particularly so to speculate about their origin and consequential fate, since myelin figures are often seen in experimental toxic injury of the liver and in hepatomas.[37] In fact, it has been speculated that some of the myelin figures seen in mirex-treated rats are the lipid precursors. A giant liposome contains a myelin-like figure, the membranes of which are beginning to lose their orderly array with their disociation into the liposomal contents (Figure 14).

In fatty liver produced by chemicals, the lipid inclusions are principally fat droplets, and myelin figures are often rare. There is a need to distinguish fatty metamorphosis from lipophanerosis. The former is a relatively simple process of deposition of fat. This has no significant effect on cellular functions from fatty degeneration produced by pesticides. The latter however, comprises fat droplets and myelin figures and is seen in highly altered liver cells, probably undergoing necrosis. In fact, mirex-treated rat has shown lipophanerosis with addition of some myelin figures into the developing liposomes.[9]

Ortega[24] observed the accumulation of lipid surrounded by several concentric layers of membranes in the liver of rat exposed to high doses of DDT. Sublethal doses of mirex showed the presence of myelin figures in the liver cells of rats. These myelin figures appear to contribute their concentric membranes to lipid droplets or vice versa. Thus, this kind of hepatic fatty metamorphosis seems to be common to both DDT and mirex.

Mirex and photomirex, for instance, did not cause a drastic effect on mitochondria, golgi complex, or bile canaliculi. The two insecticides, however, caused an increase of smooth endoplasmic reticulum. In fact, the insecticides produced whorls and stacks of parallel membranes in several liver cells. The golgi vesicles contained very low density lipoproteins.

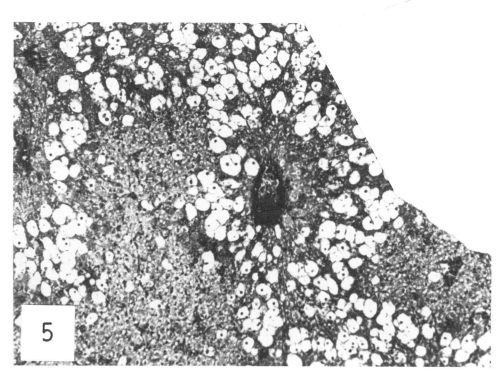

FIGURE 5. Light micrograph of liver from rat fed chlordecone in diet (10 ppm) for 15 days and with 0.1 mg/kg CCl$_4$. Note vacuolated and lipid containing hepatocytes with necrotic foci scattered throughout the lobule at 4 h. (Magnification × 190.) (From Lockard, V. G. et al., *Exp. Mol. Pathol.*, 39, 230, 1983. With permission.)

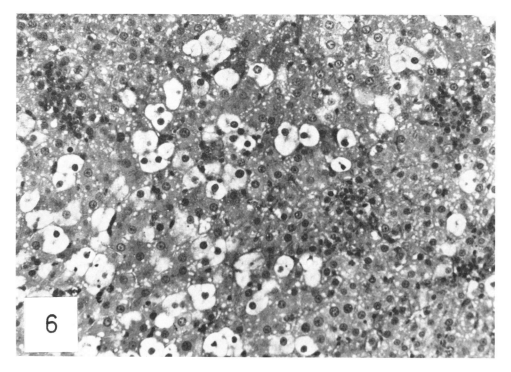

FIGURE 6. Light micrograph of liver from rat given diet containing chlordecone and injected with CCl$_4$ (0.1 mg/kg). Note increased number of well-defined nodules consisting of necrotic hepatocytes and inflammatory cells scattered throughout the lobule. (Magnification × 270.) (From Lockard, V. G. et al., *Exp. Mol. Pathol.*, 39, 230, 1983. With permission.)

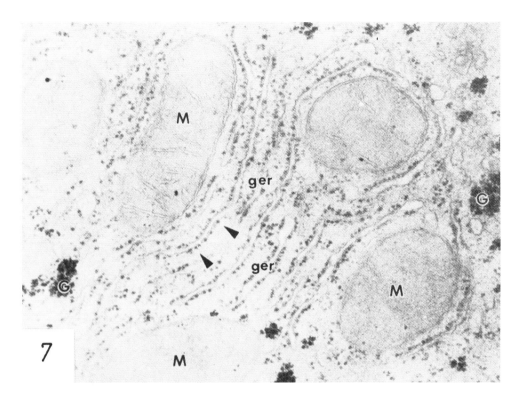

FIGURE 7.   Electron micrograph of a hepatocyte from a centrolobular zone of a control rat. Note the regularity of the granular endoplasmic reticulum (ger) with attached ribosomes (arrowheads) and deposits of glycogen rosettes (G). M = mitochondria. (Magnification × 26,000). (From Kendall, M. W., *Arch. Environ. Contam. Toxicol.*, 8, 25 1979. With permission.)

Daily feeding of technical HCH (500 ppm) in diet to mice for 2 to 8 months produced significant ultrastructural changes in liver for instance, the presence of excessive glycogen, proliferation of SER with structural changes in RER, excessive accumulation of fat, and degenerative changes in nuclear membrane and nucleoli.[38]

The ultrastructural changes produced by[17] chlordecone and CCl_4 in the rat liver include extensive damage to cellular organelles for example, accumulation of lipid droplets, disorganization of RER with loss of ribosomes and an increase in SER, dilation of the outer membrane of the nucleus, swollen mitochondria, and loss of cisternae and flocculant densities indicating grades of rupturing of cell membrane with release of cell contents to sinusoidal areas[29] (Figures 15 to 18).

IV. BIOCHEMICAL CHANGES

The biochemical changes observed in the liver of animals exposed to repeated doses of pesticides include changes in hepatic-soluble enzymes, particularly the gluconeogenic enzymes and induction of the microsomal mixed function oxidases. Pesticides also cause an increase in protein and lipid synthesis and hepatic glycogen depletion.

Exposure to pesticides cause alterations in basic metabolism which involves both anabolic and catabolic processes.[39,40] Certain soluble enzymes are used as diagnostic markers for tissue damage. Cellular changes such as necrosis, for example, are generally associated with leakage of soluble tissue enzymes into the blood. Lethal doses of DDT cause increase in serum levels of lactate dehydrogenase and glutamate pyruvate transaminase in mice.[41] Rats

157

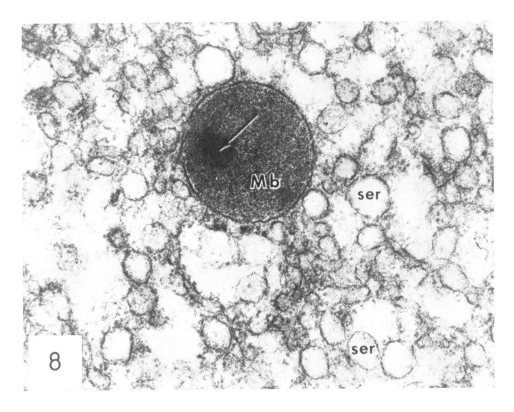

FIGURE 8. Electron micrograph of a centrolobular hepatocyte from an experimental rat. Note the immense proliferation of smooth endoplasmic reticulum (ser) and the presence of a microbody (Mb). Within each microbody is found a densely stained, eccentrically located body termed a nucleoid (arrow). (Magnification × 46,000.) (From Kendall, M. W., *Arch. Environ. Contam. Toxicol.*, 8, 25 1979. With permission.)

exposed to dietary DDT for 14 days showed a significant decrease in the serum levels of glucose-6-phosphatase (16%), glucose-6-phosphate dehydrogenase (34%), glutamate dehydrogenase (51%), lactate dehydrogenase (32%), and glucose-6-phosphatase (16%).[42]

Repeated feeding of dieldrin (50 ppm) for 8 weeks caused a significant increase in plasma and hepatic microsomal carboxylesterase activities in male and female rats. The rise in hepatic microsomal esterases has been due to an increase in microsomal protein.[43] A close correlation has been established between induction of liver enlargement and stimulation of liver microsomal enzymes during metabolism in animals exposed to pesticides.[43] For example, rats given DDT for 4 months showed increase in the activity of hepatic microsomal drug metabolizing enzymes, particularly in hexobarbital, aminopyrine, and p-nitrobenzoate metabolism.[44] Similarly, stimulation of hepatic microsomal enzymes was noticed in rats fed DDT and toxaphene.[45]

The metabolism of three substrates and NADPH cytochrome reductase, NADPH-oxidase, and cytochrome p-450 content in dieldrin-fed rats showed significant alterations. For example, both amine hydroxylase and ethylmorphine-N-demethylase were significantly induced in male rats. The mixed function oxidase components namely, NADPH-cytochrome c-reductase, NADPH-oxidase, and cytochrome p-450 were significantly elevated. The female rat showed a significant induction of aldrin epoxidation.[46] Oral administration p,p'-DDT (5 to 50 mg/kg/day) for 21 days produced a rise in the hepatic cytochrome p-450 concentration which was dose related.[47]

Treatment of male mice with dietary Kepone for 14 days produced biochemical changes for instance, kepone-induced hepatic cytochrome p-450, O- and N-demethylation of p-

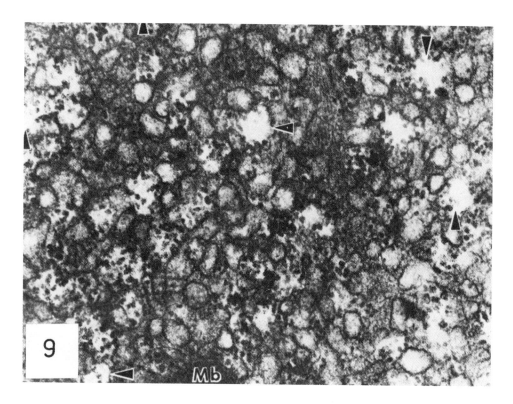

FIGURE 9.   Electron micrograph of a cytoplasmic region from a centrolobular hepatocyte showing spaces (arrowheads) that may have contained glycogen rosettes. The presence of large quantities of SER in cross-section detail the morphology of these structures. No glycogen rosette can be observed. A microbody (Mb) is found in the lower left portion of the micrograph. (Magnification × 34,500.) (From Kendall, M. W., *Arch. Environ. Contam. Toxicol.*, 8, 25 1979. With permission.)

nitroanisole and aminopyrine.[48] Similarly, Baker et al.[35] found that liver from rat fed mirex (25 ppm) for 14 days showed a significant increase in cytochrome p-450. A higher concentration of mirex (100 and 250 ppm) caused a sixfold increase in cytochrome p-450. Byard et al.[49] found that mice given mirex (90 ppm) in the diet for periods ranging from 1 to 70 weeks showed a higher activity of cytochrome p-450, N-demethylase, and 4-biphenyl hydroxylase.

Chronic exposure to insecticides have produced an increase in the key hepatic gluconeogenic enzymes. For example, DDT, endrin, heptachlor, and α-chlordane triggered the glyconeogenic enzymes. A significant increase was registered in the hepatic activities of pyruvate carboxylase, phosphoenolpyruvate carboxylase, fructose-1-6-diphosphatase, and glucose-6-phosphatase of rats exposed to these insecticides.[50-52]

Chronic treatment of mirex produced severe changes in the NADH-cytochrome-C-reductase and NADPH-cytochrome-C-reductase activities and cytochrome p-450 contents in liver microsomes of male mice. Further, the elevation of microsomal protein was consistent with the observed induction of mfo components.[53]

Prolonged exposure of squirrel monkeys to p,p′-DDT produced a significant increase in hepatic EPN hydrolysis. A significant increase was also recorded in the metabolism of p-nitroanisole.[54] Dieldrin inhibited the initial phosphorylation process of glucose by lowering the activities of glucokinase and hexokinase. The resultant inhibition of glycolysis together with the increase in the activities of hepatic lactate dehydrogenase, thus support the stimulation of gluconeogenesis by dieldrin.[55] In fact, dieldrin-mediated augmentation of hexose monophosphate shunt pathway suggests direct oxidation of glucose. The changes in the

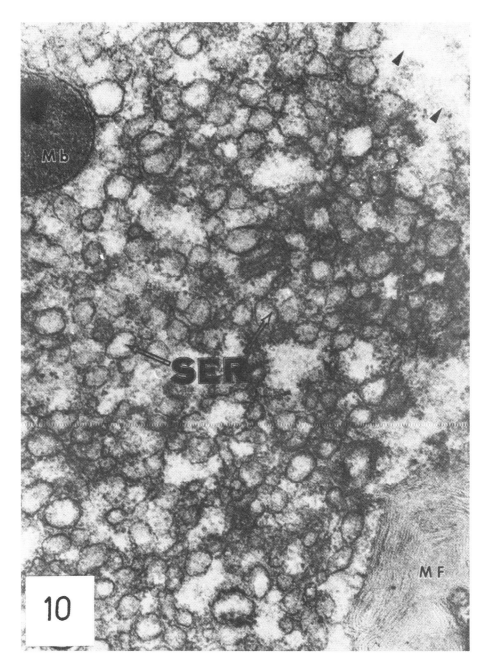

FIGURE 10.   Electron micrograph of a centrolobular hepatocyte from an experimental rat. A microbody (Mb) is found in the upper left corner and numerous vesicles of smooth endoplasmic reticulum (SER) are present. A necrotic, empty area (arrows) is found surrounding myelin figures (MF), one of which is shown in the lower right corner. The lamellae demonstrate a periodicity of 106 to 120 Å . (Magnification × 60,000.)(From Kendall, M. W., *Arch. Environ. Contam. Toxicol.*, 8, 25 1979. With permission.)

activities of hepatic alkaline phosphatase and ATPase are, thus, indicative of an impairment of liver function and altered mitochondrial morphology.[56]

Some of the OCI are known to interact with the biological membranes causing membrane perturbation which subsequently could alter membrane fluidity and transport functions.[57] For example administration of dieldrin (5 mg/kg/day) for 15 days produced significant

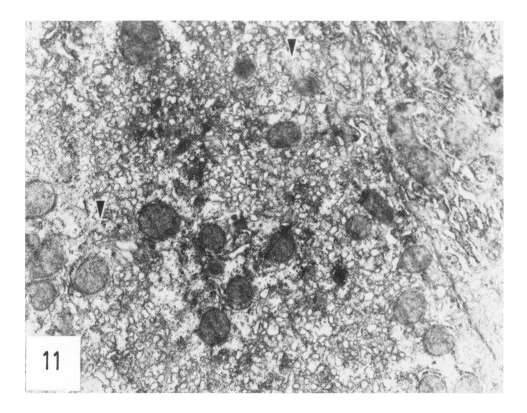

FIGURE 11.   Electron micrograph of two adjacent periportal hepatocytes. Lipid vacuoles are not evident in this particular view. Irregular RER, free ribosomes, and large proliferations of SER can be observed. Myelin figures (arrowheads) are dispersed throughout the cytoplasm. (Magnification × 8,600.) (From Kendall, M. W., *Arch. Environ. Contam. Toxicol.*, 8, 25, 1979. With permission.)

inhibition in the activities of Mg^{2+} ATPase and stimulation of 5′-necleodase and NADH-dehydrogenase in liver plasma membrane. This seems to suggest alteration of ATP-dependent transport system through altered ATP levels.[58]

Chlordecone is known to enhance the hepatotoxicity of CCl_4 in a significant manner.[59,60] However, rats pretreated with chlordecone displayed only moderately increased mfo activity and a very large shift in sensitivity to CCl_4. In fact, chlordecone increases the sensitivity of CCl_4 by either specifically inducing the subset of cytochrome p-450 species responsible for CCl_4 metabolism, or altering the affinity of constitutive p-450 species for CCl_4.[33]

The effect of a single oral dose of chlordecone (10 mg/kg) followed by a challenge of CCl_4 (i.p.) indicated increased sensitivity of liver cells to CCl_4. In fact, pretreatment of chlordecone as short as 6 h produced significant elevation in the levels of serum, GOT, GPT, and LDH. It is quite possible that chlordecone induces the specific cytochrome which activates CCl_4 since the extent of binding of label from[14] CCl_4 did not correlate with hepatotoxicity as a senstive index of activation.[61]

Despite the heterogenicity and multiplicity[23] of etiologic factors, it is of interest that in almost all cases of fatty livers, the lipid that accumulates in the liver cell is predominantly, but not exclusively, the triglyceride.[62] In fact, a fatty liver is the end product of an imbalance between the rate of synthesis and the rate of utilization of hepatic triglycerides. Fatty change or metamorphosis in the liver cells often begins with the formation of *liposomes*. The storage of fat following a single large dose of dieldrin was found to involve triglycerides only with no increase in phospholipid or cholesterol. The increase in triglycerides was accompanied by an increased incorporation of ^{14}C glucose into glyceride-glycerol but a decrease of its

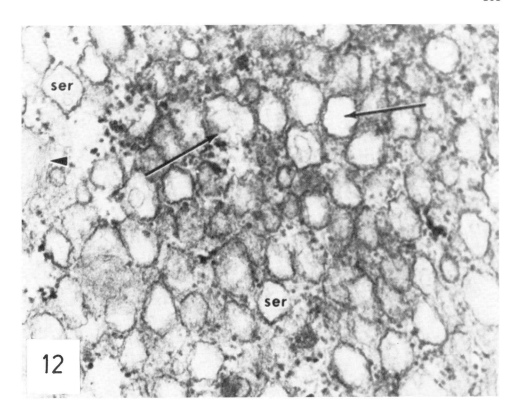

FIGURE 12.   Electron micrograph of a cytoplasmic region from a periportal hepatocyte showing a circular myelin figure (arrowhead) and large amounts of SER (arrows). No glycogen rosettes are observable. Compare with Figure 9. Membranous whorls are seen in some cross-sections of SER leading to the speculation that myelin figures may originate there. (Magnification × 34,500.) (From Kendall, M. W., *Arch. Environ. Contam. Toxicol.,* 8, 25, 1979. With permission.)

incorporation into fatty acids. It seems probable more triglyceride is formed in the presence of more glyceride glycerol.[63]

The liver of mirex-treated rats in comparison to that of normal rats contained a higher concentration of DNA and lipids while the concentration of RNA, protein, and glycogen were lower[9] (Table 1).

V. HEPATOCARCINOGENESIS

A large variety of pesticides, particularly the organochlorine insecticides have been shown to elicit carcinogenic changes in laboratory animals.[64,65] An increased incidence of liver tumors in mice fed dieldrin and HCH has been reported. However, the overall tumor incidence in rats fed aldrin (20 to 50 ppm) or dieldrin (20 to 50 ppm) was lower than the controls. Subsequent studies also show that dieldrin is hepatocarcinogenic in mice.

Rats given a diet containing mirex (50 and 100 ppm) show a dose-dependent toxicity and incidence of hepatic megalocytosis, cellular alterations, and neoplastic nodules. The hepatocellular carcinoma was seen only in male rat at the high dietary level.

Liver of mice given a daily dose of technical HCH in diet (500 ppm) showed excessive accumulation of glycogen within the cytoplasmic matrix, a factor common to various chemical carcinogens. In fact, a large amount of glycogen was seen enclosed in autophagic vacuoles during neoplastic development. The decreased activity of glucose-6-phosphatase in mice liver and the long meandering cisternae of rough endoplasmic reticulum are all suggestive of the hepatocarcinogenic potential of technical HCH.[38]

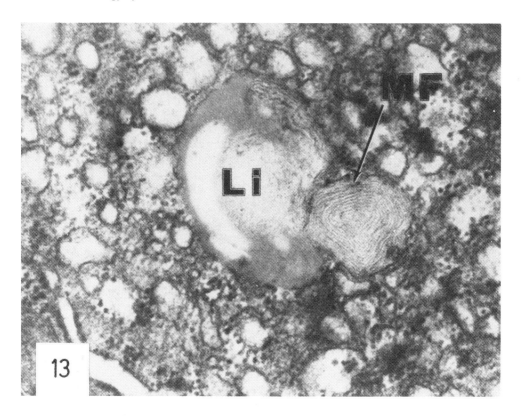

FIGURE 13.   Electron micrograph of a portion of a periportal hepatocyte showing a liposome (Li) and a circular myelin figure (MF). It is not known if the latter develops from the former of vice versa, although this figure suggests that myelin figures may contribute their membranes to the developing liposome since the myelin figure is evidently formed first within SER (See Figure 12). (Magnification × 34,000.) (From Kendall, M. W., *Arch. Environ. Contam. Toxicol.*, 8, 25, 1979. With permission.)

There is evidence that a number of OCs cause marked changes in the livers of different rodents. These changes progress to tumor formation in some species of animals, particularly the mouse.[65]

Evidence on carcinogencity has shown that the tumors produced by DDT, HCH, and several cyclodiene insecticides are peculiar to rodents.[65] Evidence to show that the tumors occur in species other than mouse is not abundant in the literature (see Table 3 in Chapter 9).

There still is no conclusive agreement regarding the carcinogenicity of several OCI. For example, the lesion caused by the classical carcinogen was very different from that caused by the OCs.[4,66,67] Details on hepatocarcinogenicity of several OCs may be found elsewhere in the literature.[68,69]

VI. CONCLUSION

Most chemicals to which man is exposed undergo biotransformation predominantly, but not exclusively, in the liver. This process makes many of the lipophilic environmental chemicals, for instance pesticides, more soluble in the aqueous mileu of urine and bile where they are excreted. It is now well-recognized that the endoplasmic reticulum of the hepatocyte is the major site for this biotransformation, which is mediated by a group of hemoprotein isoenzymes for example, cytochrome p-450 is the most widley studied hemoprotein.

The study of the hepatic organelles by electron microscopy is another method which is

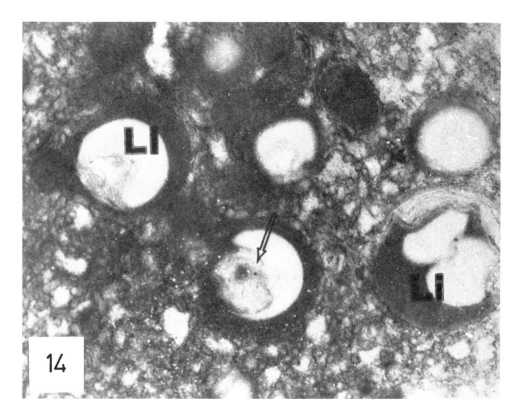

FIGURE 14.   Electron micrograph of a portion of a periportal hepatocyte showing membranes within a developing liposome (Li). Note the close association of the liposome with adjacent mitochondria. This section has been lightly stained and the lipid has been partially extracted, revealing a peripheral ring of lipid on the inside of each liposome. The center of one liposome (near the bottom center of the field) contains a myelin figure (arrow), suggesting that the middle of a liposome, when unextracted, consists of a lamellated core. (Magnification × 37,000.) (From Kendall, M. W., *Arch. Environ. Contam. Toxicol.*, 8, 25, 1979. With permission.)

useful only for limited studies in heavily exposed animals and humans with obvious clinical evidence of hepatotoxicity.

In the case of liver injury, one of the earliest changes to occur is the release of intracellular enzymes into the blood. Some of these enzymes are found preferentially in hepatocytes. For instance, aspartate aminotransferase (AST) and alanine aminotransferase (ALT). Some other enzymes, however are predominantly released from the cholangolar and ductular cells of the liver; for example, alkaline phosphatase and 5'-nucleotidase. Assay of these enzymes in blood is regularly used to detect liver damage.

ALT is relatively specific for liver injury, whereas others may be altered by injury to other organs.

In the case of alkaline phosphatase on isoenzyme fraction is possible which can specifically identify the liver isozyme. In the identification of the hepatotoxic effects of insecticides both ALT and AST have been used as markers.

Of the other liver function determinations for evaluation of hepatic injury due to chemicals the most specific and sensitive is the estimation of serum bile acid level. Bile acids are formed in liver cells excreted into the biliary tree largely in a conjugated form and later reabsorbed from the intestine following bacterial deconjugation. Serum-free bile acid levels rise in any injury which decreases the capacity of liver cells to remove other toxicants from blood and reexcrete bile acids into bile.

The biochemical changes caused by pesticide showed depletion of glycogen with the

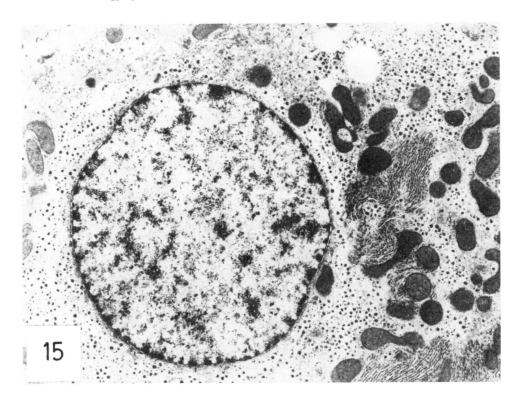

FIGURE 15.   Electron micrograph showing normal ultrastructure of a liver cell; rats were given control diet plus injection of corn oil (1 ml/kg). Mitochondria, RER, and particulate glycogen are scattered throughout the cytoplasm. (Magnification × 4200.) (From Lockard, V. G. et al., *Exp. Mol. Pathol.*, 39, 230, 1983. With permission.)

concomitant increase in the lipid content and lowering of protein/DNA and RNA/DNA values. The compensatory response exhibited by mammalian liver to pesticides and other toxic chemicals is a fascinating subject which deserves greater investigation.

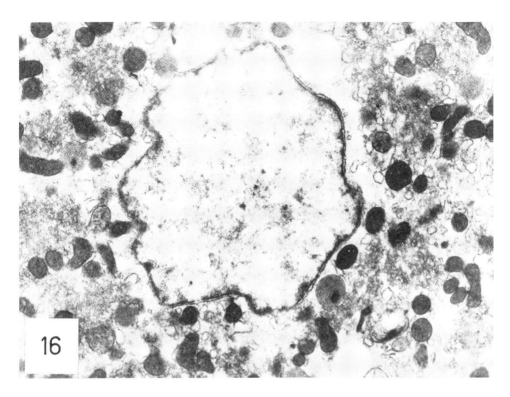

FIGURE 16. Electron micrograph of pericentral hepatocyte from rat fed a diet containing chlordecone (10 ppm) for 15 days. Note focal increase in SER at 24 h. (Magnification × 4200.) (From Lockard, V. G. et al., *Exp. Mol. Pathol.*, 39, 230, 1983. With permission.)

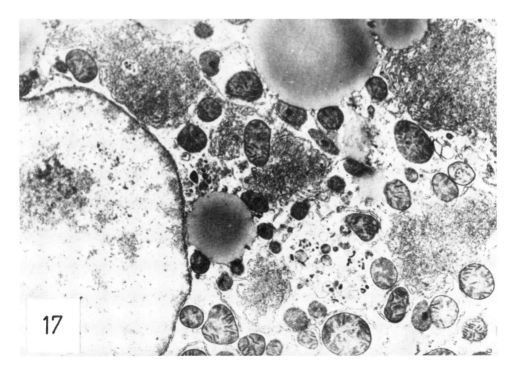

FIGURE 17. Electron micrograph of liver cell from rat given chlordecone diet and injection of CCl_4 (0.1 ml/kg). Note lipid droplets and increased SER at 4 h. (Magnification × 4200.) (From Lockard, V. G. et al., *Exp. Mol. Pathol.*, 39, 230, 1983. With permission.)

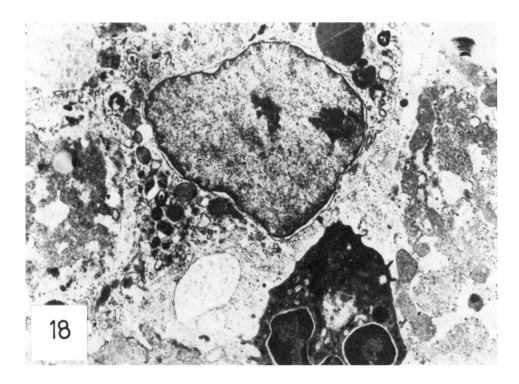

FIGURE 18.   Electron micrograph of a necrotic focus in liver of rat given diet with chlordecone and injection of 0.1 ml/kg CCl$_4$. Note hepatocyte cell membrane ruptured and degenerating Kupffer cell containing phagocytosed material. Also see the presence of a polymorphonuclear leucocyte. (Magnification × 4,200.) (From Lockard, V. G. et al., *Exp. Mol. Pathol.*, 39, 230, 1983. With permission.)

TABLE 1
Biochemical Changes in Rat Liver (Total Homogenate)

Treatment	DNA[a]	RNA[b]	Protein[b]	Glycogen[b]	Lipids[a]
Control[c]	2.57 ± 0.05	3.46 ± 0.03	74 ± 0.82	9.4 ± 0.97	48 ± 0.73
Mirex (200 mg/kg)	2.98 ± 0.10	2.00 ± 0.07	22 ± 4.27	0.2 ± 0.11	155 ± 7.96

[a]   mg/g wet liver.
[b]   mg/mgDNA.
[c]   25 rats in each group.

From Kendall, M. W., *Arch. Environ. Contam. Toxicol.*, 8, 25, 1979. With permission.

REFERENCES

1. **Sarett, H. P. and Jandof, B. J.,** Effects of chronic DDT intoxication in rats on lipids and other constituents of liver, *J. Pharmacol. Exp. Ther.*, 91, 340, 1947.
2. **Laug, E. P., Nelson, A. A., Fitzhugh, O. G., and Kunze, F. M.,** Liver cell alternation and DDT storage in the fat of the rat induced by dietary levels of 1 to 50 ppm DDT, *J. Pharmacol. Exp. Ther.*, 98, 268, 1950.
3. **Durham, W. F., Ortega, P., and Hayes, W. J. Jr.,** The effect of various dietary levels of DDT on liver functions, cell morphology, and DDT storage in the Rhesus monkey, *Arch. Int. Pharmacodyn. Ther.*, 141, 111, 1963.

4. **Wright, A. S., Potter, D., Wooder, M. F., Donninger, C., and Greenland, R. D.,** The effects of dieldrin on the subcellular structure and function of mammalian liver cells, *Food. Cosmet. Toxicol.,* 10, 311, 1972.

5. **Wright, A. S., Donninger, C., Greenland, R. D., Stemmer, K. L., and Zavon, M. R.,** The effects of prolonged ingestion of dieldrin on the livers of male rhesus monkeys, *Ecotoxicol. Environ. Safe.,* 1, 477, 1978.

6. **Kimbrough, R. D., Gaines, T. B., and Hayes, W. J. Jr.,** Combined effect of DDT pyrethrum and piperonyl butoxide on rat liver, *Arch. Environ. Health,* 16, 333, 1968.

7. **Mahendale, H. M.,** Pesticide induced modification of hepatobiliary function: hexachlorobenzene, DDT and toxaphene, *Food Cosmet. Toxicol.,* 16, 19, 1978.

8. **Krampl, V.,** Relationship between serum enzymes and histological changes in liver after administration of hepatochlor in the rat, *Bull. Environ. Contam. Toxicol.,* 5, 529, 1971.

9. **Kendall, M. W.,** Light and electron microscopic observations of the acute sublethal hepatotoxic effects of mirex in the rat, *Arch. Environ. Contam. Toxicol.,* 8, 25, 1979.

10. **Dikshith, T. S. S., Tandon, S. K., Datta, K. K., Gupta, P. K., and Behari, J. R.,** Comaprative response of male rats to parathion and lindane. Histopathological and biochemical studies, *Environ. Res.,* 17, 1, 1978.

11. **Dikshith, T. S. S., Raizada, R. B., Srivastava, M. K., Kumar, S. N., Kaushal, R. A., Singh, R. P., Gupta, K. P., and Sree Lakshmi, K.,** Dermal toxicity of HCH in rabbit, *Indian J. Exp. Biol.,* 27, 252, 1989.

12. **Zimmerman, H. J.,** *Hepatoxicity,* Appleton-Century-Crofts, New York, 1978.

13. **Mehendale, H. M.,** Application of isolated organ techniques in toxicology, in *Principles and Methods of Toxicology,* Hayes, A. W., Ed., Raven press, New York, 1982.

14. **Plaa, G. L.,** Toxic responses of the liver, in *Casarett and Doull's Toxicology. The Basic Science of Poisons,* 2nd ed., Doull, J., Klassen, C. D., and Amdur, M. O., Macmillan, New York, 1980, 206.

15. **Karl, P. I. and Yarbrough, J. D.,** A comparison of mirex-induced liver growth to liver regeneration, *Toxicol. Lett.,* 23, 127, 1984.

16. **Kendall, M. W.,** Acute histopathological alterations induced in livers of rat, mouse and quail by the fire ant poison, mirex, *Anta. Rec.,* 178, 388, 1974a.

17. **Kendall, M. W.,** Acute hepatotoxic effects of mirex in the rat, *Bull. Environ. Contam. Toxicol.,* 12, 617, 1974b.

18. **Cameron, G. R. and Burgess, F.,** Toxicity of DDT, *Br. Med. J.,* 1, 865, 1945.

19. **Cameron, G. R. and Cheng, K. K.,** Failure of oral DDT to induce changes in rats, *Br. Med. J.,* 2, 819, 1951.

20. **Ortega, P., Hayes, W. J. Jr., Durham, W. F., and Mattson, A.,** DDT in the Diet of Rat, U.S. Public Health Serv. Publ. No. 484, No. 43, Washington, D.C., 1956.

21. **Curtis, L. R., Klein, A. K. T., and Mehendale, H. M.,** Ultrastructural and biochemical correlations of the specificity of chlorodecone potentiated CCl_4 hepatotoxicity, *J. Toxicol. Environ. Health,* 7, 499, 1981.

22. **Walker, A. J. T., Steuenson, D. E., Robinson, J., Thorpe, E., and Robert, M.,** The toxicology and pharmacodynamics of dieldrin (HEOD). Two year oral exposures of rats and dogs, *Toxicol. Appl. Pharmacol.,* 15, 345, 1969.

23. **Ortega, P., Hayes, W. J. Jr., and Durham, W. E.,** Pathologic changes in the liver of rats after feeding low levels of various insecticides, *A.M.A. Arch. Pathol.,* 64, 614, 1957.

24. **Ortega, P.,** Light and electron microscopy of dichlorodiphenyl trichloroethane (DDT) poisoning in the rat liver, *Lab. Invest.,* 15, 657, 1966.

25. **Kimbrough, R. D., Gaines, T. B., and Linder, R. E.,** The ultrastructure of livers of rats fed DDT and dieldrin, *Arch. Environ. Health,* 22, 460, 1971.

26. **Jonsson, H. T. Jr., Walker, E. M. Jr., Greene, W. P., Hughson, M. D., and Henniger, G. R.,** Effects of prolonged exposure to dietary DDT and PCB on rat liver morphology, *Arch. Environ. Contam. Toxicol.,* 10, 171, 1981.

27. **Dikshith, T. S. S., Datta, K. K., Kushwah, H. S., Chandra, P., and Raizada, R. B.,** Effect of methyl demeton on vital organs and cholinesterase in male rats, *Indian J. Exp. Biol.,* 18, 163, 1980.

28. **Dkshith, T. S. S., Raizada, R. B., and Datta, K. K.,** Interaction of phosphamidon and benzene in female rabbits, *Indian J. Exp. Biol.,* 18, 1273, 1980.

29. **Lockard, V. G., Mehandale, H. M., and O'Neal, R. M.,** Chlorodecone induced CCl_4 hepatotoxicity: a light and electronmicroscopic study, *Exp. Mol. Pathol.,* 39, 230, 1983.

30. **Agarwal, A. K. and Mehendale, H. M.,** Potentiation of CCl_4 hepatotoxicity and lethality by chlordecone in female rats, *Toxicology,* 25, 231, 1983.

31. **Dikshith, T. S. S., Gupta, P. K., Gaur, J. S., Datta, K. K., and Mathur, A. K.,** Ninety day toxicity of carbaryl in male rats, *Environ. Res.,* 12, 161, 1976.

32. **Dikshith, T. S. S.,** Response of rats pretreated with carbon tetrachloride to carbaryl toxicity, unpublished data.

33. **Klingensmity, J. S. and Mehendale, H. M.,** Potentiation of CCl₄ lethality by chlordecone, *Toxicol. Lett.,* 11, 149, 1982.
34. **Klingensmity, J. S., Lockard, V., and Mehendale, H. M.,** Acute hepatotoxicity and lethality of CCl₄ in chlordecone pretreated rats, *Expt. Mol. Pathol.,* 39, 1, 1983.
35. **Baker, R. C., Cooris, L. D., Mailman, R. B., and Hodgson, E.,** Induction of hepatic mixed function oxidase by insecticide mirex, *Environ. Res.,* 5, 418, 1972.
36. **Davidson, K. L., Mollenhaur, H. H., Younger, R. L., and Cox, J. H.,** Mirex induced hepatic changes in chickens Jananese quail and rats, *Arch. Environ. Contam. Toxicol.,* 4, 469, 1976.
37. **Rouiller, C., Ed.,** Experimental toxic injury to the liver, *The Liver,* Part II, Academic Press, New York, 1964.
38. **Nigam, S. K., Lakkad, B. C., Karnik, A. B., and Thakore, K. N.,** Ultrastructural changes in liver of mice exposed to HCH, *Indian J. Exp. Biol.,* 22, 199, 1984.
39. **Darsie, J., Ghosa, S. K., and Holman, R. T.,** Induction of abnormal fatty acid metabolism and essential fatty acid deficiency in rats by dietary DDT, *Arch. Biochem. Biophys.,* 175, 262, 1976.
40. **Robinson, K. M. and Yarbrough, J. D.,** Liver protein synthesis and catabolism in mirex pretreated rats with enlarging livers, *J. Pharmacol. Exp. Ther.,* 215, 82, 1980.
41. **Luckens, M. M. and Phelps, K. I.,** Serum enzymes patterns in acute poisoning with organochlorine insecticides, *J. Pharm. Sci.,* 58, 569, 1969.
42. **Platt, D. S. and Cockrill, b. L.,** Liver enlargment and hepatotoxicity an investigation into the effects of several agents on rat liver enzyme activities, *Biochem. Pharmacol.,* 16, 2257, 1967.
43. **Temaitis, A., Oberholser, K. M., and Greene, F. E.,** Effects of acute and chronic dieldrin administration on liver and plasma esterases of the rat, *Toxicol. Appl. Pharmacol.,* 37, 29, 1976.
44. **Hart, L. G. and Fouts, J. R.,** Effects of acute and chronic DDT administration on hepatic microsomal drug metabolism in the rat, *Proc. Soc. Exp. Biol. Med.,* 114, 338, 1963.
45. **Kinoshita, F. K., Frawley, J. P., and Dubops, K. P.,** Quantitative measurement of induction of hepatic microsomal enzymes by various dietary levels of DDT and toxaphene in rats, *Toxicol. Appl. Pharmacol.,* 9, 505, 1966.
46. **Stevens, J. J., Oberholser, K. M., Wagner, S. R., and Greene, F. E.,** Content and activities of microsomal electron transport components during the development of dieldrin induced hypertrophic hypoactive endoplasmic reticulum, *Toxicol. Appl. Pharmacol.,* 39, 411, 1977.
47. **Down, W. H. and Chasseaud, L. F.,** The effect of DDT on hepatic microsomal drug metabolising enzymes in the baboon, comparison with the rat, *Bull. Environ. Contam. Toxicol.,* 20, 592, 1978.
48. **Fobacher, D. L. and Hodgson, E.,** Induction of hepatic mixed function oxidase activities in adult and neonatal mice by kepone and mirex, *Toxicol. Appl. Pharmacol.,* 38, 71, 1976.
49. **Byard, J. L., Koepke, V. Ch., Abraham, R., Golberg, L., and Coulston, F.,** Biochemical changes in the liver of mice fed mirex, *Toxicol. Appl. Pharmacol.,* 33, 70, 1975.
50. **Kacew, S. and Singhal, R. L.,** Metabolic alterations after chronic exposure to alpha chlordecone, *Toxicol. Appl. Pharmacol.,* 24, 539, 1973.
51. **Kacew, S. and Singhal, R. L.,** Adaptive response of hepatic carbohydrate metabolism to oral administration of p,p'-1,1,1-trichloro 2,2-bis (p-chlorophenyl) ethane in rats, *Biochem. Pharmacol.,* 22, 47, 1973.
52. **Kacew, S., Sutherland, J. B., and Singhal, R. L.,** Biochemical changes following chronic administration of hepatochlor epoxide and endrin to male rats, *Environ. Physiol. Biochem.,* 3, 221, 1973.
53. **Yarbrough, James, D., Chambors, Jamice E., and Robinson Keita, M.,** Alternations in liver structure and function resulting from chronic insecticide exposure, in *Effects of Chronic Exposures of Pesticides on Animal System* Chamber, J. and Yarbrough J. D., Eds., Raven Press, New York, 1982.
54. **Cranmer, M., Peoples, A., and Chadwick, R.,** Biochemical effects of repeated administration of p-p'-DDT on the squirrel monkey, *Toxicol. Appl. Pharmacol.,* 21, 98, 1972.
55. **Bhatia, S. C., Sharma, S. C., and Subramanian, T. A. V.,** Acute dieldrin toxicity biochemical changes in blood, *Arch. Environ. Health,* 24, 369, 1972.
56. **Kohli, K. K., Maggon, K. K., Subramanian, T. A. V.,** Induction of mixed function oxidases on oral administration of dieldrin, *Chem. Biol. Interact.,* 17, 246, 1977.
57. **Antunes-Madeira, M. C. and Madeiru, V. M. C.,** Interaction of insecticides with lipid membranes, *Biochem. Biophys. Acta,* 550, 384, 1979.
58. **Bandyopadhyay, S. K., Tiwari, R. K., Bhattacharyya, A., and Chatterjee, G. C.,** Effect of dieldrin on rat liver plasma membrane enzymes, *Toxicol. Lett.,* 11, 131, 1982.
59. **Curtis, L. R., Williams, W. L., and Mehendale, H. M.,** Potentiation of hepatotoxicity of CCl₄ following pre-exposure to chlordecone (kepone) in the male rat, *Toxicol. Appl. Pharmacol.,* 51, 283, 1973.
60. **Curtis, L. R. and Mehendale, H. M.,** Specificity of chlordecone-induced potentiation of carbon tetrachloride hepatotoxicity, *Drug. Metab. Dispos.,* 8, 23, 1980.
61. **Davis, M. E. and Mehendale, H. M.,** Functional and biochemical correlate of chlorodecone exposure and its enhancement of CCl₄ hepatotoxicity, *Toxicology,* 15, 91, 1980.
62. **Lambardi, B.,** Considerations on the pathogenesis of fatty liver, *Lab. Invest.,* 15, 1, 1966.

63. **Bhatia, S. C. and Subramanian, T. A. V.,** Mechanism of dieldrin induced far accumulation in rat liver, *J. Agric. Food Chem.,* 20, 993, 1972.

64. **Innes, J. R., Ulland, B. M., Valerio, M. G., Petrucelli, L., Fishbein, L., Hart, G. R., Pallotta, A. J., Bates, R. R. Falk, H. L., Gart, J. J., Klein, M., Mitchell, I., and Peters, J.,** Bioassay of pesticides and industrial chemicals for tumorigenicity in mice: a preliminary note, *J. Natl. Cancer Inst.,* 42, 1101, 1969.

65. World Health Organization, International Agency for Research on Cancer, Some Organochlorine Pesticides, IARC Monographs on the Evaluation of Carcinogenic risk of Chemicals to Man, International Agency for Research on Cancer, Lyon, 1974.

66. **Walker, A. I. T., Thorpe, E., and Stevenson, D. E.,** The toxicology of dieldrin (HEOD). I. Long-term oral toxicity studies in mice, *Food Cosmet. Toxicol.,* 11, 415, 1973.

67. **Kuwabara, N. and Takayama, S.,** Comparison of histogenesis of liver in mice administered respectively BHC, DDT and 2,7-FAA. *Proc. Jpn. Cancer Assoc.,* 33, 50, 1974.

68. **Reuber, M. D.,** Carcinomas of the liver in Osborne-Mendel rats ingesting methoxychlor, *Life Sci.,* 24, 1367, 1979.

69. **Hayes, W. J. Jr.,** *Pesticides Studied in Man,* Williams and Wilkins, Baltimore, MD, 1982.

Chapter 6

NEUROTOXICITY OF PESTICIDES

T. S. S. Dikshith

TABLE OF CONTENTS

I. INTRODUCTION

The mammalian nervous system is one of the most vulnerable parts of the animal body. The majority of the pesticides that have been in use are neurotoxic, i.e., these chemicals have the ability to attack the nervous system as the primary target. Some of the pesticides, especially the organophosphorus (OP) insecticides are harmful to the nervous system as shown by rapid neurological disturbances.

The mechanism of neurotoxicity is complex. This is because of the fact that neurotoxicity may be the result of several factors, for example, physiological, pharmacological, and biochemical reactions. Furthermore, the pesticides may selectively interfere with basic metabolic processes such as energy metabolism, lipid metabolism, protein synthesis etc.

The neurotoxic chemicals are grouped into six categories depending upon their primary toxic action. Some of the chemicals produce anoxic damage to gray matter, while others inflict damage to myelin leading to encephalopathy. The third category of toxic chemicals damages axons and peripheral nerves. Another group of toxic chemicals causes damage to synaptic junctions of the neuromuscular system. The chemicals of the sixth category produce lesions localized to the central nervous system (CNS).

The following pages discuss different aspects of pesticide-induced neurotoxicity in animals.

II. SYMPTOMS OF NEUROTOXICITY

A. ORGANOCHLORINE COMPOUNDS

Animals poisoned by organochlorine compounds (OC) first become nervous and show hyperexcitation. They show excessive blinking, cold skin, ruffled fur, muscular twitchings, and weakness. The animals subsequently indicate the onset of fine tremors which have been due to muscular fibrillation. In fact, these symptoms are clearly revealed in the heart muscle, the hind legs, and the back of the poisoned animal.

In young animals the tremors appear more rapidly than in the adults. In a similar way, females and animals under starvation exhibit more of the tremors than fully fed animals. Prolonged muscular and body tremors cause weakness and anorexia leading to loss of body weight of animals. The symptoms of pesticide poisoning eventually culminate in paralysis, clonic convulsions, and death.

In the case of humans, the onset of OC poisoning is characterized by parasthesia of the tongue, lips, and parts of the face. In very severe cases, the individual exhibits parasthesia of the extremities as well. The poisoned person subsequently shows symptoms of malaise, headache, vomiting, a sense of apprehension, disturbance of equilibrium, dizziness, and confusion. The individual also shows characteristic clonic and tonic convulsions and reveals dilated pupils reacting normally to light and accommodation. The sensitivity to touch and pain is exaggerated in areas in which the patient feels parasthesia. In severe cases of OC poisoning, death may occur during coma due to respiratory failure.

B. ORGANOPHOSPHORUS COMPOUNDS

The signs and symptoms of organophosphorus (OP) poisoning are categorized under three groups: (1) muscarinic, (2) nicotinic and (3) central nervous system.

The OP compounds pose a serious health hazard to animals and humans. Since these are esters of OP and direct inhibitors of acetylcholinesterase (AChE) the acute and chronic toxicities from these compounds are very severe.

In animals, OP compounds induce signs and symptoms of toxicity which include salivation, lacrimation, dyspnea, tremors, diarrhea, convulsions, and death. Tables 1 and 2 give the manner of OP poisoning in man.

TABLE 1
Manner of Organophosphate Pesticide Exposure and Clinical Symptoms

Level of poisoning	Clinical symptoms
Mild	Weakness, headache, dizziness, diminished vision, salivation, lacrimation, nausea, vomiting, lack of appetite, stomach ache, restlessness, miosis, moderate bronchial spasm, 60% reduction of ChEA, convalescence in 1 to 3 days
Moderate	Abruptly expressed general weakness, headache, visual disturbance, excess salivation, sweating, vomiting, diarrhea, bradycardia, hypertonia, stomach ache, twitching of facial muscles, tremor of hands, head, or other parts of the body, increasing excitement, distrubed gait and feelings of fear
	Miosis nystagmus, pain in the chest, difficult respiration, cyanosis of the mucous membrane, crepitations in the chest, 60 to 90% reduction of ChEA
	Convalescene in 1 to 2 weeks
Severe	Abrupt tremor, generalized convulsions, psychic disturbances, intensive cyanosis of the mucous membrane, edema of the lung, coma, 90 to 100% reduction of ChEA
	Death from respiratory or cardiac failure

The typical signs of OP poisoning in man are mostly secondary effects to AChE inhibition. The symptoms include headache, giddiness, nervousness, blurred vision, weakness, nausea, cramps, diarrhea and discomfort in the chest. In the case of severe poisoning from OPs many more signs are seen: for example, sweating, miosis, tearing salivation, excessive respiratory tract secretion, vomiting, cyanosis, papilledema, and uncontrolled muscle twitches followed by muscular weakness, convulsion, coma, loss of reflexes, and loss of sphincter control. In several cases cardiac arrhythmias, heart block, and cardiac arrest have been reported.[1-3]

III. BIOCHEMICAL CHANGES

Our knowledge of the precise biochemical lesions occurring in the nervous system of animals exposed to pesticides is far from complete. However, reports have shown that DDT causes stimulation of brain serotonin, glutamic acid and γ-aminobutyric acid, and a decrease in ACh level. Studies have shown the release of secondary metabolites such as alanine, lactate, pyruvate, and ammonia from the brain of rat exposed to dieldrin.[4-6] Many of the brain lipids undergo rapid turnover and have an important dynamic function in brain metabolism.[7]

DDT causes significant changes in the brain-lipid metabolism. For example, the brain of monkey treated with acute and chronic doses of DDT showed a significant decline in the level of total lipid, unesterified cholesterol, and phospholipid. The level of spingomyelin showed a significant increase. The lipids associated with the myelin sheath were more resistant to pesticide injury while cholesterol and phospholipid metabolism became affected, which eventually led to impairment of the CNS functioning in the animal.[8]

The OP compounds in acute doses produce signs of poisoning which resemble excessive stimulation of cholinergic nerves. This suggests that the biochemical basis for acute poisoning by OPs is by the inhibition of AChE of nerve tissues. Specific ChE is present in the nervous ganglionic synapses while the nonspecific ChE is present in the plasma and liver. OPs inhibit both specific and nonspecific ChE.

The acetylcholine (ACh) is the chemical transmitter of the nerve impulses. The cytoplasmic nerve ending of the synaptic membrane contains ACh in special vesicles. The ACh is synthesized by the AChE from acetyl-CoA and choline. The ACh contacts cholinergic receptor protein molecules of the postsynaptic membrane and changes its configuration enabling Na and K cations to penetrate. The transfer of the nerve impulse continues. This process is very brief and is followed by hydrolysis of ACh by ChE. The OPs act against

TABLE 2
Involvement of Different Sites in Organophosphate Poisoning

Site of action	Signs and symptoms
	Following Local Exposure
Pupils	Miosis marked, usually maximal (pinpoint), sometimes unequal
Ciliary body	Frontal headache, eye pain on focusing, slight dimness of vision, occasional nausea and vomiting
Conjuctivae	Hyperaemia
Mucous membranes	Rhinorrhea, hyperaemia
Bronchial tree	Tightness in chest, sometimes with prolonged wheezing, expiration suggestive of bronchoconstriction or increased secretion, cough
Sweat glands	Sweating at the site of exposure to the liquid
Striated muscle	Fasciculations at the site of exposure to the liquid
	Following Systemic Absorption
Bronchial tree	Tightness in chest, with prolonged wheezing, expiration suggestive of bronchoconstriction or increased secretion, dyspnea, slight pain in chest, increased bronchial secretion, cough
Gastrointestinal system	Anorexia, nausea, vomiting, abdominal cramps, epigastric and substernal tightness (cardiospasm) with "heartburn" and eructation, diarrhea, tenesmus, involuntary defecation
Sweat glands	Increased sweating
Salivary glands	Increased salivation
Lacrimal glands	Increased lacrimation
Pupils	Slight miosis (occasionally unequal), later marked
Ciliary body	Blurring of vision
Bladder	Frequent or involuntary micturition
Striated muscle	Easy fatigue, mild weakness, muscular twitching, fasciculations, cramps, generalized weakness including msucles of respiration, with dyspnea and cyanosis
Sympathetic glanglia	Pallor, occasional elevation of blood pressure
Central nervous system	Giddiness, tension, anxiety, jitteriness, restlessness, emotional lability, excessive dreaming, insomnia, nightmares, headache, tremor, apathy, withdrawal and depression, bursts of slow waves of elevated voltage in EEG especially on hyperventiliation, drowsiness, difficulty in concentration, slowness of recall, confusion, slurred speech, ataxia generalized weakness, coma with absence of reflexes, Cheyne-Stokes respiratory and circulatory centress with dyspnea, cyanosis and fall in blood pressure
Circulatory system	Bradycardia, decreased cardiac output, cardiac arrest, paralysis of vasomotor center

this hydrolysis. They produce phosphorylation of the esteric binding side of ChE and stop the hydrolysis of ACh at peripheral ganglionic and central endings (synapses) in effector organs and elevate the concentrations in plasma and intestinal fluid.

The inhibition of AChE results in accumulation of endogenous ACh in nerve tissue and effector organs with consequent signs and symptoms that mimic the muscarinic, nictoinic, and central nervous system action of ACh.

In recent years the interaction of lipophilic neurotoxicants like chlordecone and other insecticides with calmodulin, a well-recognized major calcium binding low molecular weight protein, has received greater attention. In fact, chlordecone induces changes in the enzymatic profile of various membranes and receptor activities. For instance, the insecticide triggers the Ca^{2+} ATPase inactivity in the CNS of animals.[9-12] Chlordecone produced a significant reduction in calmodulin levels in brain P_2 fraction. The brain synaptosomal Ca^{2+} ATPase in the insecticide-treated rats showed a 40% reduction which of course, was restored by exogenously supplemented calmodulin.[13]

Pesticides have often caused disturbances in the process of neurotransmissions particularly in the levels of markers such as Na^+, K^+ ATPase, AChE, and monoamine oxidase.

The synthetic pyrethroids exert their neurotoxic effects by acting at multiple targets within the CNS, for instance, through Na^+ channel[14-17] Ca^{2+} flux across membranes by affecting peripheral benzodiazepine receptors.[18,19]

The primary effects of type II pyrethroids are on sodium channels.[20] These compounds also produce disturbances in cholinergic function. For example, the type II pyrethroid-treated animals showed a decrease in acoustic and auditory startle reflexes[21] and compounds like cismethrin and deltamethrin lowered the cerebral and cerebellar acetylcholine in rats.[22]

IV. ELECTROPHYSIOLOGICAL CHANGES

In recent years electrophysiological techniques have been used extensively to detect the neurological disorders caused by several toxic chemicals. The nerve conduction within the axon takes place by means of a series of changes in the membrane electric potential. It is now known that the internal concentration of potassium ions is far more than the external concentration and the internal concentration of sodium ions in comparison to the outside concentration is much lower. The potential could be triggered by these variations in the ion concentrations across the membrane.[23] For instance, the giant axon of squid poisoned by DDT ($1 \times 10^{-4}M$ added internally) is different from the untreated axon with regard to speed of sodium inactivation.[24]

The electrophysiological assessment of peripheral nerves after treatment with OP compounds has primarily been studied in the cat,[25,26] rat,[27-29] and hen.[30] The studies were largely on measurements of conduction velocity which remained unchanged following exposure to OP compounds. Robertson et al.[31] measured electrophysiological and functional activities, particularly the relative refractory period and sensory afferent activity in hen exposed to OP compounds. In fact, the study included observations of birds for the onset conduction velocity, peak conduction velocity, action potential duration, and action potential amplitude.

The OPs caused pronounced changes in hen in two electrophysiological parameters; for example, the relative refractory period and the strength duration curve. It has been shown that the sciatic nereves become more refractory indicating that their ability to carry high frequency impulses get affected.

TOCP-treated hen displayed a significant action potential disruption in both the tibial and sciatic nerves. A decreased onset conduction velocity in the sciatic nerve and increased action potential duration in the tibial nerve was very evident.[31]

Since most OPs exert a generalized cholinergic action by inhibiting central and peripheral ChEs, there is a need to find a physiological monitor. Systemic electromyographic and neurological investigation offers valuable parameter to identify the adverse health effects due to OPs. For instance, the electromyographic response to nerve stimulation provides a sensitive, objective, and speedy method for detecting impairment of nerve and muscle functions in pesticide-poisoned workers.[32] Drenth et al.[33] found an abnormal electromyogram pattern in about 40% of 102 crop workers. In fact, these workers showed repetitive electromyogram activity in response to single stimuli, low electromyogram voltage, and also a decline in electromyogram voltage after maximal voluntary activity.

Acute poisoning from OPs has caused signs of paralysis in humans. For example, Wadia et al.[34] observed type I (bilateral pyramidal tract signs responding to atropine) and type II (proximal limb weakness and reflexa and cranial nerve palsies) in pesticide poisoned workers.

V. MORPHOLOGICAL CHANGES

Prolonged treatment of animals with pesticides induced morphological changes in the nervous system. For example, phosphamidon, quinalphos, and HCH cause degenerative

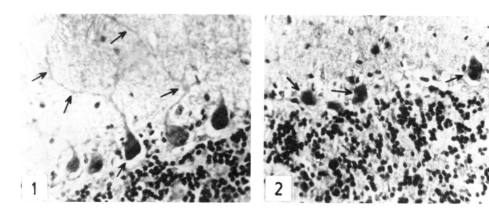

FIGURE 1.   Section of the cerebellum of normal rabbit showing intact Purkinje cells (pyriform cell) with cell body and extended dendrites projecting into the molecular layer of cortex (arrows). (Hematoxylin eosin, magnification × ca. 280.) FIGURE 2.   Section of the cerebellum of rabbit treated with technical hexachlorocyclohexane showing degenerated Purkinje cells; note damaged cell body and loss of dendrites (arrows). (Hematoxylin eosin, magnification × ca. 280.)

changes in the cerebellum of experimental animals. The Purkinje cells which constitute the boundary line between the granular layer and molecular layer underwent degeneration and resulted as deciduomatous bodies.[35-37] (Figures 1 to 4). Earlier studies have shown that chronic exposure of dogs to DDT produces changes in the anterior horn cells, and loss of Purkinje cells in the cerebellum. Changes were also seen in the neurons and in the dentate nucleus.[38]

Fenitrothion-treated white leghorn hen showed characteristic central, peripheral, and distal axonopathy although the morphological changes in the spinal cord and sciatic nerve were minimum.[39]

Besides specific neuropathological effects, pesticides do produce less well-defined effects. For instance, certain compounds are known to cause optic atrophy which includes papilloedema, and macular pigmentation.[40-43] Rabbits exposed to hexachlorocylohexane and endosulfan showed the fundal changes, which appeared more pronounced at the posterior pole associated with marked pallor of the optic disk, papilloedema, and attentuation of the blood vessels. In fact, the animals showed marked degenerative changes in the retinal tissue with reduction in ganglionic cell population.[44]

In the case of delayed neurotoxicity the initial injury is at the distal ends of both sensory and motor nerves. Studies have shown the changes in the nuclei suggesting that the initial lesions in TOCP poisoning are in the cell body which is due to disruption of the somatic cell.[45-47]

Animals exposed to TOCP show significant morphological changes. For instance, the spinal cord shows absence of organelles, aggregation and disintegration of degenerated mitochondria, neurofilaments, vesicles, and granular material with the increase in the number of synaptic vesicles and swelling.[48]

Electron microscopy of the peripheral nerves of cat and chicken exposed to TOCP showed changes in the axoplasm with aggregation, accumulation, and partial condensation of neurofilaments and neurotubules.[49,50]

VI. BEHAVIORAL CHANGES

Behavior in an animal is the outward exression of the net interaction between the sensory, motor arousal, and integrative components of the central and peripheral nervous system. Obviously, the behavioral changes, more precisely the disturbances, following the exposure

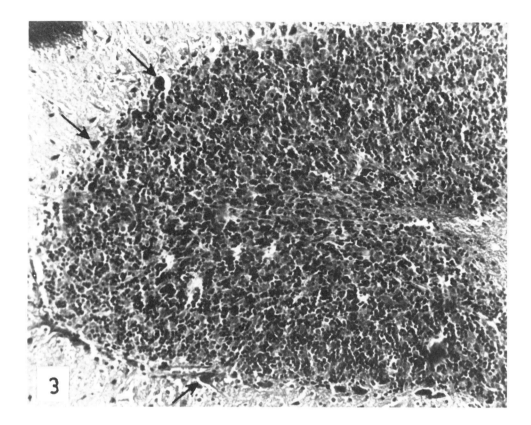

FIGURE 3.

FIGURES 3 & 4.   Sections of cerebellum of rabbit treated with phosphanidon showing damaged and distorted Purkinje cells. (Hematoxylin eosin, magnification × ca. 168.)

to pesticides are valuable indicators of neurotoxicity. Therefore, careful observation of the appearances of behavioral disturbances in the animals and humans exposed to pesticides is one of the most important methods for the early detection of neurotoxicity. In fact, the use of behavioral tests in routine toxicological study of pesticides has obvious advantages.

Pesticides cause behavioral changes such as disturbances of sensory and equilibrium functions. These changes, however, are reversible after the cessation of exposure to the toxicant.

The disturbances include several visual impairment in the poisoned animal or man, for example, fatigue, apathy, and drowsiness. The cognitive disturbances are decreased vigilance and attentional deficit; slowing of information processing, thinking, and calculation; psychomotor retardation; forgetfulness; and memory impairment. The patient also indicates language defects, like slowed speech, slurring, and intermittant pauses.

In certain specific cases, pesticides have caused mental derangement mostly during the course of recovery. For example, parathion, trichlorofon, dichlorvos, fenithioate, and dimethoate have produced delirium, combativeness, depression, and hallucinations in patients.[51]

Pyrethroids also cause significant behavioral changes in animals. For instance, the enhanced ambulation, number of rearings, stereotypic behavior, hyperactivity, aggression, and minimization of resting time to are perhaps some of the components of the motor function. These are related to the deranged functional activities particularly of GABA-nergic catecholinergic, and cholinergic activities of the nervous system.[52-54]

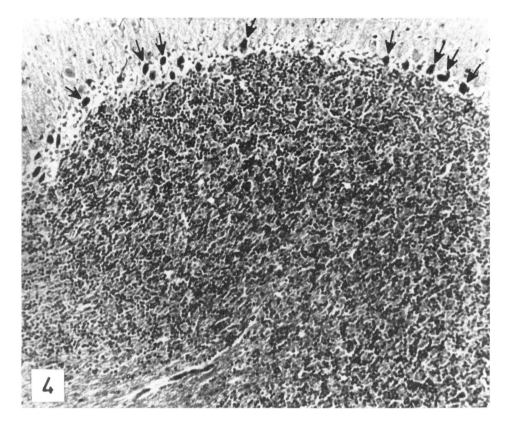

FIGURE 4.

VII. DELAYED NEUROTOXICITY

Some of the OP compounds produce persistent effects of delayed neurotoxic effects. For instance, compounds like triorthocresyl phosphate (TOCP), leptophos, and mitofox produce delayed neurotoxicity in animals and humans. In man, the delayed neurotoxicity results in a flacid paresis. This develops distally in the legs and spreads to the hand and thighs with a sensation of burning and tingling in the legs. In advanced stages, symptoms of spinal cord injury such as spasticity and ataxia become evident as the symptoms of peripheral neuropathy decline.

The latent period for delayed neurotoxicity after an acute exposure and before the onset of clinical signs normally ranges between 6 to 14 days. The pathomorphological lesions are characterized by the degeneration of the axons with subsequent secondary degeneration of myelin. The cellular damage is seen in the sciatic, peroneal, and tibial nerves, spinal cord and medulla, but not in the higher brain.

Age of animals has shown considerable preference for the development of delayed neurotoxicity; and humans are more sensitive than animals to pesticide-induced delayed neurotoxicity. More details on this aspect may be found in the reviews of Aldridge,[52] Johnson,[53] Lotti,[54,55] and Abou-Donia.[56]

In conclusion it may be stated that the nervous system is particularly vulnerable to attack by pesticides such as OCs, OPs, carbamates and organomercurial compounds. The OPs provoke neurological disturbances in animals and cause deleterious effects. In fact, certain OPs like TOCP and leptophos inhibit ChE activity and disturb nerve function and transmission profile in the poisoned animal. Some of the OPs have also been implicated in the production of delayed neurotoxicity in animals and humans. The appearance of delayed neuropathy, however, is distinguished from the action on ChE by the marked species dependency, relative insensitivity of young animals, delay in development of the lesion, and specificity of the kind of neurologic disorder. Interestingly, not all OPs have been shown to cause neuropathies in animals. It has been shown that phosphorylation of more than 80% of the neurotoxic protein by the neurotoxic OPs has been responsible for the appearance of clincial neuropathy in animals.

Diagnosis of the pesticide-induced intoxications, though difficult in mild cases, can be made out in severe cases. For example, miosis, nausea, vomiting, giddiness etc. need careful evaluation and proper follow-up remedial treatment of the patient. The subjective symptoms should be coupled with electrophysiological and behavioral studies to correctly identify the nature of poisoning. In fact, hyporeflexia has been considered as a sensitive indicator of neurotoxicity in chronic exposure to OPs. Further understanding of various facets of neuro-toxicity of pesticides is of great relevance for proper management of pesticides.

REFERENCES

1. **Chhabra, M. L., Sepaha, G. C., Jain, S. R., Bhagwat, R. R., and Khandekar, J. D.,** E.C.G. and necropsy changes in organophosphorous compound (malathion) poisoning, *Indian, J. Med. Sci.,* 2, 424, 1970.
2. **Singh, S., Balkrishan, Singh, S., and Malhotra, V.,** Parathion poisoning in Punjab. A clinical and electrocardiographic study of 20 cases, *J. Assoc. Physicians* India, 17, 181, 1969.
3. **Khandekar, J. D.,** Organophosphate poisoning, *JAMA,* 217, 1864, 1971.
4. **Peters, D. A., Hrdina, P. D., Singhal, R. L., and Lung, G. M.,** The role of brain serotonin in DDT induced hyperpyrexia, *J. Neurochem.,* 19, 1131, 1972.
5. **Hrdina, P. D., Singhal, R. L., Peters, D. A., and Lung, G. M.,** Role of brain acetylcholine and dopamine in acute neurotoxic effects of DDT, *Eur. J. Pharmacol.,* 15, 379, 1971.
6. **Hathway, D. W., Mallinson, A., and Atkintonva, D. A. A.,** Effects of dieldrin, picrotoxin and telodrin on the metabolism of ammonia in brain, *Biochem. J.,* 94, 676, 1965.
7. **Davison, A. N.,** Lipids and brain development, *UCLA Forum Med. Sci.,* 14, 365, 1971.
8. **Sanyal, S., Agarwal, N., and Subrahmanyam, D.,** Effect of acute sublethal and chronic administration of DDT (chlorophenotane) on brain lipid metabolism of Rhesus monkeys, *Toxicol. Lett.,* 34, 47, 1986.
9. **Desiah, D., Gilliland, T., Ho, I. K., and Mahendale, H. M.,** Inhibition of mouse brain synaptosomal ATPase and ouabain binding by chlordecone, *Toxicol. Lett.,* 6, 275, 1980.
10. **Mishra, S. K., Koury, M., and Desaiah, D.,** Inhibition of calcium ATPase activity in rat brain and muscle by chlordecone, *Bull. Environ. Contam. Toxicol.,* 25, 262, 1980.
11. **Desaiah, D.,** Interaction of chlordecone with biological membranes, *J. Toxicol. Environ. Health,* 8, 719, 1981.
12. **Desaiah, D.,** Biochemical mechanisms of chlordecone neurotoxicity. A review, *Neurotoxicology,* 3, 103, 1982.
13. **Desaiah, D., Chetty, C. S., and Prasad Rao, K. S.,** Chlordecone inhibition of calmodulin activation calcium ATPase in rat brain synaptosomes, *J. Toxicol. Environ. Health,* 16, 189, 1985.
14. **Gray, A J. and Soderlund, D. M.,** Mammalian toxicology of pyrethroids, in *Insecticides,* Hutson, D. H. and Roberts, T. R., Eds., John Wiley & Sons, New York, 1985, 193.
15. **Vijverberg, H. P. M. and Vanden Bercken, J.,** Action of pyrethroid insecticide on the vertebrate nervous system, *Neuropathol. Appl. Neurobiol.,* 8, 421, 1982.
16. **Vijverberg, H. P. M., Vander Zalm, J. M., Van Kleef, R. D. M., and Vanden Bercker, J.,** Temperature and structure dependent interaction of pyrethroids with the sodium channels in the frog node of Ranvier, *Biochim. Biophys. Acta,* 728, 73, 1983.
17. **Lond, A. E. and Narahasti, T.,** Kimetics of sodium channel modifications as the basis for the variation in nerve membrane. Effects of pyrethroids and DDT analogs, *Pestic. Biochem. Physiol.,* 20, 203, 1983.
18. **Ramadan, A. A., Bakry, M. N., Abdel-Salam, M. M., Elderfraur, A. T., and Elderfraur, M. E.,** Action of pyrethroids on K^+ stimulated calcium uptake by and (3H) Nimodipine binding to rat brain synaptosomes, *Pestic. Biochem. Physiol.,* 32, 114, 1988.

19. **Ramadan, A. A., Bakry, M. N., Abdel-Salam, M. M., Elderfraur, A.T., and Alderfraur, M. E.,** Action of pyrethroids on the peripheral pine receptor, *Pestic. Biochem. Physiol.,* 32, 106, 1988.

20. **Ghiasuddin, S. M. and Soderlund, D. M.,** Pyrethroid insecticides: potent, stereospecific enhancers of mouse brain sodium channel activation, *Pestic. Biochem. Physiol.,* 29, 1985.

21. **Hijzen, T. H. and Slangen, J. L.,** Effects of type I and type II pyrethroids on the startle response in the rats, *Toxicol. Lett.,* 40, 141, 1988.

22. **Aldridge, W. N., Clothiet, B., Forshaw, P., Johnson, M. K., Parker, V. H., Price, R. J., Skilleter, D. N., Verschoyle, R. D., and Stevens, G.,** The effect of DDT and the pyrethroids cismethrin and deltamethrin on the acetylcholines and cyclic nucleotide content of rat brain, *Biochem. Pharmacol.,* 27, 1703, 1978.

23. **Narahashi, T. and Haas, H. G.,** Interaction of DDT with components of lobster nerve membrane conductance, *J. Gen. Physiol.,* 51, 177, 1968.

24. **Lund, A. E. and Narahashi, T.,** Mode of action of chlorinated hydrocarbon pesticides on the nervous systems, *Neuroscience,* 6, 2253, 1981.

25. **Baker, T. and Lowndes, H. E.,** Muscle spindle function in organophosphorus neuropathy, *Brain Res.,* 18, 577, 1980.

26. **Baker, T., Lowndes, H. E., Johnson, M. K., and Sanborg, I. C.,** The effects of phenyl methanesulfonyl fluoride on delayed organophosphorus neuropathy, *Arch. Toxicol.,* 46, 305, 1980.

27. **Anderson, R. J. and Dunham, C. B.,** Electrophysiologic changes in peripheral nerve following repeated exposure to organophosphorous agents, *Arch. Toxicol.,* 58, 97, 1985.

28. **Anderson, R. J.,** Relative refractory period as a measure of peripheral nerve neurotoxicity, *Toxicol. Appl. Pharmacol.,* 71, 391, 1983.

29. **Averbook, B. J. and Anderson, R. J.,** Electrophysiologic changes associated with chronic administration of organophosphates, *Arch. Toxicol.,* 52, 167, 1983.

30. **Durham, H. D. and Ecobichon, D. J.,** The function of motor nerves innervating slow tonic skeletal muscle in hens with delayed neuropathy induced by tri-o-toyl phosphate, *Can. J. Physiol. Pharmacol.,* 62, 1268, 1984.

31. **Robertson, D. G., Schwab, B. W., Gills, R. T., Richardson, R. J., and Anderson, R. J.,** Electrophysiologic changes following treatment with organophosphorus induced delayed neuropathy-producing agents in the adult hen, *Toxicol. Appl. Pharmacol.,* 87, 420, 1987.

32. **Jager, K. W., Roberts, D. V., and Wilson, A.,** Neuromuscular function in pesticide workers, *Br. J. Ind. Med.,* 27, 273, 1978.

33. **Drenth, H. W., Ensberg, I. E. G., Roberts, D. V., and Wilson, A.,** Neuromuscular function in agricultural workers using pesticides, *Arch. Environ. Health,* 25, 395, 1972.

34. **Wadia, R. S., Sadagopan, C., Amin, R. B., and Sardesai, H. V.,** Neurological manifestations of organophosphorus pesticide poisoning, *J. Neurol. Neurosurg. Psychiatry,* 37, 891, 1974.

35. **Dikshith, T. S. S., Raizada, R. B., and Datta, K. K.,** Interaction of phosphamidon and benzene in female rabbits, *Indian J. Exp. Biol.,* 18, 1273, 1980.

36. **Berge, G. N., Nafstad, I., and Fonnum, F.,** Prenatal effects of trichlorfon on the guinea pig brain, *Arch. Toxicol.,* 59, 30, 1986.

37. **Dikshith, T. S. S., Raizada, R. B., Srivastava, M. K., Kumar, S. N., Kaushal, R. A., Singh, R. P., Gupta, K. P., and Sreelakshmi, K.,** Dermal toxicity of hexachlorocyclohexane (HCH) in rabbit, *Indian J. Exp. Biol.,* 27, 252, 1989.

38. **Haymaker, W., Ginzter, A. M., and Ferguson, R. L.,** The toxic effects of prolonged ingestion of DDT on dogs with special reference to lesions in the brain, *Am. J. Med. Sci.,* 212, 423, 1946.

39. **Durham, H. D. and Ecobichon, D. J.,** As assessment of the neurotoxic potential of fenitrothion in the hen, *Toxicology,* 41, 319, 1986.

40. **Sanborn, G. E., Selhorst, J. B., Calabrese, V. P., and Taylor, J. R.,** Pseudotumor cerebri and insecticide intoxication, *Neurology,* 29, 1222, 1979.

41. **Imai, H., Miyata, M., Uga, S., and Ishikawa, S.,** Retinal degeneration in rats exposed to an organophosphate pesticide (fenthion), *Environ. Res.,* 30, 453, 1983.

42. **Misra, U. K., Nag, D., Misra, N. K., and Krishna Murti, C. R.,** Macular degeneration associated with chronic pesticide exposure, *Lancet,* 1, 288, 1982.

43. **Misra, U. K., Nag, D., Misra, N. K., Mehra, M. K., and Ray, P. K.,** Some observations on the macula of pesticide workers, *Human Toxicol.,* 4, 135, 1985.

44. **Ahmed, M. M. and Gless, P.,** Neurotoxicity of tricresylphosphate (TCP) in slow Loris *(Nycticebus coucang coucang), Acta Neuropathol.,* 19, 94, 1971.

45. **Prineas, J.,** Triorthocresyl phosphate myopathy, *Arch. Neurol.,* 21, 150, 1969.

46. **Bischoff, A.,** The ultrastructure of tri-ortho-cresyl phosphate poisoning. I. Studies on myelin and axonal alterations in the sciatic nerve, *Acta Neuropathol.,* 9, 158, 1967.

47. **Abou-Donia, M. B. and Preissig, S. H.,** Delayed neurotoxicity of leptophos: toxic effects in the nervous system of hens, *Toxicol. Appl. Pharmacol.,* 35, 269, 1976.

48. **Prineas, J.,** The pathogenesis of dying-back polyneuropathies. An ultrastructural study of experimental TOCP intoxication in the cat, *J. Neuropathol. Exp. Neurol.,* 28, 571, 1969.
49. **Levay, S., Meier, C., and Glees, P.,** Effects of tri-ortho-cresyl phosphate on spinal ganglia and peripheral nerve of chicken, *Acta Neuropathol.,* 17, 103, 1971.
50. **Bischoff, A.,** Ultrastructure of tri-ortho-cresyl phosphate poisoning. II. Studies on spinal cord alterations, *Acta Neuropathol.,* 15, 142, 1970.
51. **Hayes, W. J., Jr.,** *Pesticide Studied in Man,* Williams and Wilkins, Baltimore, MD, 1982, 302.
52. **Aldridge, W. N. and Johnson, M. K.,** Side effects of organophosphorous compounds: delayed neurotoxicity, *Bull. World Hlth. Org.,* 44, 259, 1971.
53. **Johnson, M. K. and Lotti, M.,** Delayed neurotoxicity caused by chronic feeding of organophosphates requires a high point of inhibition of neurotoxic esterase, *Toxicol. Lett.,* 5, 99, 1980.
54. **Lotti, M. and Johnson, M. K.,** Neurotoxicity of organophosphorous pesticides: predictions can be based on *in vitro* studies with hen and human enzymes, *Arch. Toxicol.,* 41, 215, 1978.
55. **Lotti, M. and Johnson, M. K.,** Repeated small doses of a neurotoxic organophosphate. Monitoring of neurotoxic esterase in brain and spinal cord, *Arch. Toxicol.,* 45, 263, 1980.
56. **Abou-Donia, M. B.,** Organophosphorous ester-induced delayed neurotoxicity, *Annu. Rev. Pharmacol. Toxicol.,* 21, 511, 1981.

Chapter 7

EFFECTS OF PESTICIDES ON THE ENDOCRINE SYSTEM

T. S. S. Dikshith and R. B. Raizada

TABLE OF CONTENTS

I. INTRODUCTION

The endocrine system of animals consists of several important secretory glands. The glands through hormonal secretions maintain physiological balance and homeostasis and regulate body functions (Figure 1).

The endocrine system is very sensitive and highly susceptible to the toxic effects of pesticides, which are now known to disturb the regulatory function of the hormones.[1-4] Pesticides have produced changes in gonads, thyroids, and adrenals of animals. This review deals with the effects of different pesticides on the endocrine system of animals.

II. SECRETORY GLANDS

A. GONAD

The effects of pesticides on the gonadal system of animals are diverse. For example, the organochlorine insecticides (OCs) have produced estrogenic effects in rats. Administration of DDT, methoxychlor, aldrin, dieldrin, chlordecone, and lindane has produced uterotropic response and other estrogenic effects in experimental animals.[5-12]

Recent study has confirmed that chlordecone induces identical cellular and morphological changes like that of estradiol in the development of uterine and vaginal histology of mouse.[2] Administration of chlordecone or estradiol to immature chick also produces an increase in oviduct ovalbumin and canalbumin synthesis. In fact, in the avian and mammalian species chlordecone mimics the estrogenic and progesterone-like action.[13] Administration of low doses of chlordecone to weanling rats causes changes in uterine growth, precocious vaginal opening, persistent vaginal estrous, and anovulation. However, chlordecone produced no alteration in the pituitary level of the enkephaline system in experimental rats.[14,15] Chlordecone has induced abnormalities in sperm counts, morphology, and sperm mortality besides a decline in the rhythm of spermatogenesis in animals.[16]

As stated earlier, pesticides induce male sterility in animals. This has been found to be through the covalent binding of the highly reactive metabolites to the macromolecules associated with androgen activity. For instance, o,p′-DDT inhibits the binding of 5-dihydrotestosterone to specific receptor proteins in rat prostate cytosol.[17,18] In fact, multiple administration of o,p′-DDT to castrated male quail stimulated the growth of the proctodeal (foam) gland.[19] An earlier report has shown that DDT analogs cause a decrease in testicular androgen as a result of enhanced metabolism of endogenous androgens by the monooxygenase system.[20] o,p′-DDT causes alterations in the levels of testosterone, dihydrotestosterone, and androstenediol formation indicating decreased androgen biosynthesis, plasma estradiol level, and β-hydroxylase activity in rats.[21,22] Prolonged treatment of DDT has produced disturbances in spermatogenesis in rams.[23]

Disturbances in the estrogen secretion induce immunological changes. Several pesticides have produced estrogen-induced immune alterations, for instance, DDT and chlordecone did cause a decline in the antibody production as well as thymic atrophy in animals.[24-26]

Methoxychlor has reduced the reproductive performance of animals, besides producing a precocious vaginal opening in immature female rat pups. In the immature male rat, the insecticide delayed the age of preputial separation. In the adult rat, methoxychlor produced a decline in testis weight, arrest of spermatogenesis, and atrophy of ventral prostate and seminal vesicle.[27,28] It has been indicated that the reproductive effects produced by methoxychlor are mediated through the elevation of prolactin concentration and the release of which in turn influences the gonadotropic releasing hormone (GnRH) in hypothalamus.[29]

Fenaimol, a pyrimidine carbinol fungicide has been reported to block the perinatal development of male patterns of sexual behavior in association with the gonadal steroids.[30]

Dibromochloropropane (DBCP) is a known potent fumigant. Reports have shown DBCP

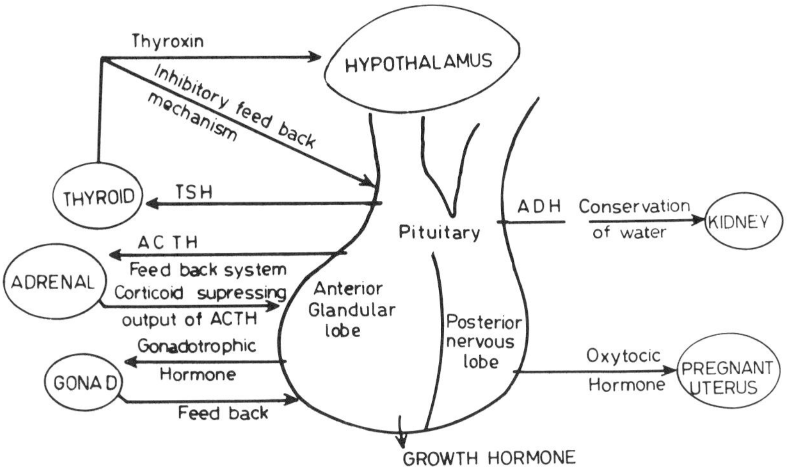

FIGURE 1. Interrelationship of hormonal function in animals.

produces testicular atrophy, decreased fertility, and a decline in sperm count.[31,32] It also causes a high rate of pregnancy wastage.[33,34] Workers exposed to DBCP have shown oligospermy and a fall in the level of testosterone.[35] DBCP has been found to interfere in spermatogenesis by disturbing the rhythm of stem cell pool and normal development and maturation of spermatogonia.[36]

Acephate has produced significant reduction in the level of plasma LH in white-footed mouse. A report has shown that several organophosphorus compounds do disturb the estrus cycle and also the gestation in animals.[37] Benomyl, besides producing gonadal changes also induces a change during prepubertal and postpubertal stages of reproduction through interference in the FSH activity in animals.[38]

B. THYROID

The thyroid gland in mammals is composed of two embryologically and functionally distinct populations of cells concerned with the biosynthesis of two types of hormones — the follicular cells secrete the iodothyronines while parafollicular cells (c-cells) produce calcitonin.[39] The thyroid hormones are necessary for growth, development, and normal body metabolism.[40] The thyroid gland is one of the most reactive organs to environmental insults.[41] For instance, in male rats DDT produces changes in the weight, morphology, and function of thyroid.[42] In fact, DDT and lindane have altered the iodine and hormone metabolism in rat. This is evidenced by the increase in thyroid mass, thyroxin, and triodothyronin level.[43]

Mirex, monohydromirex, and photomirex have also produced morphological changes in the thyroid gland of animals.[44,45]

Dithiocarbamates, a group of fungicides, undergo metabolism in the body and produce ethylene thiourea (ETU), a known potent toxicant and carcinogen.[46] ETU has been found to be responsible for the induction of certain antithyroid effects by interfering in the conversion of inorganic iodide to organic iodide in the thyroid gland.[47] In fact, similarities have been found between the molecular structure of ETU and thioamide (the known antithyroid drug).

Several dithiocarbamates have caused an antithyroid effect in animals.[48] For example, high doses of zineb produced formation of microfollicles lined with laminar cells and reduction in PAS-positive granules. An increase was also seen in the number of basophilic cells with PAS positive granules in the adenohypophysis besides significant increase (about 80%) in the radiolabeled iodine uptake in the animals.[49] Maneb, another dithiocarbamate fungicide, has produced a decline in the level of thyroglobulin in rats.[50] In male rats, for instance, a dose of zineb (1000 mg/kg/day for 30 days), increased the weight and cellularity of the thyroid, increased the weight of the pituitary, and led to seminal tubular necrosis and giant cell formation without change in the weight of the testes. The study has shown that zineb blocks the conversion of iodide to iodine.[51] Daily administration of ziram produces alterations in the iodine uptake, protein bound iodine, and histology of the thyroid gland of rat.[52]

C. ADRENAL

The adrenal cortex is the most vulnerable of the endocrine glands to chemical-induced injury.[53] However, our knowledge on the physiological regulation of adrenal cortex due to exposure of chemicals, particularly to pesticides is very inadequate. Colby and Eacho[54] have reviewed the chemical-induced adrenal injury and the role of metabolic activation. As a result of multifacet function of adrenal, there are a number of potential sites at which chemicals can interfere with adrenal homeostasis. DDT and its metabolites have been extensively studied for their possible adverse effect on the adrenal system in dogs.

HCH has produced significant hypertrophy of the adrenal with vacuolated cells in the cortex and accumulation of cholesterol-positive lipids in the adrenal cortex suggesting the inhibition of steroidogenic enzymes such as PDH and SDH.[55]

While chlordecone has shown both biochemical and ultrastructure changes in adrenal medulla of rats its nonketo analog, mirex produced a morphological effect on epinephrine or norepinephrine granules.[56]

The results show that concentrations of toxaphene of about 11.7 μg/ml added to adrenal cell *in vitro* decreased the ACTH-stimulated corticosterose synthesis by about 50%. Long-term pretreatment of rats with 1.2 ppm toxaphene in diet produced a significant inhibition of corticosteroid synthesis as compared to control rats indicating that toxaphene interferes with the ACTH-stimulated corticosterone synthesis in rat adrenal cortex *in vivo*.[57]

III. CONCLUSION

Structurally diverse compounds such as pesticides have produced physiological and biochemical changes in the endocrine system of animals; the pesticides in certain cases have mimicked the classical estrogens such as estradiol. Clear evidence is seen with o,p'-DDT and methoxychlor.

The infertility and reproductive effects produced by several pesticides in themselves are aspects of greater study. The role of several gonadotropic hormones, the biological processes of spermatogenesis, and the drastic effect of pesticides on this vulnerable system have added a new dimension to our understanding of the endocrine effects of pesticides. The fate of adrenals and thyroids to the toxic effects of pesticides needs to be known in greater detail if we are to fully delineate the action of pesticides vis à vis the endocrine system in animals.

REFERENCES

1. **Bitman, J., Cecil, H. C., Harris, S. J., and Feil, V. J.,** Estrogenic activity of o,p'-DDT metabolities and related compounds, *J. Agric. Food Chem.,* 26, 149, 1978.
2. **Eroschenko, V. P.,** Surface changes in oviduct, uterus and vaginal cells of neonatal mice after estradiol-17β and the insecticide chlordecone (kepone) treatment: a scanning electron microscopic study, *Biol. Reprod.,* 26, 707, 1982.
3. **Ousterhout, J. M., Sruck, R. F., and Nelson, J. A.,** Estrogenic activities of methoxychlor metabolites, *Biochem. Pharmacol.,* 30, 2869, 1981.

4. **Stancel, G. M., Ireland, J. S., Mukkum, V. R., and Robison, A. K.,** The estrogenic activity of DDT: *in vivo* and *in vitro* induction of a specific estrogen inducible urine protein by o,p'-DDT, *Life Sci.*, 27, 1111, 1980.

5. **Gellert, R. J.,** Kepone, mirex, dieldrin and aldrin: estrogenic activity and the induction of persistent vaginal estrus and anovulation in rats following neonatal treatment, *Environ Res.*, 16, 131, 1978.

6. **Fry, D. M. and Toone, C. K.,** DDT induced feminization of gull embryos, *Science*, 213, 922, 1981.

7. **Kupfer, D. and Bulger, W. H.,** Estrogenic properties of DDT and its analogs, in *Estrogens in the Environment*, McLachlan, J. A., Ed., Elsvier/North-Holland, New York, 1980, 239.

8. **Ireland, J. S., Mukku, V. R., Robison, A. K., and Stancel, G. M.,** Stimulation of uterine deoxyribonuclic acid synthesis by 1,1,1-trichloro-2,(p-chlorophenyl)-2-(o-chlorophenyl) ethane (o,p'-DDT), *Biochem. Pharmacol.*, 29, 1469, 1980.

9. **Bulger, W. H., Muccitelli, R. M., and Kupfer, D.,** Studies on the *in vivo* and *in vitro* estrogenic activities of methoxychlor and its metabolites. Role of hepatic mono-oxygenase in methoxychlor activation, *Biochem. Pharmacol.*, 24, 2417, 1978.

10. **Raizada, R. B., Misra, P., Saxena, I., Datta, K. K., and Dikshith, T. S. S.,** Weak estrogenic activity of lindane in rats, *J. Toxicol. Environ. Health*, 6, 483, 1980.

11. **Reel, J. R. and Lamb, J. C.,** Reproductive toxicology of chlordecone (kepone), in *Endocrine Toxicology* Thomas, J. A., Korach, K. S., and McLachlan, J. A., Ed., Raven Press, New York, 1985, 357.

12. **Bulger, W. H. and Kupfer, D.,** Estrogenic activity of pesticides and other xenobiotics on the uterus and male reproductive tract, in *Endocrine Toxicology*, Thomas, J. A., Korach, K. S., and McLachlan, J. A., Eds., Raven Press, New York, 1985, 1.

13. **Palmitter, R. D. and Muloihill, E. R.,** Estrogenic activity of the insecticide kepone on the chicken oviduct, *Science*, 201, 356, 1978.

14. **Hammond, B., Katzenellenbogen, B. S., Krauthammer, N., and McConnell, J.,** Estrogenic activity of the insecticide chlordecone (kepone) and interaction with uterine estrogen receptors, *Proc. Natl. Acad. Sci. USA*, 76, 6641, 1979.

15. **Hudson, P. M., Yoshikawa, J. K., Ali, S. F., Lamb, J. C., Reel, J. R., and Hong, J. S.,** Estrogen like activity of chlordecone (kepone) on the hypothalmo-pituitary axis, effect on pituitary enkaphalian system, *Toxicol. Appl. Pharmacol.*, 74, 383, 1984.

16. **Taylor, J. R., Sclhorst, J. B., Houff, S. A., and Matinez, A. J.,** Chlordecone intoxication in man. I. Clinical observations, *Neurology*, 28, 626, 1978.

17. **Thomas, J. A.,** Effect of pesticides on reproduction, in *Advances in Sex Hormones Research*, Vol. 1, Thomas J. A. and Singhal, R. L., Eds., University Press, Baltimore, 1975, 205.

18. **Schein, L. G., Donovan, M. P., Thomas, J. A. and Felicel, P. R.,** Effects of pesticides on ³H-dihydrotestosterone binding to cytosol proteins from various tissues of the mouse, *J. Environ. Pathol. Toxicol.*, 3, 461, 1980.

19. **Adkins-Regan, E. and Hurvitz, E. D.,** o,p'-DDT causes growth of an androgen dependent gland in *Coturnix* quail, *Experientia*, 38, 1082, 1982.

20. **Kupfer, D.,** Effects of pesticides and related compounds on steroid metabolism and function, *Crit. Rev. Toxicol.*, 4, 83, 1975.

21. **Gobbett, A.,** Endocrine modifications produced by o,p'-DDT in male adult rat, *Pestic. Biochem. Physiol.*, 14, 139, 1980.

22. **Krause, W.,** Influence of DDT, DDVP and malathion on FSH, LH testosterone serum levels and testosterone concentration in testes, *Bull. Environ. Contam. Toxicol.*, 18, 231, 1977.

23. **Biswas, R. K., Rao, A. R., and Rao, V. S. N.,** Effect of feeding DDT on semen characteristics of rams, *Indian Vet. J.*, 58, 665, 1981.

24. **Glick, B.,** Antibody-mediated immunity in the presence of mirex and DDT, *Poultry Sci.*, 53, 1476, 1974.

25. **Strect, J. C. and Sharma, R. P.,** Alteration of induced cellular and humoral immune responses by pesticides and chemicals of environmental concern: quantitative studies of immunosuppression by DDT, Arochlor 1254, carbaryl, carbofuran and methylparathion, *Toxicol. Appl. Pharmacol.*, 32, 587, 1975.

26. **Wiltrout, R. W., Ercegovich, C. D., and Ceglowski, D. S.,** Humoral immunity in mice following oral administration of selected pesticides, *Bull. Environ. Contam. Toxicol.*, 20, 423, 1978.

27. **Ball, H.,** Effect of methoxychlor on reproductive systems of the rat, *Proc. Soc. Exp. Biol. Med.*, 176, 187, 1984.

28. **Gray, L. E. Jr., Ferrell, J., Ostby, J., and Gray, K.,** A Preliminary Protocol to Assess Alterations in Reproductive Development in Rats and Hamsters: A Model for Screening Chemicals for Reproductive Effects, presented at U.S. EPA/U.S. Army Workshop to Evaluate a Protocol for Reproductive Assessment, Charleston, SC, November 1985.

29. **Goldman, J. M., Cooper, R. L., Rehnberg, C. L., Hein, J. F., McElroy, W. K. and Gray, L. E., Jr.,** Effects of low subchronic doses of methoxychlor on the rat hypothalmic pituitary reproductive axis, *Toxicol. Appl. Pharmacol.*, 86, 774, 1986.

30. **Hirsch, K. S., Adams, E. R., Hoffman, D. G., Markham, J. K., and Owen, N. V.,** Studies to elucidate the mechanism of fenaimol induced infertility in male rat, *Toxicol. Appl. Pharmacol.,* 86, 391, 1986.

31. **Barlow, S. M. and Sullivan, F. M.,** *Reproductive Hazards of Industrial Chemicals,* Academic Press, New York, 1982.

32. **Kluwe, W. M., Gupta B. N., and Lamb, J. C.,** The comparative effects of 1,2-dibromo-3-chloropropane (DBCP) and its metabolites, 3-chloro-1,2-propaneoxide (epichlorohydrin), 3-chloro-1,2-propanediol (alphachlorohydrin) and oxalic acid on the urinogenital system of male rats, *Toxicol. Appl. Pharmacol.,* 70, 67, 1983.

33. **Kharrazi, M., Potashnik, G., and Goldsmith, J. R.,** Reproductive effects of dibromochloropropane, *Ir. J. Med. Sci.,* 16, 403, 1980.

34. **Lipshultz, L. I., Ross, C. E., Whorton, D., Milby, T., Smith, R., and Joyner, R. E.,** Dibromochloropropane and its effect on testicular function in man, *J. Urol.,* 124, 464, 1980.

35. **Lantz, G. D., Cunningham, G. R., Huckins, C., and Lipshultz, L. I.,** Recovery from severe oligospermia after exposure to dibromo-chloropropane, *Fertil. Steril.,* 35, 46, 1981.

36. **Biava, C. G., Smuckler, E. A., and Whorton, D.,** The testicular morphology of individuals exposed to dibromochloropropane, *Exp. Mol. Pathol.,* 29, 448, 1978.

37. **Rattner, B. A. and Michael, S. D.,** Organophosphorous insecticide induced decrease in plasma luteinizing hormone concentration in white footed mice, *Toxicol. Lett.,* 24, 65, 1985.

38. **Carter, S. D. Hein, J. F., Renberg, G. L., and Laskay, J. W.,** Effect of benomyl on the reproductive development of male rats, *J. Toxicol. Environ. Health,* 13, 53, 1984.

39. **Capen, C. C.,** Chemical injury of thyroid: pathologic and mechanistic considerations, in Toxicology Forum: 1983 Annual Winter Meeting, Bowers Reporting Company, Washington, D.C., 1983.

40. **Netter, F. H.,** Endocrine system and selected metabolic diseases, in *The CIBA Collection of Medical Illustrations,* Vol. 4, Forsham, P. H., Ed., R. R. Donnelley & Sons, New York, 1974.

41. **Simionescu, L., Oprescu, M., Ghinea, E., Ghinea, L., Sahleanu, V., and Dimitriu, V.,** The radioimmunological measurement of thyroglobulin secretion *in vitro* under the influence of some herbicides, *Rev. Roum. Med. Endocrinol.,* 15, 243, 1977.

42. **Goldman, M.,** The effect of a single dose of DDT on thyroid function in male rats, *Arch. Int. Pharmacodyn. Ther.,* 252, 327, 1981.

43. **Seidler, H., Haertia, M., and Engst, R.,** Zur wirking von DDT und lindane auf die schilddruesenfunktion der ratle (on the effect of DDT and lindane on the thyroid function in the rat), *Nahrung,* 20, 399, 1976.

44. **Yarbrough, J. D., Chambers, J. E., Grimley, J. M., Alley, E. G., Fang, M. M., Morrow, J. T., Ward, B. C., and Conroy, J. D.,** Comparative study of 8-monohydromirex and mirex toxicity in male rats, *Toxicol. Appl. Pharmacol.,* 58, 105, 1981.

45. **Singh, A., Bhatnagar, M. K., Villeneuve, D. C., and Valli, V. E. O.,** Ultrastructure of the thyroid glands of rat fed photomirex: a 48 week recovery study, *J. Environ. Pathol. Toxicol. Oncol.,* 6, 115, 1985.

46. **World Health Organisation,** Dithiocarbamate Pesticides, ETU and PTU, A General Introduction, Environmental Health Criteria, WHO, Geneva, 1988, 78.

47. **O'Neil, W. M. and Marshall, W. D.,** Goitrogenic effects of ethylene thiourea (ETU) on rat thyroid, *Pestic. Biol. Chem. Phsyiol.,* 41, 91, 1984.

48. **Ivanova-Chemishanska, L.,** Dithiocarbamates in Toxicology of Pesticides, Interim Document No 9, World Health Organisation, Geneva, 1982, 158.

49. **Studer, H. and Grer, M. A.,** Thyroid function during the rebound phase following the discontinuation of antithyroid drugs, *Endocrinology,* 80, 52, 1967.

50. **Sabotka, T.,** Comparative effects of 60 day feeding of maneb and ethylene thiourea on thyroid electrophoretic pattern of rats, *Food Cosmet. Toxicol.,* 9, 537, 1971.

51. **Raizada, R. B., Datta, K. K., and Dikshith, T. S. S.,** Effect of zineb on male rats, *Bull. Environ. Contam. Toxicol.,* 22, 208, 1979.

52. **Pandey Mamta, Raizada, R. B., and Dikshith, T. S. S.,** 90 day oral toxicity of ziram: a thyrostatic and hepatotoxic study, *Environ. Pollut.,* 65, 1990.

53. **Ribelin, W. E.,** Effects of drugs and chemicals upon the structure of the adrenal gland, *Fundam. Appl. Toxicol.,* 4, 105, 1984.

54. **Colby, H. D. and Eacho, P. I.,** Chemical-induced adrenal injury: role of metabolic activation, in *Endocrine Toxicology,* Thomas, J. A., Korach, K. S., and Mc Lachlan, J. A., Eds., Raven Press, New York, 1985, 35.

55. **Shivanandappa, T., Krishnakumari, M. K., and Majumder, S. K.,** Inhibition of steroidogenic activity in the adrenal cortex of rats fed benzene hexachloride, *Experientia,* 38, 1251, 1982.

56. **Baggett, J. M., Thuresan-Klein, A., and Klein, R. L.,** Effects of chlordecone on the adrenal medulla of the rat, *Toxicol. Appl. Pharmacol.,* 52, 313, 1980.

57. **Mohammed, A., Hallberg, E., Rydstrom, J., and Slanina, P.,** Toxaphene: accumulation in the adrenal cortex and effect of ACTH-stimulated corticosteroid synthesis in the rat, *Toxicol. Lett.,* 24, 137, 1985.

Chapter 8

MUTAGENICITY AND TERATOGENICITY OF PESTICIDES

T. S. S. Dikshith

TABLE OF CONTENTS

I. INTRODUCTION

Man and animals are constantly being exposed to a wide variety of pesticides. Some of the pesticides, because of their alkylating properties and persistence have demonstrated genotoxic effects. These chemicals when released into the environment alter the genome and its normal function. Depending upon the ontogenetic stage of the animal, pesticides have produced teratogenic and embryotoxic effects. This chapter deals with the state of the art regarding the mutagenic and teratogenic potential of pesticides.

II. MUTAGENICITY

The spectrum of genetic effects produced by physicochemical agents in the biological system is called *mutation*. The genetic effects are broadly divided into two major categories: (1) point mutations (gene mutations) and (2) cytologically detectable chromosomal changes.

The point mutations are invisible and occur as microlesions and consist of a single gene mutation involving base pair substitution (addition or deletion) of DNA. It also involves qualitative and quantitative change in one or more nucleotide pairs.

The chromosomal changes, however are visible and cytologically detectable macrolesions involving numerical and structural changes in chromosomes. These changes may be either chromatid type or chromosome type. The changes, again, may be associated with a single chromosome, *intrachanges* or an exchange or parts between different chromosomes, *interchanges*. The types of chromosome aberrations generally seen are acentric fragments, centric and acentric rings, inversions, deletions, and translocations etc. The chromatid type of aberrations include chromatid break and gap. Different kinds of chromosomal aberrations are indicated in brief in Figure 1 and Table 1.

A mutagenic agent depending upon its target may induce either a somatic muation or a germinal mutation. This may eventually result in the formation of neoplastic tissue or terrata in the embryo culminating in the deleterious effects in the progeny.[1]

A battery of tests has been advocated for the identification of mutagenic effects of pesticides and other toxic agents.[2,3] (Table 2).

Our current knowledge regarding mutagenic potential of pesticides is both inadequate and often equivocal. For example, some workers report positive effects of certain pesticides in mouse and syrian hamsters, while others report negative results;[4-7] another example is that of DDT, which in high doses produces chromosomal aberrations in the bone marrow system of mouse.[8,9] In an *in vitro* study with rat kangaroo cell line, p,p'-DDT, DDE, and DDD produced a significant increase in chromosome abnormalities. These were seen as chromatid breaks, terminal deletions, and exchange figures (Figures 2 to 4). A high percent mitotic inhibition was recorded in cultures incubated with DDT. The o,p'-DDT and p,p'-DDT produced about 40 and 35% more inhibition respectively than did the solvent control medium. The DDD and DDE produced similar mitotic indexes of 20 to 25% below the control values. p,p'-DDA caused no mitotic inhibition[10] (Figure 5). Interestingly, there were no chromosomal changes in the Chinese hamster cell line exposed to DDT, DDE, and DDD. In fact, the rate of changes were well within the spontaneous range.[11] In contrast to these, DDE produced significant chromosome changes over those seen in control cell population of Chinese hamster cell line, whereas DDT produced no such changes.[12] Studies have shown that endosulfan, endrin, DDT, and lindane produce mild to severe chromosomal aberrations in rats.[13-15]

Daily gavage of different organochlorine insecticides in low doses (both technical grade and formulations) produced clastogenic effects in the bone marrow system of male rats. The changes included chromatid gaps, chromatid breaks, fragments, and pulverization of chromation material (Table 3). In another screening study, daily oral doses of different organ-

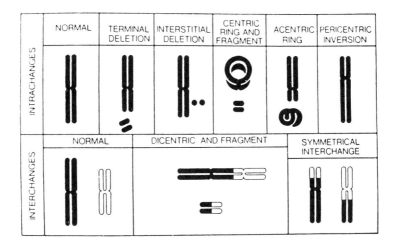

FIGURE 1.   Schematic diagram showing different types of chromosomal aberrations.

TABLE 1
Description of Chromosomal Changes

Gaps	Breaks narrower than the width of a chromatid
Chromatid break	Change seen on only one arm of chromosome
Chromosome break	Change seen on both arms of chromosome at identical sites
Break without fragment	Any chromatid separation that is wider than the arm itself but without identifiable chromatid fragments
Fragment	Any free displaced chromatid pieces seen in association or not with a parent chromatid
Exchange figure	Chromatid interchange involving two or more chromosomes with either symmetrical or asymmetrical distributions of the usual chromatid pattern
Pulverization	Extreme fragmentation of the chromatid material

TABLE 2
Mutagenicity Testing Requirements[2]

1. A test from each of three of the following classes of tests for detecting gene mutations
    A. Bacteria with and without metabolic activation
    B. Eukaryotic microorganisms with and without metabolic activation
    C. Insects (e.g., sex-linked recessive lethal test)
    D. Mammalian somatic cells in culture with and without metabolic activation
    E. Mouse-specific locus test
2. A test from each of three of the following classes of tests for detecting chromosomal aberrations
    A. Cytogenetic tests in mammals *in vivo*
    B. Insect tests for heritable chromosomal effects
    C. Dominant-lethal effects in rodents and heritable translocation tests in rodents
3. A test from each of the following classes of tests for detecting primary DNA damage
    A. DNA repair in bacteria (including differential killing DNA of repair defective strains) with and without metabolic activation
    B. Unscheduled DNA repair synthesis in mammalian somatic cells in culture, with and without metabolic activation
    C. Mitotic recombination and gene conversion in yeast, with and without metabolic activation
    D. Sister-chromatid exchange in mammalian cells in culture with and without metabolic activation

ophosphorus insecticides also produced clastongenic effects in the bone marrow system of male rats. The low doses of pesticides did not register a significant chromosomal change in the animals.[16] (Table 4).

A report of Durham and Williams has shown that pesticides produce chromosomal aberrations in species of animals.[17] Studies of Chen et al.[18] and Tezuka et al.[19] have indicated

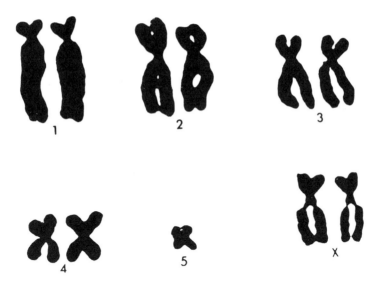

FIGURE 2.   Normal karyotype of rat kangaroo. (From Palmer, K. A. et al., *Toxicol. Appl. Pharmacol.*, 22, 355, 1972. With permission.)

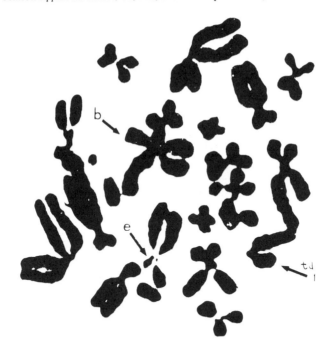

FIGURE 3.   Different types of chromosomal aberrations caused by DDT in the rat kangaroo cell line. Chromatid breaks (b), terminal deletions (d) and exchanges (e). × 1000. (From Palmer, K. A. et al., *Toxicol. Appl. Pharmacol.*, 22, 355, 1972. With permission.)

that malathion produces sister chromatid exchanges in the fibroblast of human embryonic lung and V_{79} hamster cells; parathion also produces chromosomal changes in the germinal cells of male guinea pig.[20] The bone marrow system of several animals has shown weak clastogenic effects produced by a variety of pesticides. For example, malathion produced mild clastogenic effects in mouse;[21] demeton, dichlorvos, and endosulfan produced positive effects in syrian hamsters *in vivo*.[22] The findings made from life-time cancer studies in

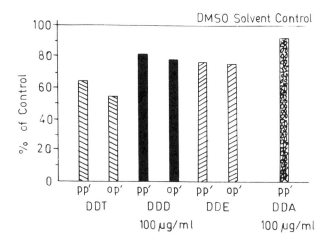

FIGURE 4. Histogram showing mitotic index of DDT compounds with respect to the solvent control. The actual value of the control was 15%. (From Palmer, K. A. et al., *Toxicol. Appl. Pharmacol.*, 22, 355, 1972. With permission.)

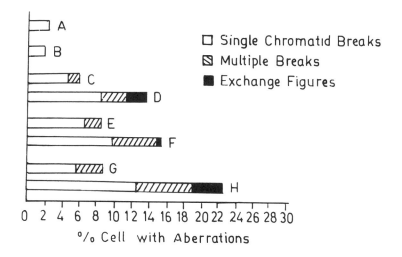

FIGURE 5. Histogram showing frequency of the various chromosomal aberrations observed after treatment with DDT compound. (From Palmer, K. A. et al., *Toxicol. Appl. Pharmacol.*, 22, 355, 1972. With permission.)

rodents show that captan is an active mutagen.[23] The administration of chlorpropham to male rats for 7 days elicited no significant chromosomal changes in the bone marrow cells.[24]

Information, though inadequate, has suggested that certain organophosphorus pesticides do produce chromosomal aberrations in the lymphocytes of severely exposed populations and occupational workers.[25-29]

While much data are needed to arrive at any meaningful conclusion it is very important to adhere to uniform test protocols to avoid contradictory observations. In fact, several animal studies with pesticides vis à vis mutagenicity are essentially not conducted in uniformity and hence demand additional confirmatory studies.

III. TERATOGENICITY

Agents that produce defects of fetal development are called *teratogens*. The complex

TABLE 3

Chromosome Aberrations in Bone Marrow Cells of the Male Rat After Oral Doses of Organochlorine Pesticides[16]

Pesticide	Purity	Dose (mg/kg/d × 5 d)	Percentage aberrations; total metaphase score = 50 metaphases			
			Gap	Chromatid break	Fragment	Pulverization
Control	Peanut oil	0.5 ml	0.4	0.6	—	0.4
Aldrin	98%	2.0 ml	0.8	—	—	0.8
HCH	Technical	5.0	1.6	—	—	0.4
DDT	99.8%	5.0	0.6	0.8	—	—
Dieldrin	98%	4.0	0.8	0.4	—	0.4
Endosulfan	93.8%	3.0	1.2	0.4	—	0.6
Endosulfan	Technical	3.0	1.0	0.6	—	0.8
Endrin	20% EC	0.5	1.2	0.8	—	1.6
Endrin	98%	0.5	1.4	1.2	—	1.2
Lindane	99.2%	5.0	1.0	0.4	0.4	1.0
Lindane	98%	5.0	1.0	0.6	1.4	0.6
Methoxychlor	Technical	5.0	0.4	0.8	0.6	1.0
Methoxychlor	25% EC	5.0	0.4	1.4	1.2	0.2

TABLE 4

Chromosome Aberrations in Bone Marrow Cells of Male Rats After Oral Doses of Organophosphorus and other Pesticides[16]

Pesticides	Purity	Dose (mg/kg/d × 5 days)	Percentage aberrations:total metaphase score = 50 metaphases			
			Gap	Chromatid break	Fragment	Pulverization
Control	Peanut oil	0.5 ml		0.4	0.2	0.8
Diazinon	95%	2.0	0.4	1.0	—	0.6
Diazinon	98.7%	2.0	1.2	0.8	0.2	0.4
Dichlorovos	94.3%	2.0	1.4	0.6	0.6	—
Malathion	95.2%	5.0	0.6	0.6	1.2	0.8
Malathion	75% EC	5.0	0.8	0.6	0.4	0.6
Malathion	50% EC	5.0	1.2	0.4	0.4	1.0
Methyl demeton	Technical	0.5	0.2	0.4	0.4	1.0
Parathion	98%	0.1	1.2	0.8	0.8	0.4
Phenothoate	Technical		0.8	0.8	0.6	0.4
Phosphamidon	Technical	0.6	0.6	0.4	1.0	0.6
Quinalphos	Technical		0.6	0.6	—	0.4
Carbaryl	99%	10.0	0.4	0.6	—	—
Thanite	Technical	5.0	1.2	0.4	0.2	0.4
Paraquat dichloride	Technical	10.0	1.0	1.6	0.2	0.8
Thiram	Technical	10.0	0.2	—	0.4	0.8
Zineb	76.6%	10.0	0.4	—	0.8	0.2

processes of embryogenesis in animals are essentially a precise sequence of cell proliferation, differentiation, migration, and finally organogenesis. In fact, embryogenesis embraces complex cellular interactions in both time and space. It is now known that susceptibility to teratogenic agents depends with the developmental phase of the embryo at the time of exposure.

Each animal has a relatively brief critical period of sensitivity to teratogens, particularly during the period of early organogenesis. This period ranges from the time of implantation

TABLE 5
Period of Gestation (In Days) and Characteristic Malformation in Laboratory Animals[30,31]

Animals	Implantation period	13 to 20 somites	End of embryonic period	End of metamorphosis	Fetal development	Parturition
Mouse	5	9	13	17	18—20	19
Rat	11	14	17	17	18—20	19
Rabbit	9	10	11	15	16—32	32
Hamster	7	9	10	14	15—16	15
Major susceptibility	Embryo lethality	Birth defects	Embryo lethality		Growth retardation, functional defects fetus death; transplacental carcinogenesis	Growth retardation; other defects

to the end of the embryonic period. In the mouse and rat the sensitive or vulnerable period ranges from day 5 through 14 of the approximately 20 days gestation period. Table 5 describes the period of gestation and characteristic malformation in species of laboratory animals.[30,31]

A. EXPERIMENTAL TERATOGENESIS

Chemical-induced teratogenic effects are dose related. A correct dosage of pesticide will produce some defective offspring, some normal offspring, and some fetal deaths. Pesticides can also produce *in utero* death followed by abortion or resorption. For example, dipterex, imidan, and hexachlorocyclohexane were embryotoxic and teratogenic in pregnant rat.[32,33]

Organophosphorus pesticides like diazinon, pirimiphos-methyl, and monocrotophos and methyl carbamates produce a variety of defects in the avian embryos. These include vertebral malformations, beak defects, and decreased hatchability.[34] Studies have shown that avian species are more susceptible to pesticides as teratogens.[35] In a recent review, Hoffman and Albers[36] reported the embryotoxic effects of several pesticides. Although the short term tests by external application of the test compound to eggs suggest the potential embryotoxicity, utilization of wild bird eggs and nest incubation are needed for better understanding of the problems.

In contrast to the avian embryo, the mammalian embryo is placental. The special advantage of maternal protection, in terms of chemical absorption, detoxification, and excretion certainly offers great benefits to the developing fetus. However, instances are reported in literature where carbaryl, diazinon, trichlorfon, phosmet, and dimethoate have produced deformities in the developing fetus. These include hydrocephaly, hypogntheia, polydactyly, and disturbances and defects in skeletal ossification etc. These changes have been seen in rat, guinea pig, rabbit, dog, cat, and miniature swine.[37-40]

IV. CONCLUSION

Our present knowledge on the mutagenicity of pesticides needs more confirmatory studies. This is particularly true because of the wide variation in test methodologies. The utility of mammalian studies is a must to determine risk of pesticides for man. In fact, the essential sites of attack of the pesticide on DNA remain to be elucidated and more studies are desired in this direction.

The existing data on teratogenicity of pesticides in mammals are very inadequate as is the case with our knowledge of mechanisms of teratogenesis after exposure to a particular pesticide. The practicality of the test dosage is yet another aspect which requires careful consideration for the meaningful delineation of the experimental data from animal to man.

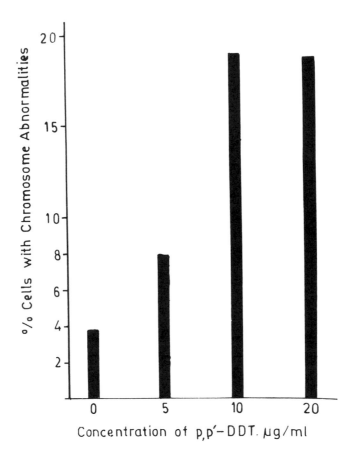

FIGURE 6.   Histogram showing dose response of the kangaroo cell line to p,p'-DDT. (From Palmer, K. A. et al., *Toxicol. Appl. Pharmacol.,* 22, 355, 1972. With permission.)

REFERENCES

1. **Miller, E. C. and Miller, J. A.,** Studies on the mechanism of activation of aromatic amine and amide carcinogens to ultimate carcinogenic electrophilic reactants, *Ann. N.Y. Acad. Sci.,* 163, 731, 1969.
2. Federal Insecticide, Fungicide, Rodenticide Act, U.S. Environmental Protection Agency, proposed guidelines for registering pesticides in the United States, Hazard Evaluation: Humans and Domestric Animals, *Fed. Reg.,* 43, 37335, August 22, 1978.
3. **Waters, M. D., Sandhu, S. S., Simmon, V. F., Mortel Mans, K. E., Mitchell, A. D., Jorgenson, T. A., Jones, D. C. L., Valencia, R., and Garrett, N. E.,** Study of pesticide genotoxicity in *Genetic toxicology* Fleck, R. A. and Hollander, A., Eds., Plenum Press, New York, 1982, 275.
4. **Seiler, J. P.,** A survey on the mutagenicity of various pesticides, *Experientia,* 29, 622, 1973.
5. **Degraeve, N. and Moutschen, J.,** Absence of genetic and cytogenetic effects in mice treated by the organophosphorous insecticide parathion, its methyl analogue and paraoxon, *Toxicology,* 32, 177, 1984.
6. **Degraeve, N., Marie-Christine and Moutschen, J.,** Cytogenetic effects induced by organophosphorous pesticides in mouse spermatocytes, *Toxicol. Lett.,* 21, 315, 1984.
7. **Singh, S., Lehmann-Grube, B., and Goedde, H. W.,** Cytogenetic effects of paraoxon and methyl parathion in cultured human lymphocytes: SCE clastogenic activity and cell cycle delay, *Int. Arch. Occup. Environ. Health,* 52, 195, 1984.
8. **Larsen, K. D. and Jalal, S. M.,** DDT induced chromosome mutations in mice: further testing, *Can. J. Genet. Cytol.,* 16, 491, 1974.

9. **Johnson, G. A. and Jalal, S. M.,** DDT induced chromosomal damage in mice, *J. Hered.,* 64, 7, 1973.
10. **Palmer, K. A., Green, S., and Legator, M. S.,** Cytogenetic effects of DDT in a cultured mammalian cell line, *Toxicol. Appl. Pharmacol.,* 22, 355, 1972.
11. **Mahr, U. and Miltenburger, H. G.,** The effects of insecticides on Chinese hamster cell cultures, *Mutation Res.,* 14, 107, 1976.
12. **Kelly Garvert, F. and Legator, M. S.,** Cytogenetic and mutagenic effects of DDT and DDE in a chinese hamster cell line, *Mutation Res.,* 17, 223, 1977.
13. **Dikshith, T. S. S. and Datta, K. K.,** Endrin induced cytological changes in albino rats, *Bull. Environ. Contam. Toxicol.,* 9, 65, 1973.
14. **Tzoneva-Maneva, M. T., Kalinova, F., and Georgieva, V.,** Influence of diazinon and lindane on the miotic activity and the caryotype of human lymphocytes, cultivated *in vitro, Bibl. Haematol.,* 38, 344, 1971.
15. **Dikshith, T. S. S. and Datta, K. K.,** Endosulfan: Lack of cytogenetic effects in male rats, *Bull. Environ. Contam. Toxicol.,* 20, 826, 1978.
16. **Dikshith, T. S. S.,** Cytogenetic effects of pesticides in the bone marrow system of male rats (unpublished data), 1982, scientific report, ITRC, Lucknow, India 1981—1984.
17. **Durham, W. F. and Williams, C. H.,** Mutagenic, teratogenic and carcinogenic properties of pesticides, *Annu. Rev. Entomol.,* 17, 123, 1972.
18. **Chen, H. H., Hsuch, J. L., Sirianni, S. R., and Huang, C. C.,** Induction of sister chromatid exchanges and cell cycle delay in cultured mammalian cells treated with eight organophosphorous pesticides, *Mutation Res.,* 88, 307, 1981.
19. **Tezuka, H., Ando, N., Susuki, R.,** Sister chromatid exchanges and chromosomal aberrations in cultured chinese hamster cell treated with pesticides positive in microbial reservation assays, *Mutat Res.,* 78, 177, 1980.
20. **Dikshith, T. S. S.,** *In vivo* effects of parathion on guinea pig chromosomes, *Environ. Physiol. Biochem.,* 3, 161, 1973.
21. **Dulout, F. N., Pastori, M. C., and Oliver, O. A.,** Malathion induced chromosomal aberration in bone marrow cells of mice: dose response relationships, *Mutation Res.,* 122, 163, 1983.
22. **Dzwoukowska, A. and Hubner, H.,** Induction of chromosomal aberrations in the syrian hamster by insecticides tested *in vivo, Arch. Toxicol.,* 58, 152, 1986.
23. **Legator, M. S.,** Mutagenicity of captan, *Mutat. Res.,* 85, 220, 1981.
24. **Dikshith, T. S. S., Carrera, G., and Mitjavila, S.,** Lack of cytogenetic effects of chlorpropham in male rats, *Natl. Acad. Sci. Lett.,* 11, 245, 1988.
25. **Yoder, J., Watson, M., and Beson, W. W.,** Lymphocyte chromosome analysis of agricultural workers during extensive occupational exposure to pesticides, *Mutation Res.,* 21, 335, 1973.
26. **Van Bao, T., Szabo, I., Ruzieska, P., and Czeizel, A.,** Chromosome aberrations in patients suffering acute organic phosphate insecticide intoxication, *Human Genet.,* 24, 33, 1974.
27. **Rabeloo, M. N., Becak, W., De Almeida, W. F., Pigati, P., Ungaro, M. T., Murata, T., and Percira, C. A. B.,** Cytogenetic study on individuals occupationally exposed to DDT, *Mutation Res.,* 28, 449, 1975.
28. **Stocco, R. D., Becak, W., Gaeta, R., and Rubelo-Gay, M. N.,** Cytogenetic studies of workers exposed to methyl parathion, *Mutation Res.,* 103, 71, 1982.
29. **Dulout, F. N., Pastori, M. C., Olivero, O. A., Cid, M. G., Loria, D., Matos, E., Sobel, N., Debujan, E. C., and Albiano, N.,** Sister chromatid exchanges and chromosomal aberrations in a population exposed to pesticides, *Mutation Res.,* 143, 237, 1985.
30. **Wilson, J. G.,** Factors determining the teratogenicity of drugs, *Annu. Rev. Pharmacol.,* 14, 205, 1974.
31. **Harbinson, R. D.,** Teratogens, *In Toxicology the Basic Science of Poisons,* Doull, J., Klaassen, C. D., and Amdur, M. O., Eds., Macmillan, New York, 1980, 158.
32. **Martson, L. V. and Voronina, V. M.,** Experimental study of the effect of a series of phosphoro-organic pesticide (Dipterex and Imidan) on embryogenesis, *Environ. Health Perspect.,* 13, 121, 1976.
33. **Dikshith, T. S. S., Srivastava, M. K., and Raizada, R. B.,** Fetotoxicity of hexachlorocyclohexane (HCH) in mice: morphological biochemical and residue evaluation, *Vet. Hum. Toxicol.,* in press.
34. **Scifert, J. and Casida, J. E.,** Mechanism of teratogenesis induced by organophosphorous and methyl carbamate insecticides, in *Progress in Pesticide Biochemistry,* Hutson, D. H. and Roberts, T. R., Eds., John Wiley and Sons, New York, 1981, chap. 5 & 219.
35. **Scifert, J. and Casida, J. E.,** Relation of yolk sac membrane kynurenine formamidase inhibition to certain teratogenic effects of organophosphorous insecticides and of carbaryl, esterine in chicken embryos, *Biochem. Pharmacol.,* 27, 2611, 1978.
36. **Hoffman, D. J. and Albers, P. H.,** Evaluation of potential embryotoxicity and teratogenicity of 42 herbicides, insecticides, and petroleum contaminants to Mallard eggs, *Arch. Environ. Contam. Toxicol.,* 13, 15, 1984.

37. **Earl, F. L., Miller, E., and Vanloon, E. J.,** Reproductive, teratogenic and neonatal effects of some pesticides and some related compounds in beagle dogs and in miniature swine, in *Pesticides and the Environment: A Continuing Contraversy* Deichman, W. B., Ed., Intercontinental Medical Book Corporation, New York, 1973, 253.

38. **Khera, K. S.,** Evaluation of dimethoate (Cygon 4E) for teratogenic activity in the cat, *J. Environ. Pathol. Toxicol.,* 2, 1283, 1979.

39. **Murray, F. J., Staples, R. E., and Schwetz, B. A.,** Teratogenic potential of carbaryl given to rabbits and mice by gavage or by dietary inclusion, *Toxicol. Appl. Pharmacol.,* 51, 81, 1979.

40. **Berge, G. N. and Nafstad, I.,** Distribution and placental transfer of trichlorfon in guinea pigs, *Arch. Toxicol.,* 59, 26,1986.

Chapter 9

CARCINOGENICITY OF PESTICIDES

T. S. S. Dikshith

TABLE OF CONTENTS

I. INTRODUCTION

The causes of cancer promotion in animals and humans vis à vis environmental chemicals are still not fully understood. The potentiality of pesticides in the induction of neoplasms in animals has remained yet another unresolved but challenging area. In fact, the data on the carcinogenicity of a large number of pesticides in animals have been found to be inadequate as they have demonstrated inconclusive and equivocal observations. For example, while DDT increases the risk of liver tumors in CF_1 mouse[1] it causes no increase in liver tumor in BALB/c mouse.[2] Further, many of the pesticides show tumorigenicity in rodents when tested only at very high doses.

At this point it is important to make a distinction between carcinogenesis and tumorigenesis. The characteristic potentiality of pesticides to cause malignancy needs special emphasis. An uncontrolled somatic cell division leading to the formation of a malignant tumor is *carcinogenesis,* while the formation of a benign tumor is *tumorigenesis.* For instance, liver carcinoma is a case of carcinogenesis, whereas hepatoma is tumorigenesis. Some of the observations in this important field in relation to pesticides are discussed here.

II. MICROSOMAL ENZYME SYSTEM

A few enzymes or enzyme systems are known to be induced by pesticides. For example, the microsomal mixed function enzymes of the liver and some other organs are produced in greater quantity in response to certain pesticides. We know today that microsomal enzymes are associated with oxidation (N-O-, and S-dealkylation, deamination, epoxidation, disulfuration, hydroxylation) of both ring and side chains, oxidation of both nitrogen and sulfur reduction of nitro groups, hydrolysis, and conjugation.

The changes produced by microsomal enzymes render lipid soluble compounds more water soluble and hence rapidly eliminated from the body. In fact, the mixed function oxidase system represents a very important detoxification mechanism; however, it also renders certain pesticides more toxic. For instance, paraoxon the metabolite of parathion is more toxic than parathion. Excellent reviews covering this subject are available in the literature.[3]

Induction of microsomal enzymes lead to marked liver changes in animals. In certain species of rodents, particularly mouse, these morphological changes have been related to tumorigenicity. Interestingly, though DDT induces microsomal enzymes in other species of animals[4] their liver does not demonstrate morphological changes akin to mouse liver.

III. CARCINOGENICITY

A. ORGANOCHLORINE INSECTICIDES

Several reports have shown that DDT induces hepatocarcinogenicity in strains of mice and Osborne-Mendel rats.[5-7] In fact, studies of Tomatis et al.[8] and Turusov et al.[9] on CF_1 mice, and Terracini et al.[10] on BALB/c mice clearly demonstrate that DDT produces liver tumors in these strains of mice. In a similar way, methoxychlor also produced liver tumor in C3H and BALB/c mice, rats, and dogs.[11-13]

Information on the carcinogenicity of some of the cyclodiene insecticides is very inadequate, for instance, aldrin, dieldrin, endrin, and heptachlor produced hepatocellular tumors in strains of mice such as CF_1, C3HeB/Fe, and $B6C_3F_1$.[14,15] These insecticides could not conclusively produce tumorigenicity in other species of animals. Mirex produces a dose-dependent increase in the incidence of hepatic megalocytosis, cellular alterations, and neoplastic nodules. Waters et al.[16a] reported a significant increase in the incidence of hepatocellular carcinoma in male rats exposed to a high dietary dose of mirex.

TABLE 1
Response of Animals to Dietary DDT and Tumors

Species	Sex	Dose (ppm)	Duration	Tumor	Ref.
Mouse CF$_1$	Male Female	250	2 generations	Liver	10
Mouse CF$_1$	Male Female	50	2 generations	Liver	8
Mouse	Male Female	140	18 months	Hepatoma	31
Mouse	Male Female	100	2 years	More liver tumors	23
Mouse-Balb/c		3	5 generations	Liver	24
Rat	—	25	2 years	No tumor	28
Rat	Male Female	500	2.9 years	Tumor	25
Dog		2000	49 months	No tumor	4
Monkey		200	7.5 years	No tumor	32

TABLE 2
Response of Animals to Dietary Dieldrin and Tumors

Species	Sex	Dose (ppm)	Duration	Tumor	Ref.
Mouse	Male Female	10	2 years	More liver tumors	33
Mouse	—	10	2 years	No liver tumor	23
Rat	Male Female	20	Lifespan	Liver tumor	34
Rat	Male Female	10	2 years	Less liver tumor	35
Dog	Male Female	0.005 to 0.05	2 years	No tumor	36
Dog	Male Female	1-3	68 weeks	No tumor	28
Monkey	—	1.75 2.5	6 years	No tumor	37

Some of the organochlorine insecticides, for example chlordane, heptachlor, lindane, and toxaphene produce thyroid tumors in rats.[17-20] These tumors have been identified as c-cell and follicular cell adenomas, follicular cell carcinomas, and squamous cell carcinomas.

It has been shown that the tumorigenic effect intensifies with the continuation of the insecticide treatment. The tumors have been shown to possess well-differentiated nodular growths, compressing, but not infiltrating the surrounding parenchyma.[8,21] In fact, reports on a multigeneration study have shown that continuous exposure of mice to DDT leads to a profound increase in hepatoma.[22-24]

In contrast with mouse, data on the tumorigenicity of DDT in rat is equivocal and often conflicting. For instance, while the study of Rossi et al.[25] reveals occurrence of liver tumor in DDT-treated rats, reports of Ortega et al.,[26] Ottoboni,[27] and Trejon and Cleaveland[28] could not confirm that DDT has carcinogenic effects in rat. Thus, our current knowledge of tumorgenicity of pesticides in species of experimental animals is still very limited and often inconclusive[29-37] (Tables 1 and 2).

The international agency for research on cancer (IARC) has reviewed the evidence on carcinogenicity of several organochlorine insecticides, carbamates, dithiocarbamates, herbicides etc. The study group felt that the data are inadequate for a large number of pesticides

TABLE 3
Status of Hepatocarcinogenicity of Pesticides[5]

Insecticide	Species of animals	Evaluation
DDT	Rat	No convincing evidence
	Mouse	Positive in both sexes, several strains
	Hamster	Negative
	Dog	Inconclusive
	Monkey	Inconclusive
DDE	Mouse	Positive
Methoxychlor	Rat	Inconclusive
Chlorobenzylate	Rat	Inconclusive
	Mouse	Positive in male of two strains
HCH	Rat	Inconclusive
	Mouse	Positive in both sexes
Heptachlor	Rat	Inconclusive
Aldrin	Rat	Negative
	Mouse	Positive in both sexes
	Dog	Inconclusive
	Monkey	Inconclusive
Endrin	Rat	1 negative and 1 inconclusive
	Mouse	Inconclusive
Mirex	Mouse	Positive in both sexes, 2 strains

to arrive at definite conclusions to show the carcinogenicity of the candidate insecticide.[38,39] For example, data on HCH in mouse are positive for both sexes, but inconclusive in rat. In a similar manner, data on dieldrin in rat, dog, and monkey are inconclusive but positive in mouse[5] (Table 3).

B. ORGANOPHOSPHORUS INSECTICIDES

Several organophosphorus insecticides have produced tumors in experimental animals. For example, reexamination of histopathological sections confirmed that malathion induces benign and malignant neoplasms in mice and rats.[40,41] In fact, malathion and malaoxon (oxygen analog of malathion) enhanced the incidence of liver tumor in B6C3F1 mice and Fisher 344 rats.[42] Dimethoate has caused benign and malignant neoplasms in the ovaries of rat.[43]

C. OTHER INSECTICIDES

The working group of IARC reported that oral administration of maneb and zineb significantly increase the incidences of lung adenomas in one strain of mouse.[38] Ethylene thiourea (ETU) the degradation product and metabolite common to the ethylene bis-dithio-carbamic acid salts, has shown carcinogenic effects in mice, hamsters, and rats. In fact, ETU behaves like a number of other thio compounds which cause thyroid carcinoma and indirectly affect the liver. However, some of the carbamate insecticides did not cause any tumorigenic effect in animals. For instance, daily administration of carbaryl and isopropyl N-methyl carbamate to mice for 18 months did not show any tumorigenic effect.[31]

Mancozeb has shown tumor initiating effects in mouse skin. For example, dermal administration of mancozeb followed by local application of 1,2-O-tetradecanoylphorbol-13-acetone (TPA) produces distinct finger-like/flat paillomatous growth and mancozeb plus TPA treatment produces a significant number of skin tumors. The study shows that mancozeb has the potentiality to initiate the mouse epidermis for neoplastic changes.

Tumors arising in hyperplastic thyroid tissue due to hormonal imbalance and the role of ethylene thiourea deserve careful evaluation while considering tumorgenicity of dithio-carbamate pesticides.

It is important to consider here some of the aspects which are closely associated with the carcinogenicity of pesticides. For example, a comparison of the lesions caused by a pesticide and also by a known carcinogen like 2,7-FAA is perhaps of relevance. The lesion caused by 2,7-FAA did not involve induction of microsomal enzymes, the pathologic change started as a hyperplastic nodule rather than isolated cell change; the animals had bile duct proliferation which were not seen in controls or in the pesticide-treated animals; the lesion produced by 2,7-FAA was hepatocellular carcinoma in contrast with the adenoma produced by DDT or HCH.[46] Although the tumors produced by pesticides are principally of the liver, tumors are also seen in lung and lymphoid organs. However, the incidence of the tumor of the lung and lymphoid over the hepatomas is relatively less.

Evidence has shown that man has failed to indicate any sort of susceptibility to the tumorigenic action of the organochlorine insecticides. For instance, no increase in the occurrence of tumors has been seen in heavily exposed populations of occupational workers who are involved in the manufacture and formulations of DDT and dieldrin.[47,48]

IV. CONCLUSION

Predicting carcinogenic effects of pesticides on humans from animal studies is very difficult. From past experience with known human carcinogens it is becoming very evident that animal data, *particularly based on only one rodent species like mouse,* are not always a reliable indicator of carcinogenic effects of pesticide on the human, the reason being that human response to a pesticide (or to any chemical agent) varies widely in different mammalian species. One aspect of this interspecies metabolic variation partially explains the differences in tumorigenic response. However, our knowledge in this area is very limited.

Epidemiologic studies have shown little evidence supporting the tumorigenic effect of pesticide among occupationally exposed populations.

While the advances made in recent years have greatly improved our knowledge of the molecular events involved in carcinogenesis of environmental chemicals, a number of important issues related to the carcinogenicity of pesticides remain unresolved.

In light of the above observations there is a need to generate additional data on the tumor promotion of pesticides because of the increasing impact of other environmental chemicals on the animal. In fact, with the validity of the tumor promotion model as a major factor in the carcinogenicity of humans, more studies should be carried out in this direction.

REFERENCES

1. **Tomatis, L., Turusov, V., Charles, R. T., Biocchi, M., and Gati, F.,** Liver tumors in CF-1 mice exposed for limited periods to technical DDT, *Z. Krebs. Forsch.,* 82, 25, 1974.
2. **Terracini, B., Testa, M. C., Cabral, J. R., and Day, N.,** The effects of long term feeding of DDT to BALB/C mice, *Int. J. Cancer.,* 11, 747, 1973.
3. **Nakatsugawa, T. and Morelli, M. A.,** Microsomal oxidation and insecticide metabolism, in *Insecticide Biochemistry and Physiology,* Wilkinson, C. F., Ed., Plenum Press, New York, 1976, 61.
4. **Lehman, A. J.,** *Summaries of Pesticide Toxicity,* Association of Food and Drug Officials of the United States, Topeka, KS, 1965.
5. **Anon.,** *IARC Monographs on the Evaluation of Carcinogenic Risk of Chemicals to Man. Some Organochlorine Pesticides,* Vol. 5, International Agency for Research on Cancer, Lyon, 1974.
5a. **Anon.,** *IARC Monographs on the Evaluation of the Carcinogenic Risk of Chemicals to Humans. Some Halogenated Hydrocarbons,* Vol. 20, International Agency for Research on Cancer, Lyon, 1979.
5b. **Anon.,** *IARC Monographs on the Evaluation of the Carcinogenic Risk of Chemicals to Humans. Miscellaneous Pesticides,* Vol. 30, International Agency for Research on Cancer, Lyon, 1983.
6. Report of an IARC working group, An evaluation of chemicals and industrial process associated with cancer in humans based on human and animal data, IARC Monographs, Vols. 1—20, *Cancer Res.,* 40, 1, 1980.

7. **Reuber, M. D.,** Carcinoma of the liver in Osborne-Mendal rats ingesting DDT, *Tumori*, 64, 571, 1978.

8. **Tomatis, L., Turusov, V., Day, N., and Charles, R. T.,** The effect of long term exposure to DDT on CF-1 mice, *Int. J. Cancer*, 10, 489, 1972.

9. **Turusov, V. S., Day, N. E., Tomatis, L., Gati, E., and Charles, R. T.,** Tumors in CF_1 mice exposed for six consecutive generations to DDT, *J. Natl. Cancer Inst.*, 51, 983, 1973.

10. **Terracini, B., Cabral, R. J., and Testa, M. C.,** A multigeneration study on the effects of continuous administration of DDT to BALB/c mice, in *Proceedings of the 8th Inter-American Conference on Toxicology, Pesticides and the Environment, a Continuing Controversy, Miami, Florida,* Diechmann, W. B., Ed., International Medical Book Corporation, New York, 1973, 77.

11. National Cancer Institute, Bioassay of methoxychlor for possible carcinogenicity, *Tech. Report Series No. 35,* U.S. Department of Health, Education, and Welfare, Washington, D.C., 1978.

12. **Reuber, M. D.,** Interstitial cell carcinomas of the testis in BALB/c male mice ingesting methoxychlor, *J. Cancer Res. Clin. Oncol.*, 93, 173, 1979.

13. **Reuber, M. D.,** Carcinogenicity and toxicity of methoxychlor, *Environ. Health Perspect.*, 36, 205, 1980.

14. **Reuber, M. D.,** Carcinogenicity of endrin, *Sci. Total Environ.*, 12, 101, 1979.

15. **Reuber, M. D.,** Carcinomas, sarcomas and other lesions in Osborne-Mendal rats ingesting endrin, *Exp. Cell. Biol.*, 46, 129, 1979.

16. **Reuber, M. D.,** Histopathology of carcinomas of the liver in mice ingesting hepatochlor or hepatochlor epoxide, *Exp. Cell. Biol.*, 45, 147, 1977.

16a. **Waters, E. M., Huff, J. E., and Gerstner, H. B.,** Mirex: an overview, *Environ. Res.*, 14, 212, 1977.

17. National Cancer Institute, Bioassay of chlordane for possible carcinogenicity, *Tech. Report Series No. 8,* U.S. Department of Health, Education, and Welfare, Washington, D.C., 1977.

18. National Cancer Institute, Bioassay of hepatochlor for possible carcinogenicity, *Tech. Report Ser. No. 9,* U.S. Department of Health, Education, and Welfare, Washington, D.C., 1977.

19. National Cancer Institute, Bioassay of lindane for possible carcinogenicity, *Tech. Report Series No. 14,* U.S. Department of Health, Education, and Welfare, Washington, D.C., 1977.

20. National Cancer Institute, Bioassay of toxaphene for possible carcinogenicity, *Tech. Report Series No. 37,* U.S. Department of Health, Education, and Welfare, Washington, D.C., 1979.

21. **Fitzugh, O. G.,** A summary of carcinogenicity study of DDT in mice, U.S. Food and Drug Administration, in FAO/WHO 1969 Evaluations of some Pesticide Residues in Foods, World Health Organization, Geneva, 1970, 61.

22. **Shabad, L. M., Kolesnichenko, T. S., and Nikonova, T. V.,** Transplacental and combined lung tumor effect of DDT in five generations of A-strain mice, *Int. J. Cancer,* 11, 688, 1973.

23. **Walker, A. I. T., Thorpe, E., and Stevenson, D. E.,** The toxicology of dieldrin (HEOD). I. Longterm oral toxicity studies in mice, *Food Cosmet. Toxicol.,* 11, 415, 1973.

24. **Tarjan, R. and Kemeny, T.,** Multigeneration studies on DDT in mice, *Food Cosmet. Toxicol.,* 7, 215, 1969.

25. **Rossi, L., Ravera, M., Repetti, G., and Santi, L.,** Long term administration of DDT or phenobarbital-Na in Wistar rats, *Int. J. Cancer,* 19, 179, 1977.

25a. **Rossi, L., Barbieri, O., Sanguineti, M., Cabral, J. R. P., Bruzsi, P., and Santi, L.,** Carcinogenicity study with technical grade dichlorobiphenyl-trichloroethane and 1,1-dichloro-2,2-bis (p-chlorophenyl) ethylene in hamsters, *Cancer Res.,* 43, 776, 1983.

26. **Ortega, P., Hayes, W. J., Jr., Durham, W. F., and Mattson, A.,** *DDT in the Diet of the Rat,* U.S. Public Health Service Monograph No. 43, PHS, 484, 1956.

27. **Ottoboni, A.,** Effect of DDT on reproduction in the rat, *Toxicol. Appl. Pharmacol.,* 14, 74, 1969.

28. **Trejon, J. F. and Cleveland, F. P.,** Toxicity of certain chlorinated hydrocarbon insecticides for laboratory animals with special reference to aldrin and dieldrin, *Agric. Food Chem.,* 3, 402, 1955.

29. **Durham, W. F. and Williams, C. H.,** Mutagenic, teratogenic and carcinogenic properties of pesticides, *Annu. Rev. Entomol.,* 17, 123, 1972.

30. **Thorpe, E. and Walker, A. I. T.,** The toxicology of dieldrin (HEOD). II. Comparative long term oral toxicity studies in mice with dieldrin, DDT, phenobarbitone, B-BHC and gamma-BHC, *Food Cosmet. Toxicol.,* 11, 433, 1973.

31. **Innes, J. R. M., Ulland, B. M., Valerio, M. G., Petrucelli, L., Fishbein, L., Hart, E. R., Pallotta, A. J., Bates, R. R., Falk, H. L., Gart, J. J., Klein, M., Mitchell, I., and Peters, J.,** Bioassay of pesticides and industrial chemicals for tumorigenicity in mice, a preliminary note, *J. Natl. Cancer Inst.,* 42, 1101, 1969.

32. **Durham, W. F., Ortega, P., and Hayes, W. J., Jr.,** The effect of various dietary levels of DDT on liver function, cell morphology, and DDT storage in the rhesus monkey, *Arch. Int. Pharmacodyn. Ther.,* 141, 111, 1963.

33. **Davis, K. J. and Fitzhugh, O. G.,** Tumorigenic potential of aldrin and dieldrin for mice, *Toxicol. Appl. Pharmacol.,* 4, 187, 1962.

34. **Deichmann, W. B., Mac Donald, W. E., Blum, E., Bevilacguce, M., Rodomski, J., Keplinger, M. L., and Balkas, M.,** Tumorigenicity of aldrin, dieldrin and endrin in the albino rat, *Ind. Med. Surg.,* 39, 426, 1970.

35. **Stevenson, D. E., Thorpe, E., Hunt, P. F., and Walker, A. I. T.,** The toxic effects of dieldrin in rats: a reevaluation of data obtained in a two-year feeding study, *Toxicol. Appl. Pharmacol.,* 36, 247, 1976.

36. **Walker, A. I. T., Stevenson, D. E., Robinson, J., Thorpe, E., and Roberts, M.,** The toxicology and pharmacodynamics of dieldrin (HEOD): two-year oral exposures of rats and dogs, *Toxicol. Appl. Pharmacol.,* 15, 345, 1969.

37. **Wright, A. S., Donninger, C., Greenland, R. D., Stemmer, K. L., and Zavon, M. R.,** The effect of prolonged ingestion of dieldrin on the livers of male rhesus monkeys, *Ecotoxicol. Environ. Safe.,* 1, 477, 1978.

38. **IARC,** *Monographs on the Evaluation of Carcinogenic Risk of Chemicals to Man,* Vol. 12, International Agency for Research on Cancer, Lyon, 1976.

39. **IARC,** *Monographs on the Evaluation of Carcinogenic Risk of Chemicals to Man,* Vol. 15, International Agency for Research on Cancer, Lyon, 1977.

40. National Cancer Institute, Bioassay of malathion for possible carcinogenicity, *Technical Report Series No. 24,* U.S. Department of Health, Education, and Welfare, Washington, D.C., 1978.

41. **Reuber, M. D.,** Carcinogenicity and toxicity of malathion and malaoxon, *Environ. Res.,* 37, 119, 1985.

42. **Huff, J. E., Bate, R., Eustis, S. L., Haseman, J. K., and McConnell, E. E.,** Malathion and malaoxon: histopathology re-examination of the National Cancer Institute's carcinogenesis studies, *Environ. Res.,* 37, 154, 1985.

43. **Reuber, M. D.,** Carcinogenicity of dimethoate, *Environ. Res.,* 34, 193, 1984.

44. **Mehrotra, N. K., Kumar, S., and Skukla, Y.,** Tumor initiating activity of mancozeb — a carbamate fungicide in mouse skin, *Cancer Lett.,* 36, 283, 1987.

45. **Yogeshwar, S., Antony, M., Kumar, S., and Mehrotra, N. K.,** Tumor promoting ability of mancozeb a carbamate fungicide, on mouse skin, *Carcinogenesis,* 9, 8, 1988.

46. **Hamada, M., Yutangi, C., and Miyaji, T.,** Induction of hepatoma in mice by benzene hexachloride, *Gann,* 64, 511, 1973.

47. **Laws, E. R., Jr., Maddrey, W. D., Curley, A., and Burse, V. W.,** Long term occupational exposure to DDT, *Arch. Environ. Health,* 27, 318, 1973.

48. **Jager, R. J.,** Kepone chronology, *Science,* 193, 95, 1976.

Chapter 10

PESTICIDE RESIDUES

T. S. S. Dikshith

TABLE OF CONTENTS

I. INTRODUCTION

The development of modern pesticides undoubtedly provided more food and fiber to the hungry millions; along with this success, pesticides also posed problems of health and hazard to man and animals. Global concern on pesticides became more and more evident with the identification of pesticide residues in air, water, food products[1,2] nay, even in the tissue of the unborn child.

Reports have shown that pesticides cause short term and long term health effects in man and animals. The persistent insecticides, for example, DDT, HCH, dieldrin, chlordecone, mirex, and toxaphene etc., have been shown to produce neurological, reproductive, carcinogenic, and genotoxic effects in animals and humans.[3-5] Reviews have been published on several of the pesticides and interested readers may refer to the literature.[3-6]

In the light of the current literature available on pesticides there is a wide gap in terms of quantitation of residues in animals vis-à-vis their health status. The present chapter, which is an overview of the published reports, attempts to delineate the status of pesticide load in the body of animals and humans. The information, hopefully, will be of value in understanding the body burden of pesticides in animals which may help for the better management of pesticides.

II. LABORATORY STUDIES

A. ORGANOCHLORINE INSECTICIDES

Among the modern insecticides, DDT ranks at the top. The effectiveness of DDT in controlling a wide variety of insect pests ushered in a new era and helped in the eradication of major pests.

Reports have shown that animals with an abnormal liver store more residues. For example, rats with a damaged liver show more residues of DDT and methoxychlor[7,8] than normal animals.

Prolonged exposure to pesticides has not only led to accumulation of residues in the body but also produced adverse effects in animals. For instance, male and female mice maintained on dietary HCH (500 ppm) for 6 months showed liver enlargement and neoplastic nodules.[9,10] In a similar way, daily treatment of rabbits for 30 days led to accumulation of HCH residues in blood and vital organs of the animals. It is of significance to know that animals become susceptible when HCH is painted on the groin region of the body rather than other areas, i.e., the ventral or dorsal area of the body[11] (Figure 1).

Information on the residue build up of endosulfan and chlordane is limited. Rats exposed to different doses of endosulfan for 30 days showed residues in the vital organs.[12] The study showed that female rat accumulates more (0.73 ppm) residues than the male (0.29 ppm).[13,14] Sprague-Dawley rats and mice (C57B1/6 JX) were exposed to ^{14}C chlordane (1.0 mg/kg). The animals showed peak tissue residues within 4 h after treatment. For instance, the blood level of the compound after 15 min was 14.1 and 3.4 ppb in rat and mouse respectively. The peak blood level for rat was 81 ppm after 2 h and for mouse 113 ppb after 8 hr.[15] The study revealed the differential metabolism and disposition of chlordane in rat and mouse, an important factor in the delineation of health effects of pesticides.

A single oral dose of mirex (6 mg/kg) showed accumulation of the chemical in vital tissues of experimental rat. For instance, the levels in fat (28%), muscle (3.2%), liver (1.8%), and kidney (0.09%) indicate the preferential storage or residue in the fat.[16,17] ^{14}C photomirex (20 mg/kg) 20 μCi) was administered intravenously to squirrel monkey to find the tissue distribution of the compound. It was found that the residue was highest in perirenal fat followed by pancreas, liver, and adrenals. Substantially high levels of residues were noticed in the sciatic nerve. Interestingly, a high residue of the compound was seen in skin and subcutaneous fat after 34 and 52 weeks.[18]

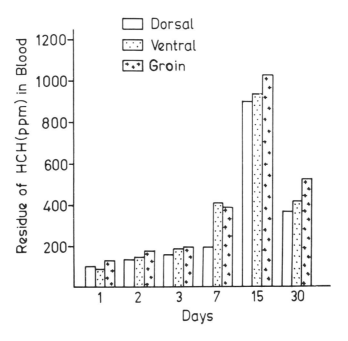

FIGURE 1. Histogram showing the residues of HCH (total) in blood of
male rabbit exposed through dorsal, ventral, and groin regions of the skin.
(From Dikshith, T. S. S., et al., *Indian J. Exp. Biol.*, 27, 252, 1989.
With permission.)

Robinson and Yarbrough[19] studied the disposition of mirex in the liver of rat. They
identified high residues in liver after 2 days, which however gradually declined by day 4
through 14. In another study Gaille et al.[20] investigated the residues of mirex in rats which
showed dose-related residue storage in liver, kidney, fat, and plasma. A comparison of
tissues revealed accumulation of more residue in plasma than in other tissues.

Administration of chlordecone to ovariectomized rats for 4 months showed residues in
liver, fatty tissue, and brain.[21] Similar observations have been made by other workers. For
instance, Guzelinan[22] and Egle et al.[23] reported accumulation of residues in liver, fatty tissue,
lung, and adrenal glands of rats. It is apparent from the foregoing observations that lipophilic
insecticides settle into fatty tissues after a certain period of time. A continuous daily dosing
of pesticides leads to gradual accumulation in the fat which, of course, approaches a plateau
after some period of time.

B. ORGANOPHOSPHORUS INSECTICIDES

The organophosphorus insecticides (OPs) account for about 35% of the synthetic pesticides that are used for pest control programs. The OPs are excellent inhibitors of cholinesterases. The OPs are highly toxic compounds and have very low acute LD_{50} values as
exemplified by parathion, TEPP, EPN etc. The OPs are used as contact and systemic
insecticides in the control of pests.

Tomokuni and Hasegawa[24] showed that administration of diazinon (20 and 100 mg/kg)
to rats results in the accumulation of residues in blood, liver, kidney, and brain within 8 h
of treatment. The residue level was maximum in blood within 1 to 2 h (Figure 2). While
the residue level in blood declined significantly within 24 h, it persisted for a longer time
in other tissues with maximum accumulation in kidney[25] (Figures 3 and 4).

Accumulation of pesticide residue in the body tissues of animals has been modulated
by different factors. For instance, hormonal, biochemical, and physiological body conditions

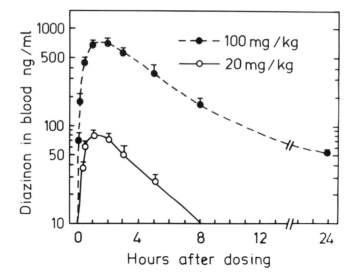

FIGURE 2.   Graph showing the blood level of diazinon in male rats after different periods of dosing (20 and 100 mg/kg body wt.). (From Tomokuni, K. et al., *Toxicology,* 37, 91, 1985. With permission.)

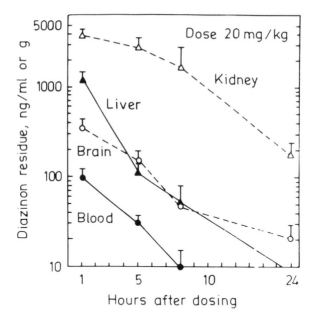

FIGURE 3.   Graph showing residue of diazinon in kidney, liver, brain, and blood of male mice treated with diazinon (20 mg/kg). (From Tomokuni, K. et al., *Toxicology,* 37, 91, 1985. With permission.)

do favor the storage of pesticide residues. Weitman and co-workers[26] studied the relationship between virgin and pregnant mice particularly on day 19 of gestation, comparing the susceptibility of pregnant animals, the activity of cholinesterase in brain and plasma, and the storage of parathion. These workers showed that the level of parathion in the blood and brain of pregnant mice was much higher than that in virgin[26] (Figures 5 and 6).

Recent studies of Berge and Nafstad[27] using ^{14}C trichlorofon also confirmed that pregnant

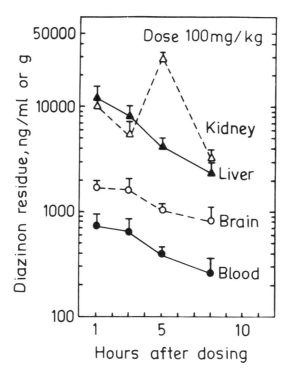

FIGURE 4. Graph showing residues of diazinon in kidney, liver, brain, and blood of male mice treated with diazinon (100 mg/kg). (From Tomokuni, K. et al., *Toxicology*, 37, 91, 1985. With permission.)

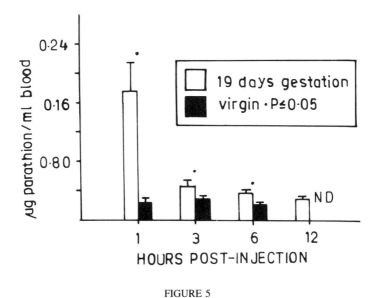

FIGURE 5

FIGURES 5 and 6. Histograms showing residues of parathion in blood and brain of pregnant and virgin mouse. (From Weitman, J. D. et al., *Toxicol. Appl. Pharmacol.*, 71, 215, 1983. With permission.)

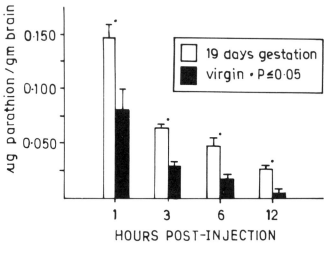

FIGURE 6

guinea pigs do rapidly store residues in liver and kidney. In fact, a comparison of maternal tissues and fetuses suggested more residues in the former than in the latter.

III. RESIDUES IN FIELD ANIMALS

Pesticides can come into contact with a variety of farm and field animals either by accident or through the food chain. Although the storage of residues in the animals through the food chain appears insignificant, no correlation has been made about the possible chronic exposure to persistent pesticides. There is much controversy concerning accumulation of pesticides in larger animals. For instance, reports of Durham et al.,[28] Gilbert,[29] Lambscher,[30] Benson and Smith,[31] Franson et al.,[32] and Kutz and George[33] showed that the level of DDT in animals like monkeys, shrews, voles, elk, black bear, white-tail deer and mule deer indicates a wide range of variation. In most cases the levels detected in big game are in the ppb range. In fact, the total DDT residue in the fat of black bear also ranged from 0.3 to 3 ppb with another instance being that of mule and white-tail deer where the DDT level ranged from 29 to 107 ppb in the fat.

It was of interest to note that the DDT level in some of the field animals showed a decline over the years. Studies of Krieger et al.[34] demonstrated a dose-dependent absorption and storage of DDT in the fat of rhesus monkeys (Figures 7 and 8). These findings are of great significance in the light of the earlier observations reported by Durham and co-workers[28] who also observed that prolonged feeding of DDT to monkeys failed to show larger accumulation of DDE.

Identification of pesticide residues in marine animals has caused concern. High levels of DDT have been demonstrated in the blubber of beluga whales in eastern and Arctic Canada.[35-37] Information on the storage of residues in marine mammals is still limited and more data are required to correlate the impact of residues on marine life.

IV. RESIDUES IN HUMANS

A. RESIDUES IN TISSUES

In spite of the apparent uniformity of pesticide residue levels in the common population within a country, the available data suggest variation in the residue levels among specific and distinct segments of the population. In fact, the importance of race differences in a

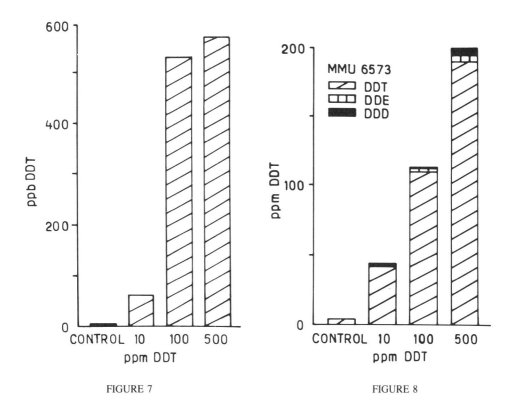

FIGURE 7   FIGURE 8

FIGURES 7 and 8   Histograms showing the level of DDT in the fat of Rhesus monkey. (From Krieger, R. I. et al., *Fate of Pesticides in Large Animals*, Ivie, G. W. and Dorough, H. W., Eds., Academic Press, New York, 1977, 77. With permission.)

population has been found to be statistically significant in several cases. For example, a statistically significant variation is seen in the residue levels of DDT and HCH in the autopsy samples of black and white populations. Another example is seen in the residue levels in blood samples of Indians in Utah which was lower than that in the caucasian samples.

The lipophilic property of pesticides, specifically the OCs has resulted in the accumulation and storage of residues in the fatty tissues. In fact, DDT, HCH, and their metabolites are stored in high concentrations.[39] The important source of residues for OCs at the equilibrium is the adipose tissues. Evidence has shown a definite correlation between the fat content of the tissue in question and the level of storage of the OCs.

Varied levels of residues are seen in the human populations from the same country and different countries.[38,40] For example, the general population of the north eastern, the southern, the north central, and the western parts of U.S. has shown different levels of residues of DDT and HCH. In fact, the level of DDT has been found to be highest in the western parts than in other parts of the U.S. Similar observations have been reported from the general population of Latin American countries and cities: namely Terreon, Mexico City and Puebla,[41] Canada,[42] and Norway.[43] Readers may refer the literature for more details.[44-46]

It has been shown that pesticides cross the placental barrier and are present in the neonate at levels normally lower than those of the mother. Bazulic et al.[47] found significant residues of DDT and HCH in the serum of mothers and newborn.

Pesticides have been implicated with several human diseases such as leukemia, agramlocytosis, aplastic anemia, allergy, etc. However, it has been reported that careful analysis has not shown any relationship to the epidemiological problem;[48] yet it needs careful consideration because of the fact that the scarce data on epidemiology of pesticides neither incriminate nor exonerate the pesticides. For instance, leptophos and chlordecone have produced debilitating diseases among occupational workers. A recent study of Runhaar et al.[49] showed that the levels of endrin and dieldrin in the adipose tissue of patients was much higher. In fact, the adipose tissue showed more residues than blood. It was also reported that the blood plasma of hospital patients had lower levels of OCs like DDT and HCH than those of the outdoor patients.[50]

A health survey of pesticide formulators in India showed that a majority of formulators (73% of 160) exhibited symptoms of pesticide poisoning. These occupational workers were associated with the formulation of malathion, parathion, DDT, HCH, and phorate. Because of the involvement of several pesticides and multiple exposures no clear cut and specific conclusion could be made to health status and the insecticide associated thereof.[51]

A comparison of total HCH in the serum of control population, nonhandlers, and handlers of pesticides showed that handlers show significantly high concentrations of HCH in their serum than other groups. While the mean level of HCH in the control group showed 0.051 ppm, that of the nonhandlers and handlers was found to be 0.266 and 0.604 ppm respectively. Occupational workers exposed to HCH show paresthesis of face and extremities, headache, giddiness, apprehension, confusion, tremors, loss of sleep, and vomiting. About 60% of the formulations exposed to phorate show symptoms of poisoning during the second week of exposure. The workers complained of gastrointestinal (50%), neurobehavioral (45%), and ocular (55%) types of disorders. These workers however, showed no ECG abnormalities although bradycardia was recorded in about 40% of the workers.[51]

B. RESIDUES IN MILK

The chemical nature of OCs is such that it persists in nature and the lipophilic properties help their movement to living tissues. For instance, insecticides like DDT, HCH, and dieldrin accumulate in fat, and it was soon discovered that with the use of DDT on animal feeds, etc. the residues were identified in products like milk and poultry. In fact, the problem today has become critical because milk and milk products are a major food source, particularly for the young, the aged, and sick persons. Any contamination of such an important food item with OCs is a matter of serious concern.

Studies have shown the presence of DDT and HCH in the milk of cows and milk products in Greece, Germany, and The Netherlands.[52] Recently Kalra et al.[53] reported that the milk of buffalos which were exposed to DDT contain appreciable levels of DDT. In fact, these workers demonstrated a maximum level of 1.2 ppm of DDT in the milk collected 2 h after treatment.

Any discussion of pesticide residues in humans would be incomplete without the mention of residues in the milk of nursing mothers. Analysis of the milk samples from the nursing mothers revealed different values. In fact, a wide variation is seen in the values reported from different countries. For example, the Hawaiian mothers showed a very high residue (2.16 ppm) of DDT in milk,[54] while the same in the milk of Finnish mothers was very low (0.031 ppm).[55] The level of DDT in mothers' milk from other countries fell between these two extreme values. For instance, China, India, Mexico, Germany, Japan, Yugoslavia, Spain, United States, Sweden, Norway, and Canada showed the DDT content as 1.8, 1.1, 0.7, 0.25, 0.21, 0.18, 0.17, 0.1, 0.1, 0.09, 0.082, and 0.039 respectively[56-59] (Figures 9 and 10).

With the presence of such residues in mother's milk, the infant is bound to become exposed to some quantities of DDT during its growth period. The important question for us to answer is whether or not such exposures to DDT through mother's milk represents a potential hazard to the growing child. Unfortunately, this has not been well established. There is no evidence in the literature of any illness in babies attributable to the intake of OCs with mother's milk as a source. In view of this, extensive studies are required to prove breast-fed babies imbibe excess amount of pesticide residues through mothers' milk.

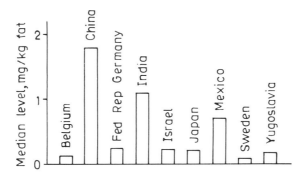

FIGURE 9.   Median levels of p,p'-DDT in milk fat of lactating
mothers in different countries. (From Slorach, S. A. and Vaz, R.,
Assessment of Human Exposure to Selected Organochlorine Compounds through Biological Monitoring, Swedish National Food
Administration, Uppsala, 1983. With permission.)

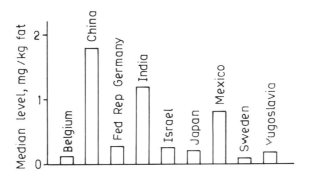

FIGURE 10.   Median levels of p,p'-DDT in milk fat of primi-
parous mothers in different countries. (From Slorach, S. A. and
Vaz, R., Assessment of Human Exposure to Selected Organochlorine Compounds through Biological Monitoring, Swedish National
Food Administration, Uppsala, 1983. With permission.)

In conclusion, one is tempted to observe that despite the problems, the data available
on pesticide residues indicate interesting trends with respect to the movement of pesticides
through animal and human populations. Although the major factor determining the distribution of pesticides in the body is fat content, there are several other factors modulating the
final distribution of residues. Besides fat, the susceptible sites for the storage of pesticide
residues could be the nervous system, reproductive organs, and more importantly the mother-
child or mother-fetus transfer of pesticides via milk or placental transport processes. More
information is necessary to identify the effects of residues in these vulnerable systems of
animals and humans.

REFERENCES

1. **Abbott, D. C., Harrison, R. B., Tatton, J. G., and Thomson, J.,** Organochlorine pesticides in the
atmosphere, *Nature,* 211, 259, 1966.
2. **Eichelberger, J. W. and Lichetenberg, J. J.,** Persistence of pesticides in river water, *Environ. Sci.
Technol.,* 5, 541, 1971.

3. **Van Asperen, K.,** Interaction of the isomers of benzene hexachloride in mice, *Arch. Int. Pharmacodyn. Ther.,* 99, 368, 1954.

4. **Ware, G. W. and Good, E. E.,** Effects of insecticides on reproduction in the laboratory mouse. II. Mirex, telodrin, and DDT, *Toxicol. Appl. Pharmacol.,* 10, 54, 1967.

5. **Virgo, B. B. and Bellward, G. D.,** Effects of dietary dieldrin on offspring viability, maternal behaviour, and milk production in the mouse, *Res. Commun. Chem. Pathol. Pharmacol.,* 17, 399, 1977.

6. **Reuber, M. D.,** Carcinogencity of kepone, *J. Toxicol. Environ. Health,* 4, 895, 1978.

7. **Grant, D. L. and Phillips, W. E. J.,** The effect of liver damage on the storage of p,p'-DDT in the rat, *Bull. Environ. Contam. Toxicol.,* 7, 284, 1972.

8. **Laugh, E. P. and Kunze, F. M.,** Effect of carbon tetrachloride on toxicity and storage of methoxychlor in the rat, *Fed. Proc.,* 10, 318, 1951.

9. **Nigam, S. K., Karnik, A. B., Lakkad, B. C., and Venkatakrishna, and Bhatt, H.,** Distribution of isomers of BHC and related histopathology of liver in hexachlorocyclohexane (technical grade BHC) fed mice, *Arch. Environ. Health,* 37, 156, 1982.

10. **Thankore, K. N., Nigam, S. K., Karnik, A. B., Lakkad, B. C., Bhatt, D. K., Aravinda Babu, K., Kashyap, S. K., and Chatterjee, S. K.,** Early changes in serum protein and liver LDH isoenzymes in mice exposed to technical grade hexachlorocyclohexane (BHC) and their possible relationship to liver tumors, *Toxicology,* 19, 31, 1981.

11. **Dikshith, T. S. S., Raizada, R. B., Srivastava, M. K., Kumar, S. N., Kaushal, R. A., Singh, R. P., Gupta, K. P., and Sree Lakshmi, K.,** Dermal toxicity of hexachlorocyclohexane (HCH) in rabbit, *Ind. J. Exp. Biol.,* 27, 252, 1989.

12. **Nath, G., Datta, K. K., Dikshith, T. S. S., Tandon, S. K., and Pandya, K. P.,** Interaction of endosulfan and metapa in rats, *Toxicology,* 11, 385, 1978.

13. **Dikshith, T. S. S., Raizada, R. B., Kumar, S. N., Srivastva, M. K., and Kaphalia, B. S.,** Response of rats to repeated oral administration of endosulfan, *Ind. Health,* 22, 295, 1984.

14. **Dikshith, T. S. S., Raizada, R. B., Kumar, S. N., Srivastva, M. K., Kaushal, R. A., Singh, R. P., and Gupta, K. P.,** Effect of repeated dermal application of endosulfan to rats, *Vet. Hum. Toxicol.,* 30, 219, 1988.

15. **Ewing, A. D., Kadry, A. M., and Dorough, H. W.,** Comparative disposition and elimination of chlordane in rats and mice, *Toxicol. Lett.,* 26, 233, 1985.

16. **Mehendale, H. M., Fishbein, L., Fields, M., and Matthenws, H. B.,** Fate of ^{14}C mirex in the rats and plants, *Bull. Environ. Contam. Toxicol.,* 8, 200, 1972.

17. **Ivie, G. W., Gibson, J. R., Bryant, H. E., Begin, J. J., Barnett, J. R., and Dorough, H. W.,** Accumulation, distribution and excretion of mirex-SSM, ^{14}C in animals exposed for long periods to the insecticide in the diet, *J. Agric. Food. Chem.,* 22, 646, 1974.

18. **Chu, I., Villeneuve, D. C., and Viau, A.,** Tissue distribution and elimination of photomirex in squirrel monkeys, *Bull. Environ. Contam. Toxicol.,* 29, 434, 1982.

19. **Robinson, K. M. and Yarbrough, J. D.,** Liver response to oral administration of mirex in rats, *Pesticide Biochem. Physiol.,* 8, 65, 1978.

20. **Gaille, G., Plaa, G. L., and Vezina, M.,** Gas-liquid chromatographic determining of chlordecone and mirex in biological specimens, *J. Toxicol. Clin. Exper.,* 7, 21, 1987.

21. **Reel, J. R. and Lamb, W. C. J.,** Reproductive toxicity of chlordecone (kepone), in *Endocrine Toxicology,* Thomas, J. A., Korach, K. S., and McLachlan, J. A., Eds., Raven Press, New York, 1985.

22. **Guzelian, P. S.,** Comparative toxicology of chlordecone (kepone) in humans and experimental animals, *Annu. Rev. Pharmacol. Toxicol.,* 22, 89, 1982.

23. **Egle, J. L., Jr., Fernandez, S. B., Guzelian, P. S., and Borzelleca, J. F.,** Distribution and excretion of chlordecone (kepone) in rat, *Drug. Metab. Dispos.,* 6, 91.

24. **Tomokuni, K. and Hasegawa, T.,** Diazinon concentrations and blood cholinesterase activities in rats expoxed to diazinon, *Toxicol. Lett.,* 25, 7, 1985.

25. **Tomokuni, K., Hasegawa, T., Hirai, Y., and Koga, N.,** The tissue distribution of diazinon and the inhibition of blood cholinesterase activities in rats and mice receiving a single intraperitoneal dose of diazinon, *Toxicology,* 37, 91, 1985.

26. **Weitman, S. D., Vodicnik, M. J., and Lech, J. J.,** Influence of pregnancy on parathion toxicity and disposition, *Toxicol. Appl. Pharmacol.,* 71, 215, 1983.

27. **Berge, G. N. and Nafstad, I.,** Distribution and placental transfer of trichlorofon in guinea pigs, *Arch. Toxicol.,* 59, 26, 1986.

28. **Durham, W. F., Ortega, P., and Hayes, W. J., Jr.,** The effect of various dietary levels of DDT on liver function, cell morphology and DDT storage in the rhesus monkey, *Arch. Int. Pharmacodyn.,* CXL 1, 111, 1963.

29. **Gilbert, F. F.,** Physiological effects of natural DDT residues and metabolites on ranch mink, *J. Wildl. Mgmt.,* 33, 933, 1969.

30. **Stickel, L. F.,** Pesticide residues in birds and mammals, in *Environmental Pollution by Pesticides,* Edward, C. A., Ed., Plenum Press, New York, 1973, 254.

31. **Benson, W. W. and Smith, P.,** Pesticide levels in deer, *Bull. Environ. Contam. Toxicol.,* 11, 379, 1974.

32. **Franson, J. C., Dahm, P. A., and Wing, L. D.,** Chlorinated hydrocarbon insecticides in adipose, liver and brain samples from Iowa mink, *Bull. Environ. Contam. Toxicol.,* 11, 379, 1974.

33. **Kurtz, D. A. and George, J. L.,** DDT metabolism in Pennsylvania white-tail deer, in *Fate of Pesticides in Large Animals,* Ivie, G. W. and Dorough, H. W., Eds., Academic Press, New York, 1977, 193.

34. **Krieger, R. I., Miller, J. L., Gee, S. J., and Clark, C. R.,** Comparative metabolism and an experimental approach for study of liver oxidase induction in primates, in *Fate of Pesticides in Large Animals,* Ivie, G. W. and Dorough, H. W., Eds., Academic Press, New York, 1977, 77.

35. **Adison, R. F. and Brodie, P. F.,** Occurrence of DDT residues in Beluga whales *(Delphinpterus leucas)* from the Mackenzie delta, N.W.T., *J. Fish. Res. Board Canada,* 30, 1733, 1973.

36. **Martineau, D., Beland, P., Desjardins, C., and Lagace, A.,** Levels of organochlorine chemicals in tissue of Beluga whales *(Delphinpterus leucas)* from St. Lawrence Estuary, Quebec, Canada, *Arch. Environ. Contam. Toxicol.,* 16, 137, 1987.

37. **Beland, P., Martimeau, D., Robichand, R., Plante, R., and Greendale, R.,** unpublished data, 1987.

38. **Kalayanova, S. F. and Fourmier, E.,** *Les Pesticides et 11 Homme,* Masson et Cie, Paris, 1971.

39. **Doyuchi, M.,** Chlorinated hydrocarbons in the environment in the Kanto plain and Tokyo bay, as reflected in fishes, birds and man, *Proc. Int. Symp., Japan* 1973.

40. **Kutz, F. W., Yobs, A. R., Johnson, W. G., and Wiersma, G. B.,** Pesticide residues in adipose tissue of the general population of the United States, Fy 1970 Survey, *Bull. Soc. Pharmacol. Environ. Pathol.,* 11, 1974.

41. **Albert, L., Mendez, F., Cebrian, M. E., and Portales, A.,** Organochlorine pesticide residues in human adipose tissue in Mexico. Result of a preliminary study in three Mexico cities, *Arch. Environ. Health,* 5, 262, 1980.

42. **Mes, J., Davies, D. J., and Turton, D.,** Polychlorinated biphenyl and other chlorinated hydrocarbon residues in adipose tissue of Canadians, *Bull. Environ. Contam. Toxicol.,* 28, 97, 1982.

43. **Tuvery, J. M. and Sande, H. A.,** Organochlorine pesticides and polychlorinated biphenyls in maternal adipose tissue, blood, milk and cord blood from mothers and their infants living in Norway, *Arch. Environ. Contam. Toxicol.,* 17, 55, 1988.

44. **World Health Organisation,** Environmental Health Criteria for DDT, Document No. 9, WHO, Geneva, 1979.

45. **Dikshith, T. S. S.,** DDT — the problems of residue and hazard, *J. Sci. Ind. Res.,* 37, 316, 1978

46. **Hayes, W. J., Jr.,** *Pesticide Studied in Man,* Williams and Wilkins, Baltimore, 1982.

47. **Bazulic, O., Stampar-Plasaj, B., Bujanovic, V., Stojanovski, N., Nastev, B., Rudelic, I., Sisul, N., and Zuzek, A.,** Organochlorine pesticide residues in the serum of mothers and their new borns from three Yugoslav towns, *Bull. Environ. Contam. Toxicol.,* 32, 265, 1984.

48. **Rathus, E. M.,** The effect of pesticide residues on humans, in *Pesticides and the Environment: A Continuing Controversy,* Deichmann, W. B., Ed., Intercontinental Medical Book Corp., New York, 1973, 23.

49. **Runhaar, F. A., Sangster, B., Greve, P. A., and Voortman, M.,** A case of fatal endrin poisoning, *Human Toxicol.,* 4, 241, 1985.

50. **Kaphalia, B. S. and Seth, T. D.,** Isomers and metabolites of DDT and BHC in blood plasma, adipose tissue and cerebro spinal fluid (CSF) in persons of Lucknow, *Indian J. Biochem. Biophys. Suppl.,* 15, 79, 1979.

51. **Kashyap, S. K.,** Health surveillance and biological monitoring of pesticide formulators in India, *Toxicol. Lett.,* 33, 107, 1986.

52. **Fytianos, K., Vasilikiotis, G., Weil, L., Kavlendis, E., and Laskaridis, N.,** Preliminary study of organochlorine compounds in milk product, human milk and vegetables, *Bull. Environ. Contam. Toxicol.,* 34, 504, 1985.

53. **Kalra, R. L., Chawla, R. P., Joia, B. S., and Tiwana, M. S.,** Excretion of DDT residues into milk of the Indian Buffalo, *Bubalus bubalis (L.)* after oral and dermal exposure, *Pest. Sci.,* 17, 128, 1986.

54. **Takei, G. H., Kauahikaua, and Leong, G. H.,** Analysis of human milk samples collected in Hawaii for residues of organochlorine pesticides and polychlorobiphenyls, *Bull. Environ. Contam. Toxicol.,* 30, 606, 1983.

55. **Wickstrom, K., Pyysalo, H., and Silmes, M. A.,** Levels of chlordane, hexachlorobenzene PCB and DDT compounds in Finnish human milk in 1982, *Bull. Environ. Contam. Toxicol.,* 31, 251, 1983.

56. **Slorach, S. A. and Vaz, R.,** Assessment of Human Exposure to Selected Organochlorine Compounds through Biological Monitoring, prepared for United National Environment Programme and the World Health Organisation in Swedish National Food Administration, Uppsala, 1983.

57. **Baluja, G., Hernandez, L. M., Gonzalez, M. A. J., and Rico, M. A. C.,** Presence of organochlorine pesticides, polychlorinated biphenyls and mercury in Spanish human milk samples, *Bull. Environ. Contam. Toxicol.,* 28, 573, 1982.

58. **Heyndrick, A. and Maes, R.,** The excretion of chlorinated hydrocarbon insecticides in human mother's milk, *J. Pharm. Belg.,* 24, 459, 1969.
59. **Mes, J., Davies, D. J., and Miles, W.,** Traces of mirex in some Canadian human milk samples, *Bull. Environ. Contam. Toxicol.,* 19, 564, 1978.

Chapter 11

PESTICIDES AND REGULATORY MEASURES

Fina P. Kaloyanova-Simeonova and T. S. S. Dikshith

TABLE OF CONTENTS

I. INTRODUCTION

The application of pesticides for agriculture and public health makes them one of the most commonly used chemicals in the world. In fact, the deliberate use of pesticides in high concentrations to kill pests, movement of pesticides in the environment, and the interference of pesticides in the normal body function of man and animals besides causing human poisoning and fatalities are some of the characteristic features that separate pesticides from other toxic chemicals. These characteristics indicate the need for regulating the use of pesticides both for the safety of man and the environment. We present here some of the regulatory measures that are necessary in the overall management of pesticides.

II. ROLE OF INTERNATIONAL ORGANIZATIONS IN THE REGULATION OF PESTICIDES

A. FOOD AND AGRICULTURAL ORGANIZATION (FAO)

More than 30 international organizations are concerned with the regulation of pesticides. The Food and Agriculture Organisation of the United Nations (FAO) plays an important role in the regulation of pesticides since more than 90% of pesticides over these years are used for agriculture. In fact, the main task of the FAO pesticide program has been to help to increase agricultural production of food by advising UN member countries regarding the safe and efficient application of pesticides. For this purpose a set of guidelines has been prepared dealing with the registration and control, environmental criteria for registration, packing and storage, labeling, disposal, quality control, etc.

Special attention may be drawn to the work of the experts panel on Pesticide Residues in Food and the Environment which usually holds joint meetings with the World Health Organization Expert Committee on Pesticide Residues. Their long standing joint activity is reflected in the publication of a number of monographs on assessment of pesticides, determination of acceptable daily intake (ADI) of more than 200 compounds, and maximum residues limits (MRL) of pesticides in different agricultural products. These safety norms are important both for individual countries and for international trade in food products. FAO resolutions are not obligatory for member countries. They have been proposed for use as well as for further discussion in the Commission for Pesticides of the Codex Alimentarius.

The international code of conduct on the distribution and use of pesticides has been drawn up by FAO along with other agencies of the United Nations and international organizations which are concerned with pesticides. The issue of such a document had become necessary because of the emergency situations which had arisen in the last few years as a result of application of pesticides in some countries in which a well-organized preliminary control on pesticides registration was lacking as well as the donation of pesticides not corresponding to established safety standards to developing countries.

The code is aimed to identifying the possible hazards in the distribution and application of pesticides, establishing behavioral standards and determining the responsibilities of persons engaged in the regulation, distribution, and application of pesticides. It is a collection of rules for the guidance of individuals and organizations concerned with pesticides and defines the responsibility of each of them — government, agricultural industry, interested organizations, users, and the general population.

B. WORLD HEALTH ORGANIZATION (WHO)

In the World Health Organization, there is a unit for the development and safe use of pesticides under the Vector Biology and Control (VBC) division. This division is mainly concerned with those pesticides meant for public health application. Its activity in general covers classification of pesticides according to hazard, preparation of educational materials, data sheets (issued together with the FAO), preparation of guidelines, standards, protocols and technical documents, technical reports, etc. Data sheets for more than 70 pesticides have been published so far by the WHO.

The documents of WHO also deal with the following information: restrictions on availability; transportation and storage; handling; disposal and/or decontamination of containers; selection, training and medical supervision of workers; additional regulations sprayed from aircraft; and residues in food.

Useful information is also contained in Document 5 of the World Health Organization — European Bureau, entitled Legislation and Administration, in which the situation in regard to regulation of pesticides in almost all European countries is described. The book, *Control of Pesticides*[2] presents an analysis of the legislation in 11 countries. Valuable information can be obtained also from the data profiles of the International Register for Potential Toxic Chemicals (IRPTC)[3] as well as from the Environmental Health Criteria (EHC), documents issued by the International Programme on Chemical Safety.[4]

In the Council of Mutual Economic Assistance (CMEA) no rigid regulations valid for all member countries have been proposed and the practical application of pesticides is based on a common scientific conceptual background for minimizing the risk to workers, general population, and environment.

The brochure *Pesticides*[5] issued by the European Council contains advice and recommendations to be followed by national and other authorities as well as by manufacturers concerned with registration of agricultural and nonagricultural pesticides.

In the U.S. the application of pesticides is regulated by the Federal Insecticide, Fungicide and Rodenticide Act (FIFRA)[6] and other documents of the U.S. Environmental Protection Agency (EPA).[7,8] In fact, there are no big differences in the regulation of pesticide usage in different countries.[9]

III. MEASURES FOR PRELIMINARY CONTROL

A. NOTIFICATION FOR CLEARANCE

The introduction of a new pesticide is preceded by a thorough hygiene toxicological study in order to give a basis for prediction of its effects upon humans and the environment. In this matter the toxicologist and other related specialists have a great responsibility for generating scientific data taking into account contemporary developments in all sciences, whose methods are used in toxicological analysis.

1. Good Laboratory Practice (GLP)

For more than a decade, a private company engaged in toxicological investigation of a newly synthesized chemical compound submitted false data without conducting any toxicological investigations in animals. As a consequence of this serious lapse, the U.S. Food and Drug Administration (FDA) introduced a system called Good Laboratory Practice (GLP) as well as a program for inspection of laboratories carrying out toxicological investigations in order to assess to what extent they observe the rules and requirements of this system.

The requirements of GLP cover different laboratory processes and operations. A special unit for quality assurance carries out periodic checking of the laboratory to make sure that all experiments are carried out according to the requirements. The properties of substances to be investigated should be well characterized. Only preliminary investigations for acute toxicity may be performed without full characterization, in view of the fact that some chemicals may prove to be highly toxic and undesirable for further development. Special requirements are given regarding the protocol of investigations as well as the care of animals in respect of their isolation, health control, etc. Requirements of the storage of specimens for further investigation are also specified. Some proposals have been made for changes in the requirements included in the scheme of GLP because some of the requirements significantly raise the cost of the investigation and take much time without justification.[10] Regarding the reliability and corrections of the data produced in different private laboratories and used in international trade, the companies and the notifier should have the complete responsibility.

B. NOTIFICATION DATA SCHEME

The data necessary for registration of pesticides is given below.

1. General Information

Name and address of applicant and manufacturer
Trade name of the product formulation

Type of product (insecticide, fungicide, herbicide, etc.)
Type of crop to be treated, type of pests to be controlled, materials to be protected
Methods of application (high volume, ultra low volume (ULV), fumigation, etc.)
Working solutions of pesticide
Application rate, number and time of applications (season or stage of growth)

2. Identity and Chemical and Physical Properties of the Product

Chemical name in IUPAC nomenclature, common and trade name, code number, etc.
Empirical and structural formula
Physical state, color, odor, and formulation
Molecular weight, melting point, boiling point, flash point
Specific gravity, vapor pressure, solubility in water and in organic solvent
Degree of purity, nature of impurities or additives, and their percentage
Thermal decomposition — hazardous products
Stability under other conditions

3. Experimental Data on Toxicity in Animals

a. Acute Toxicity

LD_{50} in rats (oral)
LD_{50} (approximate) in other animals (oral)
LD_{50} in rabbits and rats (dermal)
LC_{50} in rats (inhalation)
Skin irritation in rats and guinea pigs
Eye irritation in rabbits

b. Repeated Dose Toxicity (One Month)

Oral toxicity — oral application in two species of animals, one of them not rodent; coefficient of accumulation with three doses, one of which is toxic
Percutaneous toxicity with three doses in three groups of rabbits or rats and the same number of controls
Inhalation toxicity at three doses, one of them toxic
Tests for delayed toxicity in case of organophosphates and carbamates

c. Subchronic Toxicity (Three Months)

Oral, percutaneous, and inhalation

d. Long-Term (Chronic) Toxicity

Oral application in at least two species, one of which not rodent, 1 to 2 years
Three doses, one of them nontoxic
Inhalation toxicity with three concentrations, 4 months
Determination of the threshold concentration

e. Metabolic Studies

Information on metabolism of pesticides and their transformation products in the treated plants, metabolites, or other products of transformation. If the products of transformation are different from the metabolites in test animals, data of the chronic toxicological investigations of the metabolites of other products of transformation may be required.
Toxic effects of metabolites or impurities, data in two species of animals; penetration through organism, distribution, metabolic transformation, excretion

f. Reproduction Studies

Three generation test at three dose levels, one with toxic effect. Two offspring of each generation are preferred. Both male and female should be treated for a period of 60 days from the period of growth; second and third generations are treated from the moment of cessation of suckling through the whole period of growth.

g. Teratogenicity
Three dose levels, one with toxic effect to the mother

h. Mutagenicity
Gene mutation in bacteria, chromosomal aberration in *in vivo* cytogenetic tests in animals; dominant lethal effects

i. Carcinogenicity
Three dose levels, the highest being the maximum tolerated dose, duration of treatment for the normal life span

4. Observation in Man
Industrial and agricultural exposure, accidental poisoning and suicide as well as controlled experiments on volunteers in special cases
Diagnosis, specific signs of poisoning, clinical tests
Treatment, first-aid measures

5. Residues in Treated Crops
Principle residues (parent compound, breakdown products, and metabolites) in edible crops, food or fodder
Suggested metabolite analysis
Information on accuracy, precision (including recovery data), specificity, sensitivity, limit of determination, and applicability
Residue data in named edible crops, food or fodder
Degradation rates in plants
Residues in products of domestic animal origin (fed on treated plants) — meat, milk, eggs

6. Behavior in the Environment and Ecotoxicological Effects
Persistence in the soil and water; period of decomposition and mode of inactivation; identification of major metabolites; mobility and transport; bioaccumulation.
Toxicity to birds, fish, and bees

7. Measures for the Safe Use of Pesticides
Labeling information
Safety during storage, transportation, and application
Personal protective clothes and equipment
Maximum permissible levels
Reentry period/waiting period before harvest
Disposal of surplus pesticide and pesticide containers
Clearance and conditions of clearance in the country of the producer and in other countries

C. HAZARD CLASSIFICATION OF PESTICIDES
There exist numerous classifications of toxic substances including pesticides in which the data on lethal doses by oral and dermal routes are mainly taken into consideration.
The most widely used classification is that of the World Health Organization[14,15] approved by its general assembly in 1975 and completed later with guidelines in 1978, 1979, 1980,

TABLE 1
WHO Classification of Pesticide by Hazard

| | LD$_{50}$ for the rat (mg/kg body weight) | | | |
| | Oral | | Dermal | |
Class	Solids[a]	Liquids[a]	Solids[a]	Liquids[a]
I[a] Extremely hazardous	4 or less	20 or less	10 or less	40 or less
I[b] Highly hazardous	5—50	20—200	10—100	40—400
II Moderately hazardous	50—500	200—2000	100—1000	400—4000
III Slightly hazardous	Over 500	Over 2000	Over 1000	Over 4000

[a] The terms "solids" and "liquids" refer to the physical state of the product or formulation being classified.

1982, and 1984 (Table 1). The classification of WHO includes LD$_{50}$ in rats by oral and dermal application. The substances are divided into solids and liquids although this classification is based only on acute toxicological parameters, in the lists added to it later for grouping the technical products into different classes. This shortcoming is corrected by taking into consideration other effects of the substances. Depending on these effects, a given formulation is referred to as either more toxic or less toxic respectively. For example, calcium cyanide is assigned class I A type since on contact with moisture it generates hydrogen cyanide. Arsenous oxide has also been kept in category class IA because the minimum lethal dose for humans is 2 mg/kg body weight, although for animals it is 180 mg/kg. Leptophos, which is known for its delayed neurotoxicity, has been assigned the most hazardous class. Anticoagulants are often highly toxic to rats; however, in humans they do not represent a hazard since the anticoagulative effect is known to manifest after multiple oral application of definite doses.

Pesticides depending upon their hazard are classified as follows:

Extremely hazardous
Highly hazardous
Moderately hazardous
Slightly hazardous

The LD$_{50}$ values for technical products are taken into consideration in these lists. Classification of any product also depends on its formulation. For example, the smaller is the percentage of pesticide in the formulation the lower is the class to which it is assigned. If such data are not obtainable, proportional calculation for LD$_{50}$ values of the technical ingredient is made according to the formula:

$$\frac{LD_{50} \text{ active ingredient} \times 100}{\text{Percentage of active ingredient in formulation}}$$

The question of classification of mixtures of pesticides has also been considered in WHO classification, where several possibilities are given. For instance, if an oral and dermal LD$_{50}$ are available for the mixtures, the classification is performed on the basis of those data. The other method is to classify the pesticide according to the most hazardous constituent of the mixture as if that constituent was present in the same concentration in all active constituents, and as a third possibility a formula is given on the basis of which LD$_{50}$ for the mixture can be calculated.

$$\frac{C_a}{LD_{50}(a)} + \frac{C_b}{LD_{50}(b)} + \frac{C_n}{LD_{50}(n)} + \frac{100}{LD_{50}(\text{mixture})}$$

where C = the % concentration of constituent a,b. . . . . n in the mixture.

Our classification of pesticide by hazard is a modification and further development of the hygienic toxicological classification proposed by Medved et al.[13] The necessary information for an integral assessment and evaluation of pesticides from a health and environmental point of view is also available.[14,15] The new version deals with the WHO classification to differentiate substances into solid and liquid, as well as to include additional criteria (Table 2).

D. DATA ASSESSMENT AND CLEARANCE

Permission for application from the point of view of health and environment protection is issued after investigation and assessment of the detailed toxicological characterization, as well as after making other studies on the behavior of the substances in the environment. Only such a pesticide should have a clearance which, if correctly applied, would not pose a hazard for humans, animals, and the environment. No pesticide should be registered for sale and application without prior completion of all necessary tests which makes possible an integral assessment of the eventual negative effects upon human health and the environment. While it is in the process of development, the pesticide may be given permission for limited application with a view to assess its efficiency.

The assessment of data with a view to decision making for application of a pesticide becomes even more difficult. Nevertheless, the results obtained in scientific research are a solid basis for decision making, although some investigations may often be incomplete or not sufficiently predictive for the eventual negative effects upon human health and environment, and for the possibility of their appearance, type, and strength. This question should be considered in dynamics, during a given period of time, since new data concerning different effects are gathered continually, especially delayed effects, and the methods of determination of pesticides in environment become stringent.

According to Truhaut,[16] assessments should be based on such data, which are not only results of a rigid protocol, but are obtained in clearly directed investigations with particular reference to the structure of the physicochemical properties and the conditions of the use and exposure to pesticides. Of great significance is the biochemical panorama of the investigations, which makes possible the understanding of adsorption, distribution in the fluids, organs, and tissues of the body, excretion, and toxicokinetics of pesticides. This is important in order to make a qualitative and quantitative assessment of the mechanism of pesticide action and its difference among species. When a decision is to be made, the social benefit from the use of a chemical should be assessed applying the classical benefit/risk criterion. For example, in some cases, the fungicide applied can be very useful in inhibiting the development of mycotoxins, which are more dangerous than fungicides.

1. Trial Clearance

Such permission is given only for a definite period and for a limited quantity of the chemical to be applied by highly qualified personnel of the company producing and developing the respective pesticide formulation. Permission of this category is usually given for a minimum of 100 kg of the pesticide with LD_{50} less than 100 mg/kg, and 1000 kg of the pesticide with LD_{50} less than 100 mg/kg. In these cases if the treated plants are to be used for consumption by animals or man, a special permission from the regulatory body is required.

2. Provisional Clearance

The pesticide may be given a provisional clearance for a period of 1 to 2 years when the complete toxicological information for that pesticide is available and only some data concerning the environmental effects upon wild animals in particular, and data on residues, as well as the results for delayed effects are incomplete or have not been evaluated. The

TABLE 2
Classification of Pesticides by Hazard for the Purpose of Regulation

Factors		Class I (extremely hazardous)	Class II (highly hazardous)	Class III (moderately hazardous)	Class IV (slightly hazardous)
LD_{50} for rat (perorally)	Liquid	Up to 450 mg/kg	50—100 mg/kg	100—1000 mg/kg	Above 1000 mg/kg
	Solid	Up to 10 mg/kg	10—30 mg/kg	30—300 mg/kg	Above 300 mg/kg
LD_{50} for rat (percutaneous)	Liquid	Up to 100 mg/kg	100—500 mg/kg	500—2000 mg/kg	Above 2000 mg/kg
	Solid	Up to 30 mg/kg	30—150 mg/kg	150—600 mg/mg	Above 600 mg/mg
LC_{50} for rat 4 hr inhalatory exposure		Up to 200 mg/m³; the concentration of saturation is higher or equal to the toxic dose, provokes heavy acute poisonings	200—1000 mg/m³; the concentration of saturation is higher than the threshold	1000—5000 mg/m³; the concentration of saturation causes slight effect and is about threshold	Above 5000 mg/m³; the concentration of saturation provokes no effect
Coefficient of accumulation (K) $K = \dfrac{nDL_{50}}{DL_{50}}$		K = under 1	K = 1—3	K = 3—5	K = above 5
Persistence in the environment, period of decomposition, bioaccumulation, nitrozation		Very persistent above 1 year	Persistent 6 months to 1 year, bioaccumulation, nitrozation in the environment	Moderately persistent, 1—6 months, no accumulation, no nitrozation	Slightly persistent under 1 month
Blastomogenicity		Proven human cancerogens, strong cancerogens for test animals	Slightly cancerogenic for test animals; effect in less than 20% of the animals with maximum nontoxic doses; suspected cancerogen	No cancerogenic effect	No cancerogenic effect
Teratogenicity		Proven human abnormalities, reproducible in test animals; teratogenic activity in animals with doses not in practice	Strong teratogens; affect more than 50% of the offspring of test animals at doses not toxic to the mother. Polytropic adverse effects. Effect in more than one type of test animal	Provokes anomalies in less than 50% of offspring with doses not toxic for mother; teratogenic effect in one type of test animal; affects single organ or system; effective dose above 1/10 LD_{50}	No teratogenicity

TABLE 2 (continued)
Classification of Pesticides by Hazard for the Purpose of Regulation

Factors	Class I (extremely hazardous)	Class II (highly hazardous)	Class III (moderately hazardous)	Class IV (slightly hazardous)
Embryotoxicity	Not recorded in the assessment	Selective embryotoxicity manifested with doses nontoxic for the mother	Moderate embryotoxic effect manifested with doses toxic for mother	No embryotoxic effect
Character of intoxication	Acute heavy poisonings possible in practical application; pronounced specific irreversible effects	Probable acute poisoning and specific irreversible effects	Acute poisonings only in exceptional conditions	Acute poisonings are not probable
Therapeutic possibility	No special treatment; poor therapeutic possibility	Fair therapeutic possibility; antidotes available	Good therapeutic possibility; antidotes available	Good therapeutic possibility; specific treatment
Irritation of the skin	Very strong irritant; chemical burning; acute toxic dermatitis from concentrated formulations; toxic dermatitis from working solutions	Strong irritant; speedy development of symptoms; toxic dermatitis from concentrated formulations; cumulative effect of working solution	Irritant; cumulative dermatitis from concentrated formulation	Practically nonirritant
Irritation of the eyes and upper respiratory organs	Working solutions have irritant effect	Working solutions have slightly irritant effect	Formulation with irritant effect	Formulation and working solution with no practical irritant effect
Allergic sensitization	Allergic and photosensibilizing effect in humans; positive evidence of sensibilization of guinea pigs	Allergic effect in humans; negative sensitizing test in guinea pigs	Presumed sensitizing effect on the basis of chemical structure	No sensitizing effect

Notes: 1. When decision on preliminary sanitary control is being made, some pesticides may be put in an adjacent class of hazard. In addition to the limiting criteria, the remaining toxicological properties, type of formulation, and economic importance are considered.

2. The criterion of inhalation toxicity is taken as limiting if in practical application of pesticides there are conditions for creating vapors, liquids, or solid aerosol concentrations of the pesticide near to those mentioned in the classification.

provisional clearance usually does not impose limitation on the quantities of the formulation to be used. It is supposed that for the period of this clearance, additional data will be obtained and submitted for revision of this clearance and eventually for the issue of permanent clearance. In some countries, including Bulgaria, a provisional clearance is given in cases when all necessary data are presented, but some fears exist for acute intoxication in the course of the application of the pesticide, or if some of the presented data should be repeated. A period of 1 or 2 years is necessary for precise specification of these questions.

3. Permanent Clearance

A permanent permission for the use of a pesticide means that it may be applied in unlimited quantities for an unlimited period of time. Nevertheless, some limitation may exist with regard to the plants to which the chemical may be applied, as well as to the percentage solution which may be used and the formulation permitted for use. For example, a pesticide with high toxicity may be prohibited for use as emulsion and may be permitted for use in the form of granules. The permanent clearance is also subject to reasessments in connection with new information for the negative effects of the pesticide on the one hand, and eventually for a more wide application upon other cultures if the data for the substances are favorable, on the other hand. Together with the issue of clearance the necessary preventive measures and hygienic norms and requirements are recommended, and if the clearance is permanent — the label of the pesticide formulation is approved.

Different practices exist for issue of clearance to new pesticide formulations which are to be introduced, or to old products intended to be registered for other purposes. A dominating practice is that the clearances which are issued from the point of view of pesticide safety are given regardless of the decision of the agricultural bodies for their respective application. That means that the body which is authorized to deal with the question of the safe use of pesticides has the right of veto its application. In other countries, however, the decision for a pesticide's registration from the point of view of its efficiency is made simultaneously with that for its safety. Most often this is performed by a commission within the frames of the Ministry of Agriculture. In such cases the priority of the health and environmental criteria cannot always be guaranteed. It is necessary that a list of the permitted pesticides be issued every year with a full statement of their conditions of application and prevention.

E. SOME SPECIAL PROBLEMS
1. Impurities and the Need for Specification

The necessity of a precise specification of the products and the regulation of the contents of the different contaminants have been evoked in the recent years especially in connection with some accidents. Specification of the chemicals used for public health is performed by the WHO,[17] while for those used in agriculture by FAO. The specifications contain a description of the formulation and its constituent requirements with regard to its physical and chemical properties.

Pesticides in the form of a ready-to-be-used formulation are usually a mixture of a technical substances and a number of solvents and additives (stabilizers, dyes, surfactants etc.), some of which could be of toxicological importance. According to Rosival and Batora,[18] the source of impurities can be divided into main and secondary sources.

The source material for pesticide production may initially contain impurities. The amines used to produce alkyl amine salts of phenoxyalkane carboxylic acids may contain nitrosoalkylamines. In addition, the manufacturing technology includes reactions which inevitably result in pesticides containing by-products. For instance, ethylene thiourea (ETU) is formed in ethylene bis-dithiocarbamate, N-nitrate-alkylamines appear in dinitroaniline herbicides such as trifluralin, and TCDD and other dioxins occur in chlorophenoxy herbicides and pentachlorphenol.

Secondary sources include the unsuitable formulation of technical grade active ingredients, for example, the isomerization of organophosphorus thioates and dithioates. Unsuitable storage of pesticides may also lead to the physicochemical transformation of the product.

Information about the composition of certain technical grade pesticides or their formulation (toxaphene, chlorinated terpenes, HCH) is very often inadequate. There are some pesticides which are produced by several manufacturers, and this leads to variations in the consumption of technical products, especially with respect to contaminants.

The impurities of organophosphate (OP) compounds with their high toxicity are of great importance. Although it has been known since the 1950s that the interaction of malathion with other OP compounds potentiates the toxicity of the latter and that the toxicity of malathion can be influenced by impurities in the technical products,[19] the role of OP impurities in malathion formulations for field application and the consequent increased toxicity was not fully recognized. A major poisoning incident occurred in 1976 in Pakistan during a malaria control program in which large amounts of different brands of commercial malathion were dispersed. About 2800 of the 7500 sprayers became ill, and five deaths occurred. It was found that the toxic isomerization product of malathion, namely, isomalathion together with poor application practice were responsible for the intoxications.[20,21] The specification for malathion has been changed in accordance with the recommendation of the WHO Expert Committee[22] to include a test which limits the formation of isomalathion content. A summary of the toxicity of malathion and some trimethyl phosphorothioates is presented in a recent report of a WHO study group.[23]

During the manufacture of 2,4,5-trichlorphenol precursors, 2,3,7,8-tetrachlordibenzo-p-dioxin (TCDD) is formed as a contaminant. It is found as an impurity in 2,4,5-T and pentachlorphenol in concentrations up to 0, 25 mg/kg and represents an environmental problem. There are data on chronic intoxications with TCDD among workers occupationally exposed during production of herbicides.[24,25] The workers showed chloracne, liver metabolic functional disturbances, focal neurological, and psychic disorders and EMG abnormalities.

Nitrosamines are a large class of compounds and some of them are known to be highly carcinogenic in animals. Nitrosamine contaminants in certain pesticide formulations have been established, and formation of nitrosamines during manufacturing is reported. The presence of nitrosodipropylamine (NDPA) contaminants in dinitroaniline herbicides (trifluralin) results from nitrosation of the dipropylamine with residual nitrogen oxides present in the reaction mixture from previous nitration steps. Other dinitroanilines manufactured by similar processes also contain nitrosamines as impurities.[26]

Formation of nitrosamines is also possible during storage of the formulated pesticide. For example, the substituted phenoxy and benzoic acids are often formulated as amine salts (dimethylamine, diethylamine) and stored in metal containers treated with nitrite as an anticorrosive agent. The problem could be solved by using other corrosive inhibitors. Up to 640 ppm of nitrosodimethylamine was detected in a formulation of 2,3,6-trichlorobenzoic acid. The above examples clearly demonstrate the necessity of regulation of all main and secondary sources of impurities in pesticides which pose a danger to humans and the environment.

2. Ecotoxicology

Ecotoxicology is concerned with the toxic effects of chemical and physical agents on living organisms, especially on population and communities within defined ecosystems; it includes the transfer pathways of those agents and their interaction with the environment.[27]

Ecotoxicology in brief has four aspects of study: the first is concerned with the quantity, forms, and sites of release of the toxic substance into the environment; the second aspect deals with the transport in a biotic geographic environment and biotic media both of the substances and their metabolites which could have different behavior in the environment and different toxic properties; the third part deals with the assessment of the exposure with evaluation of the nature of the target and type of exposure; while in the fourth part estimation is made of the responses of the individual organism within a population or community for the appropriate time to the specific contaminant.[28] In order to obtain a meaningful toxicological assessment, the combination of these four stages should be studied in a quantitative and integrated way. It is evident that in such an assessment many uncertainties and errors may lie, and an evaluation should be made of the investigation which should be performed in the future for the solution of these problems.

All these considerations are especially valid with regard to pesticides which disperse in the environment in large quantities. It is difficult to decide to what extent investigations could be performed for prediction of the behavior of the substances and their exotoxicological effects. The schemes existing up till now envisage such investigations upon fish, the aquatic environment, birds, mammals, and bees, and for phytotoxicity upon definite kind of flora, upon useful insects, and soil organisms.

In our opinion, when there is talk about ecotoxicological investigation, the effects upon communities should be borne in mind — either aquatic or terrestrial. So, laboratory conditions would not be suitable in imitating and modeling the conditions as they exist in the environment. The study of wild animals, only during a trial assessment of pesticides in the field could hardly be sufficient for making a final decision on the perspectiveness of the application of a given pesticide. Maybe in the future, it would lead to further development of regulatory activities to identify the effects on pesticides upon definite ecosystem. In recent years, efforts have been made to develop methodologies to ecotoxicological investigation, modeling, and predicton of a variety of toxic chemicals including pesticides.[29-31]

3. Effects on Humans

It is a practice, that on the basis of animal data, predictions can be made for eventual effects on man, and the recommendations are normally outlined for safe work and application of the pesticides. Although this practice generally proves to be correct, it would be useful to test such extrapolation from animals to man by means of medical observations upon people who are occupationally exposed to pesticide during different stages of their development. The necessity of data for human exposure obtained in conditions of current application of pesticide is well underlined by Copplestone.[32]

IV. MEASURES

A. LABELING, TRANSPORT, AND STORAGE
1. Requirements for Labeling

The label contains printed information which is found in or on each container. It contains detailed information and instruction for use of the pesticide. Labeling is important for prevention of intoxicants. The label should be written in the language of the user country. All labels should contain the following information: name and address of manufacturer; name of the pesticide (trade, common or chemical name); registered use of product; physical nature of the formulation; percentage of the active ingredients; additives; direction for use; pests to be controlled; crops or animals to be treated; weight or volume of the pack; dosage and method of application; warning to protect the user and the environment; the statement Keep Out of Reach of Children indications for toxicity group; and appropriate warning of risk and symbols according to the accepted practice in the country. The label should also state what protective clothing and equipment are required during pesticide application, the reentry periods, and first-aid instructions etc.

2. Transport

During the past years the practice of simultaneous transportation of pesticides together with food stuffs in ships and other vehicles has been the cause of a number of poisonings.[14] There are many international plans which are the basis for transportation of pesticide by air, road, rail, inland water ways, and sea. Important protective measures to avoid accidents are the use of safe containers of the pesticides and the correct labeling of the container with indication of the content and the necessary warning signs.

3. Storage

Regulation for the storage of pesticide should be specified for different levels of management. They are usually well stored and the respective accommodations are well organized at the national or district levels. However, at the place of application of a pesticide the practice differs depending upon the country. In private farms, for example, in The Netherlands, the owners have separate storehouses for pesticides. In this country, farms are usually specialized producing monocultures, and the owners have special agricultural education, hence the danger of poisoning and abuse of pesticides is minimum. However, in countries where agriculture is at a lower level of development and agricultural workers have little or no education the use of pesticides on private farms should be considered hazardous.

In the villages of some countries such as Egypt, the local authorities have organized the agricultural centers where warehouse equipment and pesticides for the whole village are stored; the pesticides are usually applied by specialized workers and rarely by the farmers themselves. In countries with agricultural cooperatives, such as Bulgaria, for example, warehouses are specially equipped to store pesticides for the whole village or group of villages. They are in the vicinity of the rooms for working and have facilities for decontamination and personal hygiene.

The proper labeling and arrangement of the chemicals in the warehouse is especially important, because the labels may sometimes come off or become dirty, or some packing may break. Besides, the locking and surveillance of pesticides by specially trained persons is of great importance in order to avoid indiscriminate use of pesticides by unreliable persons.

B. USE AND DISPOSAL

1. Use of Pesticides

The use of pesticides which are highly toxic to man should be entrusted to specialists. Specialization can readily be achieved in collective organizations. It is more difficult, but not impossible, in the case of an individual organization. In this case, a body (the status of which will vary with the country concerned) may be responsible for the use of products and have adequate personnel to deal with the situation.

The specialized personnel has the advantage of knowing the technical utilization and the risk involved. They will also have available means for correct application and may be acquainted with emergency action such as evacuation of workers from the zone of accident, if any.

The selection and training of workers is of a decisive importance, particularly for preventing poisoning. The agricultural use of pesticides should be regulated and workers engaged in applying hazardous pesticides should be subjected to regular surveillance. In fact, a well-organized system should be established in every country for this purpose.

In the prevention of occupational poisoning with pesticides the mode of their application is of particular significance. Because of this, the apparatus and equipment for treating plants with pesticides are also subject to regulation. These equipments are submitted to thorough hygienic assessment at regular intervals.

The improvement of the equipment for pesticide spraying may reduce the worker's contact with pesticides. In this respect, the practice shows that highly efficient machines do not always possess the necessary qualities from the point of view of health. Technical improvements should not be approved *a priori* from the hygienic standpoint without investigations under actual agricultural conditions. Obviously, in addition to engineering specifications the toxicity of the formulation must be kept in mind when a machine is being selected. For example, knapsack sprayers are unsuitable for work with organophosphorus formulations which have high mammalian toxicity. Machines capable of performing the maximum volume of work and number of operations with less people engaged in them are given perference. Such machines are, of course, the aircrafts for agricultural aviation which perform a large volume of work. Among the ground machines, preference is given to those, which do not require additional personnel besides the driver, with all other operations are performed by spraying devices. At the present stage of development of plant protection, it is unallowable to use hand apparated equipment for treating plants. Such practice might be allowed only for small lots and with low toxicity compounds.

Of special importance is the right cleaning and maintenance of the apparatus. A full harmonization in the preparation of the solutions and their transfer into containers/sprayers is necessary.

Another important feature, relevant to labor hygiene, is the application of such methods, which requires less pesticide for treatment of a given area. The role of the formulation of a safe use of pesticides has been stressed by many authors.[18]

In the case of agricultural aviation a strict regulation and definition of responsibility is needed to avoid pollution of dams, lakes, reservoirs, and canals, as well as to protect flagmen and to avoid flying over busy roads. The role of aviation consists basically of fulfilling the operation in a safe and correct way. All other work connected with supplying chemicals, their storage, preparation of solutions, loading the plane with the chemical, and cleaning and washing up the plane and equipment should be performed by persons specially assigned for the purpose. Especially dangerous is the work of the flagmen who shows the pilot from the ground the limits within which he should fly. The flagman should be very well provided with the necessary personal protective means.

The equipment of the plane should be maintained in perfect condition, so that the spray of pesticides will reach only places to which they are assigned.

Most often, the pesticides are applied in liquid form, and rarely as dust or granules when a plane is used. In particular, the aerial dusting is a disappearing technique in view of the risk of environmental pollution connected with it. High skill and competence of the pilot is required for flying at the necessary height and with the adequate speed, carefully weighing the wind, so as to direct pesticides to the right area. For the development of legislation and regulatory measures in connection with the aerial application of pesticides a very good cooperation between the bodies responsible for agriculture, aviation, and public health is necessary.

2. Disposal of Pesticides

The question of disposal of pesticides, disqualified and undesirable for agriculture, as well as of pesticide containers, is very difficult to resolve. The wrong practice of locating polluted containers near and performing decontamination of the machines and equipment near the vicinity of water should be strictly prohibited. Burning of pesticide contaminated bags should not be carried out in a neighborhood or settlement. The best alternative would be to send back the empty containers for recycling whenever this is possible. The current opinion is that the best method to treat pesticide residues is simply to continue their application on soil and plants in low concentration, so that degradation of the pesticide occurs in the natural environment.

C. REENTRY PERIODS

Group intoxications are often observed in people who have worked in areas treated (usually by plane) with organophosphorus pesticides at different reentry periods after application of the pesticide.

Depending upon the crops cultivated and the climatic conditions, the disintegration of the pesticide and its formulations take place with different speed. Therefore, it is necessary to determine the reentry period for each pesticide depending on its concentration and the plant sprayed so that agricultural workers might be allowed to work in such areas without any hazard for their health.

Determination of the reentry period is important when vegetable material treated with organophosphorus or carbamate pesticides are handled by a large group of people. Such periods are established for tobacco plantations, orchards, citrus and vegetable gardens, greenhouse cultures etc. In fact, a special method for a reentry period determination has been developed by Kaloyanova and Izmirova.[35] Minimum reentry period is defined as the minimum interval in days after treatment necessary for degradation of the pesticide in the plant to such an extent that the contact with the latter would not be toxic to workers.

The theoretical basis of this new norm is directly connected with the other hygienic norms. In it, too, the medical criteria are given priority. The main criterion is the full security that the workers health will not be impaired while working with pesticides if such exposure continues during the whole working day. The minimum reentry periods for safe work can be efficient if plates showing the data of the reentry period are placed at some distances on the edge of the treated area.

The method for determination of reentry periods includes (1) study of the dynamics of degradation of pesticides and (2) determination of the residues of pesticides on the plants which do not produce any effect upon a human being. For this purpose the effect of organophosphorus pesticides is observed by means of periodic examination of the level of the cholinesterase activity (AchE) in serum in workers exposed to plant material treated with these compounds, as well as by the level of pesticide quantity on the surface of the plant material (mg/kg) being determined simultaneously. The aim is to establish the level of residues which does not cause a decrease in AchE activity after a few days of contact with the plant material earlier treated with an organophosphorus pesticide.

Determination of the reentry periods for safe work is possible after observations are carried out in field conditions.

Independent of the established initial quantity of pesticides upon the surface of the vegetable material different reentry periods are determined.

However, if equal quantities of a given pesticide are used/sprayed with the same technique, the plants contain similar quantities of the pesticide upon their leaves and fruits. It is possible, therefore, to avoid analysis of the washings each time, and to determine the reentry period on the basis of existing initial investigations.

Reentry period is often influenced by other factors such as degradation speed in soil and air, temperature and humidity of the environment, wind speed etc. Besides these, the capacity of the pesticide to accumulate in the body and to produce delayed effects, is certainly of importance. The dynamics of degradation of the pesticide and its respective effects upon AchE activity in the workers should be studied.

D. MEDICAL SUPERVISION AND PERSONAL PROTECTION
1. Medical Supervision

Persons who work with pesticides should be subjected to close and regular medical examination. The medical supervision should be designed to perform preliminary medical examinations to determine the persons who are not to be allowed to work with pesticides because of illness; to carry out the necessary periodic examinations or tests for detection of any potential harmful effects at the earliest possible stage; to advise and to organize first-aid and medical care assistance in cases of emergency; and to train special staff who could be of help in such exigencies. The medical supervision should be directed by a doctor with knowledge of occupational health.

2. Health Education

The prevention of poisoning by pesticides calls for important education of the occupational workers in particular and the public in general. The danger of fatal poisoning of children calls for special attention. For example, Watanobe[36] showed that in 17 of 50 children who on their way to school passed through a farm sprayed with parathion the level of AchE showed reduction with the presence of paranitrophenol in the urine. In fact, about 80% of the children suffered parathion-induced poisoning.

3. Personal Hygiene and Individual Protection

In order to protect workers from pesticide induced toxicity due to dermal contact or respiratory exposure, it is necessary to use protective means, which include respirators, gloves, aprons, special clothes, boots, hats, and goggles. They should be maintained in a working condition and be decontaminated every time after work.

Clothes and under garments should be washed everyday after use. The personal protective equipment must also be decontaminated each time after use. If protection by respirators is necessary, the expiring terms of such equipment should be strictly observed.

In agriculture the problem of designing special clothing and means of individual protection is greater than in industry. For instance, in hot climates, great difficulties arise because the worker finds it hard to use special clothing. Rearrangement of the working day could help to minimizing the hazard. In well-organized farms the washing of the workers is performed in a special complex of sanitary-filter type, where underwear and clothes are changed which will reduce the hazard to a considerable extent.

V. MANAGEMENT OF PESTICIDES IN DEVELOPING AND DEVELOPED COUNTRIES

Agricultural practices have become more and more complex due to intensive monoculture and development of newer molecules of pesticides to contain pests in different agro- and geoclimatic regions of the world. A need has arisen for the proper management of regulatory activities at state, national, and international levels. Regulatory Acts such as FIFRA 1947 and its Amendment in 1978 (U.S.), Insecticide Act, 1968 (India), Pesticide Act (No. 33) 1980 (Sri Lanka), and others in different countries have helped to ensure proper management of pesticides.[2,6,37-42]

Products of agricultural farming have been of great importance in international trade and in recent years they have taken on political as well as economic significance. Concern for the health effects of pesticide residue has resulted in a major United Nations (UN) effort to establish internationally recognized tolerance for different pesticide residues. This is a tremendous task which involves different concepts to determine acceptable levels. Each country has to decide for itself whether or not to accept the recommendations, known as Codex Alimentarius of the UN group. In fact, this group recommends quality standards for trade in pesticides. This has an inevitable effect upon other countries, and suggests the desirability for some kind of compatibility between countries in the regulation and management of pesticides.

A. BANGLADESH

Bangladesh is an agricultural country. Agriculture is the mainstay of its national economy. Pesticides have been in use in Bangladesh since 1956. At first, the government used to import and distribute pesticides to farmers free of cost. This system continued for about

24 years. In 1979 with a view to improving the plant protection activities in the country, government handed over the pesticide trade to the private sector. However, the use of pesticides in Bangladesh is regulated by the Agricultural Pesticides Amendment Act, 1980.

At present there is only one pesticide manufacturing unit, the DDT factory at Chittagong, managed by Bangladesh Chemical Industry Corporation. The factory manufactures Technical DDT which is used as DDT 75% W.P. for malaria eradication. The annual production capacity of technical DDT is 1500 M.T., while that of DDT 75% W.P. is 2000 M.T.[43]

B. BURMA

The activities of agricultural pest control in Burma are managed by the Agricultural Corporation which looks after (1) research on pest control techniques; (2) advice to farmers on appropriate pest control techniques; (3) assistance in pest control activities; and (4) procurement and distribution of agro-pesticides and application equipment. The Department of Health is responsible for the activities in the field of public vector control.

1. Supply and Distribution System of Pesticides

Interestingly, Burma neither manufactures nor formulates pesticides. In fact, all pesticides used in the country are imported as formulated products. There are about 9000 distribution points all over the country which supply the agropesticides to the farmers. The Department of Health is responsible for the procurement and distribution of insecticides required for public health and vector control program.

In Burma, many elements of pesticide regulation and management are nonexistent. For example, there are no acts to govern the management of agrochemicals and no list to restrict the use of highly toxic pesticides. In fact, the quality control, licensing, and distribution of pesticides by qualified agents and professional applicators are completely lacking.[44]

C. INDIA

A variety of pesticides are manufactured and used in India for purposes of controlling crop pests and vectors of diseases. With the intensive agricultural practices and because of agro- and geoclimatic variation in the country, the demands for more pesticides have also increased.

The occurrence of pesticide poisoning in some parts of India during 1958 and similar cases in the rest of the world like the United Kingdom, United States, Burma, and Turkey around the same time necessitated India to streamline the regulation of pesticides.

The government of India accordingly constituted a high power committee to advise the measures of legislation. This resulted in the promulgation of regulations in the form of the Insecticides Act, 1968, which includes several schedules and related sections for the safe handling, transportation, manufacture, and use of pesticides in India.[40] There are 38 sections under the Insecticide Act, some of which are

- The Central Insecticides Board
- Registration committee
- Secretary and other officers
- Registration of insecticides
- Appeal against nonregistration or cancellation
- Power of revision of central government
- Licensing officers
- Grant of license
- Revocation, suspension, and amendment of officer
- Appeal against the decision of a licensing officer
- Central Insecticide Laboratory

- Prohibition of sale, etc. of certain insecticides
- Insecticide analysis
- Powers of insecticide inspectors
- Procedure to be followed by insecticide inspectors
- Persons bound to disclose place where insecticides are manufactured or kept
- Report of insecticide analyst
- Confiscation
- Notification of poisoning
- Prohibition of sale, etc. of insecticides for reasons of public safety
- Notification of cancellation of registration etc.
- Offenses and punishment
- Defenses which may or may not be allowed in prosecutions under the Act
- Cognizance and trial of offenses
- Magistrate's power to impose enhanced penalties
- Offenses by companies
- Power of central government to give directions
- Protection of action taken in good faith
- Power of central government to make rules
- Power of the state government to make rules

The Central Insecticides Board constituted by the Ministry of Agriculture, Government of India acts as an apex body and is the regulatory authority for pesticides. All pesticides, both technical and formulated, are to be registered with the Central Insecticides Board before introduction into the market.

The registration of pesticides is based on the good points of the U.K. and U.S. systems and keeping in view the standard practices followed elsewhere, including EPA guidelines. Further FAO, WHO, and EPA guidelines are given due consideration by the registration committee to meet the national requirements.

The laboratory-based toxicological and other data are accepted by the Registration Committee. Data on bioefficacy and residue should however, be generated under Indian conditions. For registration purposes, the data are required to be generated under local conditions for each product in accordance with the recommendations of the Gaitonde Committee[45] (one of the authors, T. S. S. Dikshith was a member of this subcommittee on Pesticide Toxicology, 1978). These are somewhat similar to the measures suggested in Section III.D of this chapter.

1. Provisional Registration

Provisional registration of a pesticide is normally granted to products which are being introduced for the first time in India, or under such conditions as the Registration Committee may feel proper. But provisional registration is granted only for a period of 2 years during which time the registration holder is expected to complete all the data required for the registration of the pesticide. A regular registration is granted after submitting all the data requirements to the registration committee.

2. Inspection

After the registration, the manufacture or import of the pesticide is monitored regularly. Insecticide inspectors appointed by the government examine the records maintained by manufacturers/importers/dealers; the inspectors are also authorized to take samples for inspection. These samples are sent to the pesticide analyst for testing. The Central Insecticide Laboratory (CIL) controls this function. The CIL has facilities to counter check the data furnished by applicants for registration and also for the regular checking of registered products. In addition to CIL, there is at least one pesticide laboratory in all the states and union territories of India to carry out the tests on the pesticide samples. Besides these government laboratories, regular monitoring of pesticides is carried out by the Indian Standards Institution (ISI) for those who choose ISI as a third party guarantee regarding quality.

D. SOUTH KOREA

Pesticides in South Korea have become essential for a good crop yield as in other developing countries. An expected cultivation of high yielding varieties, dense planting, heavy application of chemical fertilizers, and other related cultural practices have resulted in the changing pattern and outbreaks of major diseases and insect pests. Korea has 20 pesticide manufacturing industries of which 11 units manufacture formulations while 9 units produce technical pesticides.[46]

E. NEPAL

Agricultural practices in Nepal are very diverse in view of its geoclimatic positions. Nepal has the influence of (a) subtropical monsoon climate, (b) temperate monsoon climate, and (c) cool temperate climate. More than 90% of the total population of Nepal depends on agriculture.

During the early years, pesticides like DDT and HCH were imported in the formulation forms for purposes of mosquito control program. During 1977, Nepal initiated indigenous production of pesticides and formulations.

In view of the bulk import of pesticides from India primarily by the Agriculture Corporation and semi-government organizations, no legislative control measures are being taken to pass pesticides acts so far. However, attempts are being initiated in this context and it is hoped that the law regarding the various aspects of pesticides will be in operation in the country. The Pesticides Board is in action which has all the responsibility for import recommendations, distribution, and control of pesticides.[47]

F. PAKISTAN

Regulation and registration of pesticides in Pakistan are controlled under the Agricultural Pesticide Ordinance. The rules and regulations under this ordinance were promulgated during 1973. The Agricultural Pesticides Technical Advisory Committee (APTAC) approves the registration of pesticides as per set procedures of the Act. It has been observed that in Pakistan more than 80% of the pesticides trade is controlled by the multinationals and foreign firms. However, a plant for manufacturing insecticides was set up in Pakistan at Nowshera in the Northwestern Frontier Province as early as 1955 with the assistance of UNICEF.[48]

G. PHILIPPINES

The pesticide industry in the Philippines is entirely managed by the private sector. In fact, the industry is built around 20 companies under the trade organization named Agricultural Pesticide Institute of the Philippines (APIP). APIP is responsible for 95% of the pesticide sales in the country. The fertilizer and pesticide authority was created in 1977 by virtue of Presidential Decree 1144. This is the sole agency whose function is to regulate all aspects of the pesticide industry such as import, export, manufacture, formulation, distribution, sale, transport, storage, use, and disposal of pesticides. Monitoring activities of formulation plants, and organization of training programs for plant workers, are geared towards upgrading standards of safety in formulation plants.[49]

H. SRI LANKA

In Sri Lanka, control over the supply, distribution, and use of pesticides came into force during the 1960s. In fact, a draft on Act on Poisons Used in Agriculture was prepared and forwarded to the legal legislation in 1964. However, it was only in the 1970s that the government of Sri Lanka took definite steps, through the advise of FAO for the establishment of a national organization. This has helped the official control of pesticides through pesticide legislation.

Pesticide Act, 1980 — The government of Sri Lanka introduced Pesticide Act No. 33 gazetted in 1980 to bring the use of pesticides under its control.[50,51] A comparison of the Insecticide Act 1968 of India and the Pesticide Act 1980 of Sri Lanka shows major similarities.

I. THAILAND

Thailand is one of the southeast Asian countries, where the majority of the population is involved in agriculture. Since Thailand is located in the tropics, there is abundant rainfall and the climate is warm throughout the year, an ideal weather condition for the multiplication of insect pests.

Thailand uses large quantities of pesticides for the control of crop pests and vectors of diseases. The Agricultural Toxic Substances Division, under the Department of Agriculture has come into being since 1982. This division is responsible for the overall management, quality control, and research activities related to pesticides in Thailand.[52]

In contrast to the developing countries, regulatory measures in other countries such as Canada, the Federal Republic of Germany, Japan, the United Kingdom, and the United States, offer varied approaches for the management of pesticides.

J. CANADA

In Canada, as in most developed countries, legislation exists controlling the use of pesticides. It is mandatory that all pesticides must be registered under the Pest Control Products Act administered by the Department of Agriculture prior to their being cleared for use. In fact, the legislation requires the manufacturer or petitioner to provide the Department of Agriculture with extensive data regarding the efficacy of the pesticide under Canadian conditions of use. This includes data to show whether or not pesticide residues exist on food products that may be consumed by humans.

In Canada, it is possible for pesticides to be registered on a negligible residue basis in cases where the residue on food products is considered to be of no toxicological significance. The Health Protection Branch of the Department of National Health and Welfare conducts a number of monitoring programs designed to determine the degree of compliance with established tolerances. In Canada, the provincial authorities are involved in issuing licenses to spray operators and restricting pesticide use whenever a potential hazard to either the applicator or by-stander is anticipated.[53]

K. FEDERAL REPUBLIC OF GERMANY

In the Federal Republic of Germany (FRG) pesticides are registered with the Federal Institute of Biology for Agriculture and Forestry (BBA). According to the legislation in FRG, it is mandatory that the data on pesticide residues contain results obtained from official trials carried out in West Germany in accordance with the approved guidelines of the government.

L. JAPAN

In Japan the regulation of pesticides is covered by the following laws:

1.   Agricultural Chemical Law
2.   The Poisons and Deleterious Substances Control Law
3.   The Food Sanitation Law

These are mandatory and product registration requires generation of toxicity and residue data in the approved and recognized laboratories in Japan.

M. UNITED KINGDOM

In the United Kingdom there is no direct legislation to control pesticides. However, the pesticide industry and agriculture and health departments of the government work closely to regulate safe use of pesticides. The Pesticide Safety Precautions Scheme deals with toxicology, safety, and environmental aspects of pesticides where the Agricultural Chemical Scheme looks after the biological efficacy of pesticides.

N. UNITED STATES

In the United States previous restrictions on the use of pesticides were the responsibility of the Plant Pest Control Division and the Forest Service of the United States Department of Agriculture (USDA); their regulatory functions, in fact, were based on the Federal Insecticide, Fungicide and Rodenticide Act of 1947. (FIFRA was amended in 1959 to include other pesticides.)

The United States Department of Health, Education and Welfare (USDHEW) is responsible for protecting people from pesticidal contamination and from epidemics. This department works in cooperation with national agencies like the Communicable Disease Center, the Public Health Service, and international agencies like the WHO. Interestingly this department has no control over the use of pesticides. In view of these and the need for a national approach to regulate the use of pesticides for the protection of man, wildlife, and other animals from accumulation of low level residues of pesticides, the President's Science Advisory Committee was organized in 1963. In 1969, a committee headed by E. Merck presented a report appraising the situation for proper use of pesticides and the need for studies on rational approaches to pesticide use.[54]

Because of the increasing public concern over environmental pollution, the U.S. Environmental Protection Agency (EPA) was created by the President's Council of Executive Organization on July 9, 1970.[55] The EPA has become an independent agency for example like the Federal Water Quality Administration (FWQA, Department of Interior), Bureau of Water Hygiene National Air Pollution Control Administration, and Bureau of Solid Waste Management (HEW). The EPA has the authority to license and monitor pesticides (earlier managed by USDA) and thus to regulate the proper use of pesticides according to FIFRA. In this way EPA has consolidated the functions of several agencies relating to the environment in order to improve regulatory performance.

To ensure that legislation and regulations are properly implemented, interaction and harmonized function of different departments, and national and international agencies are important. Regular monitoring, periodic counseling, and active participation of the industry and general public provide good measures essential for safe use of pesticides.

VI. CONCLUSION

Pesticides are required for the increased production of food and fiber products; they are also required for our protection from vector-borne diseases. To ensure this, pesticides must be handled with due care and caution, essentially because pesticides are highly toxic chemicals to man and his living environment. Legislation and regulations are, therefore, necessary for the proper and judicious use of pesticides.

Legislation for the management of pesticides varies among different nations. This is particularly so with reference to the organizations/agencies responsible for the implementation of regulatory measures such as registration, imposing restrictions on the sale, distribution, phasing out, and banning of the product. These regulatory measures provide procedures which help the judicious use of pesticides by man for his own good and for the protection of the environment.

REFERENCES

1. **World Health Organization,** European Cooperation on Environmental Health Aspects of the Control of Chemicals, *Interim Document 5,* Legislative and Administrative Procedures for the Control of Chemicals, World Health Organization, Regional Office for Europe, Copenhagen, 1982.

2. **World Health Organization,** Control of Pesticides, A Survey of Existing Legislation, World Health Organization, Geneva, 1970.

3. **Huismans, I. W.,** The International Register of Potentially Toxic Chemicals (IRPTC): Its Present Activity and Future Plans in Preventive Toxicology, IRPTC Centre of International Projects, GKNT, Moscow, 1984, 357.

4. **Mercier, M. and Gounar, M.,** The International Programme of Chemical Safety (IPCS), in *Preventive Toxicology,* IRPTC Centre of International Projects, GKNT, Moscow, 1984, 372.

5. *Pesticides,* 5th ed., Council of Europe, Strasburg, 1981.

6. **Environmental Protection Agency,** The Federal Insecticide, Fungicide and Rodenticide Act as amended, U.S. EPA Office of Pesticide Program, Washington, D.C., 1978.

7. **Environmental Protection Agency,** Part V, Special Reviews of Pesticides, 40 CFR Parts 154 and 162, 40 CFR Part 155, *Fed. Reg.,* March 27, 1985.

8. **Environmental Protection Agency,** Data requirement for pesticides, Part II. Registration final rule, 40 CFR Part 158, *Fed. Reg.,* October 24, 1984.

9. **United Nations Pesticide Safety Precautions Scheme,** Agreed between Government Departments and Industrial Associations United Nations, Rev., New York, 1979.

10. **James, G. W.,** Food and Drug Administration's good laboratory practice regulations at home and abroad, in *Safety Evaluation and Regulation of Chemicals,* Hamburger, F., Ed., S. Karger, Basel, 1985.

11. **World Health Organization,** Recommended classification of pesticides by hazards, *WHO Chronicle,* 29, 379, 1975.

12. **World Health Organization,** The WHO recommended classification of pesticides by hazard, guidelines to classification, 1988-89, *WHO/VBC,* 88, 953, 1988.

13. **Medved, L. I., Kagan, I. S., and Spinu, E. I.,** Pesticides and problems of public Health, *J. Vsesojusnogo Chim. Obstest. Mendel.,* 263, 1968.

14. **Kaloyanova-Simeonova, F.,** *Pesticides Toxic Action and Prevention,* Bulgarian Academy of Sciences, Sofia, 1977.

15. **Kaloyanova, F.,** Evaluation of pesticide toxicity for sanitary registration, in *Toxicology of Pesticides,* WHO/EURO, Copenhagen, 1982, 265.

16. **Truhaut, R.,** The need for an integrated approach in toxicological evaluation, in *Safety Evaluation and Regulation of Chemicals,* Vol. 3, Hamburger, F., Ed., S. Karger, Basel, 1986, 118.

17. **World Health Organisation,** *Specifications for Pesticides used in Public Health: Insecticides — Molluscicides — Repellents, Methods,* 1st ed., World Health Organisation, Geneva, 1979.

18. **Rosival, L. and Batora, V.,** Consequences for field exposure of impurities in pesticide formulations, in *Field Worker Exposure During Pesticide Application,* Tordoir, W. F. and Heemstra-Leguin, E. A. H., Eds., Elsevier, Amsterdam, 1980, 163.

19. **Pelegrini, G. and Santi, R.,** Potentiation of toxicity or organophosphorus compounds containing carboxylic esters functions toward warm-blooded animals by some organophosphorus impurities, *J. Agric. Food Chem.,* 20, 944, 1972.

20. **Aldridge, W. H., Miles, J. W., Mount, D. L., and Verschoyle, R. D.,** The toxicological properties of impurities in malathion, *Arch. Toxicol.,* 42, 95, 1979.

21. **Talcott, R. E.,** Hepatic and extrahepatic malathion carboxylesterases. Assay and localization in the rat, *Toxicol. Appl. Pharmacol.,* 47, 69, 1979.

22. **WHO Technical Report,** Chemistry and specification of pesticides, 2nd Rep. of the Expert Committee on Vector Biology and Control Series, No. 620, WHO, Geneva, 1978.

23. WHO Technical Reports, Recommended health-based limits in occupational exposure to pesticides: Report of WHO Study Group, Series No. 674, Geneva, 1982.

24. **Pazderova-Vejluphova, J.,** Chronic poisoning by 1,2,3,8-TCDD (Abstracts), III, Congress on Industrial Neurology, Prague, 1979.

25. **Gilioli, R.,** Neurological monitoring of workers exposed to TCDD with special reference to the study of motor unit parameters (Abstracts), III, *Congress on Industrial Neurology, Prague,* 1979.

26. **Kearney, P. C.,** Nitrosamines and pesticides: a special report on the occurrence of nitrosamines as terminal residues resulting from agricultural use of certain pesticides, *Pure Appl. Chem.,* 52, 499, 1980.

27. **Butler, G. C., Ed.,** *Principles of Ecotoxicology,* Scope 12, John Wiley & Sons, New York, 1978.

28. **Truhaut, R.,** Ecotoxicology: objectives, principles and perspectives, in *Evaluation of Toxicological Data for the Protection of Public Health,* Hunter, W. J. and Smeets, J. G. M., Eds., Pergamon Press, Oxford, 1977, 339.

29. UNESCO, Methods and Problems of Ecotoxicological Modeling and Prediction, *Proc. Workshop UNESCO Programme Man and Biosphere,* Puchchino, 1979.
30. **Moriarty, F.,** Ecological implications of pesticides, in *Toxicology of Pesticides,* WHO/EURO, Copenhagen, 1982, 100.
31. **Black, I. F. and Koeman, I. H.,** Future hazards from pesticide use — with special reference to West Africa and South East Asia, *Int. Union for Conservation of Nature and Natural Resources,* 1984.
32. **Copplestone, I. F.,** Methods for field assessment of exposure to pesticides, in *Field Worker Exposure During Application,* Tordoir, W. F. and van Heenstre, E. A. H., Eds., Elsevier, Amsterdam, 1980, 17.
33. **Speight, B.,** Effects of formulation upon safe use during pesticide application, in *Field Worker Exposure during Application,* Tordoir, W. F. and van Helmstre, E. A. H., Eds., Elsevier, Amsterdam, 1980, 29.
34. **Kaloyanova-Simeonova, F.,** Prevention of intoxication by pesticides in Bulgaria, Whiter rural medicine in Proc. Fourth Int. Congr. Rural Med., Usuda, Tokyo, 1970, 35.
35. **Kaloyanova, F. and Izmirova, N.,** Determination of minimum period for safe work with pesticides, in *Preventive Toxicology,* Kaloyanova, F., Ed., Medizina i Fizkultura, 329, 1985.
36. **Watanobe, S.,** Systematic study of poisoning of parathion in pesticides, 3, Shiter Rur, Med., *Proc. Fourth Int. Congree Rur. Med. Usuda,* 1969 Tokyo, 1970, 45.
37. Pesticide Program, Guidelines for registering pesticides in the United States, *Fed. Reg.,* 40, (123), 26802, 1975.
38. **Glasser, R. F.,** Pesticides: the legal environment, in *Pesticides and Human Welfare,* Gunn, D. L., and Stevens, J. G. R., Eds., Oxford University Press, New York, 1976, 228.
39. **Ontario Pesticides Act,** Ontario, Canada, 1973.
40. **Insecticides Act,** Government of India, New Delhi, 1968.
41. **Index Phytosannitaire,** *Acta Products, Insecticides, Fungicides, Herbicides, Association de Coordination technique Agricole,* Paris, 1980.
42. **Amin, M. R.,** Resistance of insecticides used in agriculture and public health, *International Workshop on Resistance of Insecticides in Public Health Agric.,* February 22, 1982.
43. **Miah, M. A. J.,** Pesticide formulation and its industry in Bangladesh, *Proc. International Workshop on Pesticides, Formulation,* UNIDO/UNDP/HIL, New Delhi, India, February 6, 1984.
44. **Tin, M. M.,** Insecticide usage in Burma, Rep. Int. Workshop in Resistance in Insecticides used in Public Health and Agric., February 22, 1982, Columbo, Sri Lanka.
45. Report of The Sub-Committee on Pesticide Toxicology (Gaitonde Committee), Ministry of Agriculture and Irrigation, Government of India, New Delhi, 1978.
46. **Byung-Youloh,** The status of pesticide formulation in Korea, Proc. Int. Workshop on Pesticides Formulation, UNIDO/UNDP/HIL, New Delhi, India, February 6, 1984.
47. **Gupta, M. P.,** Proc. International Workshop on Pesticide Formulation, UNIDO/UNDP/HIL, New Delhi, February 6, 1984.
48. **Baig, M. M. H.,** Resistance to pesticides used in public health in Pakistan, FAO's International Workshop on Resistance to Insecticides used in Public Health & Agriculture, February 22, 1982, Colombo, Sri Lanka.
49. **Dimaunahan, E. V.,** Status of pesticide formulation industry in the Philippines, Proc. Int. Workshop on Pesticides Formulation, UNIDO/UNDP/HIL, New Delhi, India, February 6, 1984.
50. Control of Pesticides Act, No. 33 of 1980, Supplement of Part II of Gazette of the Democratic Socialist Republic of Sri Lanka, October 3, 1980.
51. **Wickremasinghe, N. and Elikawela, Y.,** Pesticide usage and induction of resistance in pests and vectors, Int. Workshop on Resistance to Insecticides in Public Health and Agric., Colombo, Sri Lanka, February 22, 1982.
52. **Malikul, S. and Phanthumachinda, B.,** Pesticide usage and resistance of pests and vectors of pesticides, Workshop on Resistance to Insecticides used in Public Health and Agriculture, Colombo, Sri Landa, February 22, 1982.
53. **Urewski, D., Clayson, D., Collins, B., and Munro, I. C.,** Toxicological procedures for assessing the carcinogenic potential of agricultural chemicals, in *Genetic Toxicology,* Fkeck, R. A. and Hollander, A., Eds., Plenum Press, 1982, 461.
54. **Mrak, E. M.,** *Report of the Secretary's Commission on Pesticides and Their Relation to Environmental Health,* Part I and II, U.S. Government Printing Office, Washington, D.C., 1969.
55. Reorganization Plan No. 3, H.R. Document No. 91-364, Washington, D.C., 1970.

INDEX

A